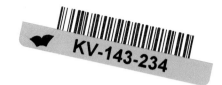

Topics in Palliative Care
Volume 1

Series Editors
Russell K. Portenoy, M.D.
Eduardo Bruera, M.D.

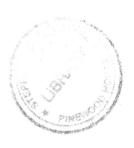

TOPICS IN PALLIATIVE CARE

Volume 1

Edited by

Russell K. Portenoy
Memorial Sloan-Kettering Cancer Center
Cornell University Medical College

Eduardo Bruera
Grey Nuns Community Health Centre
University of Alberta

New York   Oxford
OXFORD UNIVERSITY PRESS
1997

Oxford University Press

Oxford   New York
Athens   Auckland   Bangkok   Bogota   Bombay   Buenos Aires
Calcutta   Cape Town   Dar es Salaam   Delhi   Florence   Hong Kong
Istanbul   Karachi   Kuala Lumpur   Madras   Madrid   Melbourne
Mexico City   Nairobi   Paris   Singapore   Taipei   Tokyo   Toronto

and associated companies in
Berlin   Ibadan

Copyright © 1997 by Oxford University Press, Inc.

Published by Oxford University Press, Inc.
198 Madison Avenue, New York, New York 10016

Oxford is a registered trademark of Oxford University Press

Library of Congress Cataloging-in-Publication Data
Topics in palliative care / edited by Russell K. Portenoy, Eduardo Bruera.
p. cm.—(Topics in palliative care : v. 1)
Includes bibliographical references and index.
ISBN 0-19-510244-4
1. Cancer—Palliative treatment.
I. Portenoy, Russell K.
II. Bruera, Eduardo.
III. Series.
[DNLM: 1. Palliative Care.   2. Neoplasms—drug therapy.
3. Pain—drug therapy.
WB   310   T674   1997]   RC271.P33T664   1997
616.99'406—dc20   DNLM/DLC   for Library of Congress   96–22250

9 8 7 6 5 4 3 2 1

Printed in the United States of America
on acid-free paper

To our wives,
Susan and Maria,
whose love and support
make our work possible.

Preface

Palliative Care, a series devoted to research and practice in palliative care, was created to address the growing need to disseminate new information about this rapidly evolving field.

Palliative care is an interdisciplinary therapeutic model for the management of patients with incurable, progressive illness. In this model, the family is considered the unit of care. The clinical purview includes those factors—physical, psychological, social, and spiritual—that contribute to suffering, undermine quality of life, and prevent a death with comfort and dignity. The definition promulgated by the World Health Organization exemplifies this perspective.*

> Palliative care is the active total care of patients whose disease is not responsive to curative treatment. Control of pain, of other symptoms, and of psychological, social and spiritual problems is paramount. The goal of palliative care is the achievement of the best possible quality of life for patients and their families.

Palliative care is a fundamental part of clinical practice, the "parallel universe" to therapies directed at cure or prolongation of life. All clinicians who treat patients with chronic life-threatening diseases are engaged in palliative care, continually attempting to manage complex symptomatology and functional disturbances.

The need for specialized palliative care services may arise at any point during the illness. Symptom control and psychological adaptation are the usual concerns during the period of active disease-oriented therapies. Toward the end of life, however, needs intensify and broaden. Psychosocial distress or family distress, spiritual or existential concerns, advance care planning, and ethical concerns, among many other issues, may be considered by the various disciplines that coalesce in the delivery of optimal care. Clinicians who specialize in palliative care perceive their role as similar to those of specialists in other disciplines of medicine: referring patients to other primary caregivers when appropriate, acting as primary caregivers (as members of the team) when the challenges of the case warrant this involvement, and teaching and conducting research in the field of palliative care.

*World Health Organization. Technical Report Series 804, Cancer Pain and Palliative Care. Geneva: World Health Organization, 1990:11.

With recognition of palliative care as an essential element in medical care and as an area of specialization, there is a need for information about the approaches used by specialists from many disciplines in managing the varied problems that fall under the purview of this model. The scientific foundation of palliative care is also advancing, and similarly, methods are needed to highlight for practitioners at the bedside the findings of empirical research. *Topics in Palliative Care* has been designed to meet the need for enhanced communication in this changing field.

To highlight the diversity of concerns in palliative care, each volume of *Topics in Palliative Care* is divided into sections that address a range of issues. Various sections address aspects of symptom control, psychosocial functioning, spiritual or existential concerns, ethics, and other topics. The chapters in each section review the area and focus on a small number of salient issues for analysis. The authors present and evaluate existing data, provide a context drawn from both the clinic and research, and integrate knowledge in a manner that is both practical and readable.

We are grateful to the many contributors for their excellent work and their timeliness. We also thank our publisher, who has expressed great faith in the project. Such strong support has buttressed our desire to create an educational forum that may enhance palliative care in the clinical setting and drive its growth as a discipline.

New York, N.Y.   R. K. P.
Edmonton, Alberta   E. B.

Contents

Contributors

LINDA J. BEENEY, PH.D.
Medical Psychology Unit
Department of Surgery
University of Sydney
Sydney, Australia

CLAUDIA BORREANI, PH.D.
Division of Psychological Research
National Cancer Institute
Milan, Italy

WILLIAM BREITBART, M.D.
Cornell University Medical
  College, and
Psychiatry Service
Memorial Sloan-Kettering Cancer
  Center
New York, New York, USA

EDUARDO BRUERA, M.D.
Palliative Care Program
Grey Nuns Community Health
  Centre
Edmonton, Alberta, Canada

PHYLLIS N. BUTOW, PH.D.
Medical Psychology Unit
Departments of Endocrinology
  and Medical Oncology
Royal Prince Alfred Hospital
Sydney, Australia

AUGUSTO CARACENI, M.D.
Division of Pain Therapy and
  Palliative Care
National Cancer Institute
Milan, Italy

SUSAN DERBY, R.N., M.A., C.G.N.P.
Pain Management
Department of Nursing
Memorial Sloan-Kettering Cancer
  Center
New York, New York, USA

NOÉMI D. DE STOUTZ, M.D.
Onkologische Palliativstation
Klinik C für Innere Medizin
Kantonsspital St. Gallen
St. Gallen, Switzerland

STEWART M. DUNN, PH.D.
Medical Psychology Unit
Departments of Endocrinology
  and Medical Oncology
Royal Prince Alfred Hospital
Sydney, Australia

PERRY G. FINE, M.D.
Department of Anesthesiology, School
  of Medicine, and
Pain Management Center
University Hospitals and Clinics
University of Utah Health Sciences
  Center
Salt Lake City, Utah, USA

MICHAEL E. GAUTHIER, M.D.
Department of Anesthesiology, School
  of Medicine, and
Pain Management Center
University Hospitals and Clinics
University of Utah Health Sciences
  Center
Salt Lake City, Utah, USA

JANE INGHAM, M.B.B.S., F.R.A.C.P.
Department of Medicine
Lombardi Cancer Center
Georgetown University Medical Center
Washington, D.C., USA

LINDA J. KRISTJANSON, R.N., PH.D.
Faculty of Nursing
University of Manitoba, and
St. Boniface Hospital Research Centre
Winnipeg, Manitoba, Canada

ARTHUR G. LIPMAN, PHARM.D.
College of Pharmacy and Pain
   Management Center
University Hospitals and Clinics
University of Utah Health Sciences
   Center
Salt Lake City, Utah, USA

MARY JANE MASSIE, M.D.
Cornell University Medical College
and
Barbara White Center for Psychological
   Counseling
Memorial Sloan-Kettering Cancer
   Center
New York, New York, USA

MICHAEL J. MCCABE, PH.D.
Sacred Heart Parish
Petone, Lower Hutt, New Zealand

SEBASTIANO MERCADANTE, M.D.
Department of Anesthesia and
   Intensive Care
Buccheri La Ferla Fatebenefratelli
   Hospital, and
Pain Relief and Palliative Care
Società per L'Assistenza al Malato
   Oncologico Terminale
Palermo, Italy

RUSSELL K. PORTENOY, M.D.
Department of Neurology
Cornell University Medical College
and
Pain and Palliative Care Service
Department of Neurology
Memorial Sloan-Kettering Cancer
   Center
New York, New York, USA

CARLA RIPAMONTI, M.D.
Division of Pain Therapy and
   Palliative Care
National Cancer Institute
Milan, Italy

CARLOS RODRIGUEZ, M.D.
Pain Therapy and Palliative Care
   Division
National Cancer Institute
Santafé de Bogotá, Colombia

PER SJØGREN, M.D.
Multidisciplinary Pain Center
Bispebjerg Hospital
Copenhagen, Denmark

FRITZ STIEFEL, M.D.
Division Autonome de Médecine
   Psychosociale
Centre Hospitalier Universitaire
   Vaudois
Lausanne, Switzerland

MARCELLO TAMBURINI, PH.D.
Division of Psychological Research
National Cancer Institute
Milan, Italy

MARTIN H. N. TATTERSALL, M.D.
Department of Cancer Medicine
University of Sydney
Sydney, Australia

SHARON WATANABE, M.D.
Palliative Care Program
Grey Nuns Community Health Centre
Edmonton, Alberta, Canada

I

DELIRIUM IN CANCER PATIENTS

Introduction: Critical Issues in the Assessment of Delirium

RUSSELL K. PORTENOY

Delirium is a prevalent disorder in populations with progressive disease. Although it may occur at any time, the prevalence of delirium rises in the setting of advanced disease and is common in patients near death. As it evolves, delirium may signal a new and serious medical complication, contribute to intercurrent problems (for example, by worsening dehydration), markedly impair the functioning and comfort of the patient, and increase the family's distress.

Guidelines for the management of delirium, which are described by several authors of the chapters that follow, derive largely from an extensive clinical experience. In routine practice, outcomes are compromised by poor recognition of the disorder and a lack of scientific findings related to epidemiology, pathophysiology, clinical manifestations, and treatment. Much research is needed to redress these deficiencies and provide a scientific foundation for the diagnosis and management of this condition.

Even if research provides this scientific foundation, however, the management of delirium in the palliative care setting will be challenging. The clinical vagaries of progressive medical diseases and the ever-present possibility of imminent death complicate patient assessment and increase the difficulty of therapeutic decision making. As a consequence, assessment of the delirious patient in the palliative care setting raises issues that extend beyond medical concerns alone.

Patients who eventually die of a progressive medical disease typically develop confusion or somnolence immediately before death. The duration of this period of cognitive impairment is variable and may be as short as hours or as long as weeks. Regardless of duration, this period of cognitive decline is usually considered to be part of the normal dying process. The constellation of symptoms and signs may fulfill diagnostic criteria for delirium, but the therapeutic response when the imminence of death is acknowledged is limited to symptomatic therapy, if needed to ensure comfort.

In contrast, the occurrence of delirium earlier in the course is usually perceived to reflect a disease process with serious implications. In addition to symptomatic management, it is important to identify and reverse underlying causes. Management is often intensive and may include withdrawal of nonessential, centrally acting drugs and specific treatments for potentially reversible metabolic or structural disease.

Thus, the challenge posed by the management of delirium derives from a remarkable dichotomy in clinical perception, in which the symptoms and signs consistent with this diagnosis are considered a serious pathological state in one set of circumstances and part of a normal process in another. Palliative care clinicians, whose efforts are focused on patient comfort and quality of life throughout the course of progressive medical disease, are uniquely situated to address this challenge. When the ongoing assessment—the foundation of good palliative care—determines that physical and psychosocial functioning is still a relevant goal of care, the occurrence of delirium is usually perceived to be pathologic and should precipitate an aggressive clinical response based on a careful medical and psychiatric evaluation of potential etiologies.[1,2] When death is perceived to be imminent and comfort is the overriding goal, the burdens placed on the patient and the family by this assessment may not be justifiable and symptom management alone is warranted.

Unfortunately, the lack of science and deficiencies in clinical practice hamper the clinician's ability to draw these distinctions. The scientific data do not permit prediction of the time of death, and although assessment of symptom distress and other quality of life concerns by palliative care clinicians could improve prognostication,[3] the level of accuracy is still inadequate for the types of clinical judgments that must be applied to a patient who has become delirious.

Furthermore, the assessment of delirium itself is yet rudimentary. Although validated measures have been developed, none assess the severity of delirium,[4] and neither severity nor the pattern of findings in delirious patients have been empirically evaluated as potential predictors of clinical outcome. Although it is possible that the type and severity of the delirium could provide additional insights into prognosis, and thereby influence decisions about interventions at the end of life, the information required for this is lacking.

Given the high prevalence of delirium prior to death, there is a risk of a counterproductive tautology in current practice: If delirium commonly occurs just before death, then the presence of delirium may mean that death is imminent. If death is imminent, there is no reason to intervene intensively to reverse the delirium. If no interventions are offered, the potential reversibility of the delirium will never be known. In the absence of data, this tautology may be a trap for some patients, leading clinicians to foreclose on aggressive management that may indeed have the potential to work.

Until prognostication improves and much more is learned about the predictive aspects of delirium itself, it is best to be cautious in the interpretation of cognitive deterioration at the end of life. Before assuming that a delirium reflects an inevitable decline toward death, there must be a comprehensive understanding of the patient's medical status. Simple therapeutic trials, such as reducing or eliminating nonessential drugs or switching opioids, might be considered as a low-risk means of acquiring more information about the potential reversibility of the syndrome. These interventions could be followed by more aggressive strategies if any improvement occurs. Other interventions that are minimally invasive, such as hydration (which can be performed subcutaneously if there is no venous access) or oxygen therapy with measurement of pulse oximetry, may also be conceptualized as therapeutic trials in some settings.

The decision to forgo any further effort to evaluate or reverse a delirium may be the correct one for many patients, but given current limitations in the science of assessment, the clinician must be assured that the information available is sufficient to support that decision. This information can also clarify the decision making for the family, whose concerns and desires must be addressed as part of the overall palliative strategy.

References

1. Lipowski AZ. Update on delirium. *Psychiatr Clin North Am* 1995; 15:335–346.
2. Bruera E, Miller L, McCallion J, et al. Cognitive failure (CF) in patients with terminal cancer: a prospective study. *J Pain Symptom Manage* 1992; 7:192–195.
3. Degner LF, Sloan JA. Symptom distress in newly diagnosed ambulatory cancer patients and as a predictor of survival in lung cancer. *J Pain Symptom Manage* 1995; 10:423–431.
4. Smith MJ, Breitbart WS, Platt MM. A critique of instruments and methods to detect, diagnose, and rate delirium. *J Pain Symptom Manage* 1995; 10:35–77.

1

Epidemiology and Clinical Features of Delirium

JANE INGHAM AND WILLIAM BREITBART

Delirium is defined as a transient organic brain syndrome characterized by the acute onset of disordered attention (arousal) and cognition, accompanied by disturbances of psychomotor behavior and perception.[1] Delirium may complicate any of a large number of disorders and can be highly aversive to patients. Untreated delirium may increase patient morbidity and family distress, and foster conflict between staff and families.[2,3] Studies in medical populations suggest that delirium is underrecognized by medical and nursing staff.[4–6] Although often treatable and reversible, etiologic factors are often missed and treatment strategies that may be highly beneficial are neglected. Appropriate assessment of delirium is imperative, and requires knowledge of the prevalence, diagnostic criteria, and assessment methodology.

Prevalence and Predictors

The prevalence of delirium in hospitalized medical and surgical patients is approximately 10%,[6,7] and the prevalence in hospitalized cancer patients ranges from 8% to 40%.[8–10] A higher prevalence, ranging in some studies up to 50%, characterizes specific medical inpatient subpopulations, including the elderly and patients in the postoperative period.[1,7]

The variability in prevalence rates for delirium reflects differences in the diagnostic criteria and the populations studied. A higher prevalence has been found in cancer populations with advanced disease, particularly those in the last week of life.[10,11] Unfortunately, this group of patients is rarely studied and strict diagnostic criteria for delirium have often not been applied. Surveys of the last few weeks of life frequently cite "confusion" as a problem, but this does not provide diagnostic specificity.

In contrast to prevalence, the incidence of delirium in cancer patients has not been investigated. Two studies of terminally ill cancer patients have found that delirium developed prior to death in over 80%, suggesting that the incidence is very high at the end of life.[11,12] In elderly patients with medical illnesses and those in the postoperative period, the incidence of delirium is in the range of 25% to 41%.[7,13,14]

Sociodemographic and disease-related factors associated with the onset of delirium have not been documented in cancer patients. Predictive models developed for delirium in the hospitalized elderly and in patients prior to surgery highlight the importance of the following risk factors: advanced age, prior cognitive impairment, symptomatic infection and severe illness, visual impairment, fracture on admission, and a history of significant alcohol use prior to admission.[13–16] Medications that have been demonstrated to be risk factors for delirium include neuroleptics, opioids, and anticholinergic drugs.[14,16,17] Although it is likely that these and other factors may predict the occurrence of delirium in cancer patients, further studies need to be undertaken to clarify this issue.

Clinical Features

The symptoms and signs of delirium fluctuate and, therefore, the diagnosis may be overlooked if careful attention is not given to the mental status examination. Although the clinical presentation of delirium is often extremely varied, the diagnosis can be established on the basis of new-onset disturbances of cognitive function, accompanied by a disturbance of arousal or clouding of consciousness. Symptoms of delirium may be protean, which complicates the assessment. A patient may be restless, anxious, depressed, irritable, angry, or emotionally labile; however, these symptoms are highly prevalent in advanced cancer[18–20] and are not specific for a diagnosis. Such symptoms may be manifestations of adjustment disorders or may represent symptoms of an organic mood disturbance secondary to any of a large number of causes. Only when the patient is assessed in the context of the spectrum of concurrent symptoms and signs can a diagnosis of delirium be made.

Although all delirious patients have new-onset impaired cognition, the type of arousal disturbance can be variable. Three clinical variants of delirium have been described based on the type of arousal disturbance: hypoalert-hypoactive, hyperalert-hyperactive, and mixed type (fluctuations from hypoalert to hyperalert).[21,22] It has been suggested that this phenomenology may be related to specific etiologic factors. One small study found that patients with hepatic encephalopathy were more likely to be hypoalert or somnolent, whereas those in whom fever was the main etiologic factor were equally likely to have a somnolent (hypoalert) or a hyperactive (hyperalert) delirium.[23] This study also demonstrated a trend toward a hyperactive delirium in patients with alcohol withdrawal, an observation consistent with clinical experience.[24] The phenomenology of delirium in cancer patients has not yet been described, but the diagnosis of delirium may be overlooked if the existence of differing phenomenological subtypes, particularly the less apparent hypoactive delirium, is not recognized.

To establish a diagnosis of delirium, specific criteria must be met (see below). These criteria reflect disturbances in behavior that may involve cognition, affective state, perception, or arousal and responsiveness. Disturbances in thinking may be reflected in memory impairment or confusion. Affective disturbances may range from dysphoria to hypomania. Perception may be impaired with illusions or hallucinations. Arousal may be increased or decreased, or the patient may merely be distractible or less responsive. Delirium may be an appropriate diagnosis if an acute change in arousal or responsiveness is accompanied by a change in one or more of these areas of function. Most patients have disturbances in multiple aspects of cognition and behavior, but the interpatient variability is very large.

Some patients experience an isolated disturbance that can be related to an organic cause but does not fulfill the criteria for diagnosis of delirium. For example, a patient may experience hallucinations or a mood disturbance in the absence of any other evidence of cognitive dysfunction. Such problems must be fully assessed and monitored over time. If other disturbances occur later, the criteria for a diagnosis of delirium may then be met.

Diagnostic Criteria

The diagnosis of delirium requires that the patient meet the published criteria recently outlined by the American Psychiatric Association in the *Diagnostic and Statistical Manual* (DSM) IV.[25] Prior to the development of these criteria, the DSM-IIIR criteria had formed the basis of delirium diagnosis.[26] The DSM criteria for delirium have been considered the "gold standard" for diagnosis, but it is important to note that "these diagnostic criteria and the DSM-IV classification of mental disorders reflect a consensus of the current formulations of evolving knowledge in our field but do not encompass all the conditions that may be legitimate focuses of treatment or research efforts."[27] The problems with inconsistent terminology that have characterized both the study of delirium and diagnosis in clinical practice may be minimized by the use of DSM criteria.

Essential elements for the diagnosis of delirium that have been incorporated, in some form, into both the earlier DSM-IIIR and the recent DSM-IV criteria are:

• Impairment in responsiveness and alertness as manifest by fluctuating inability to maintain or shift attention to external stimuli.

- Cognitive dysfunction of recent onset that is not accounted for by preexisting dementia.
- Development of the disturbance over a short period of time (usually hours or days).
- Evidence from history, physical examination, or laboratory findings of a general medical condition or organic factor judged to be etiologically related to the disturbance.

For a DSM-IIIR diagnosis of delirium at least two of the following were required. These criteria symptoms are no longer required as essential criteria in the DSM-IV:

- Reduced level of consciousness.
- Perceptual disturbances.
- Disturbance of the sleep–wake cycle.
- Increased or decreased psychomotor activity.
- Disorientation to time, place, or person.
- Memory impairment.

The DSM-IIIR diagnostic criteria may be ambiguous in patients with advanced malignancy. For example, it may be difficult to attribute a symptom such as irritability or sleep disturbance to delirium rather than an intercurrent process, such as pain. In part to address this problem, the DSM-IV criteria for delirium are more simple than those used previously and facilitate the detection of milder forms of delirium.[25] These criteria emphasize that disordered attention (arousal) and cognition are the most essential elements of the delirious state, which is characteristically of acute onset and has an organic etiology.

Evaluation Instruments

To improve diagnostic accuracy, a number of approaches to the assessment and evaluation of delirium have been developed (Table 1.1). Smith and colleagues have recently extensively reviewed these instruments, along with other evaluation methods, and have grouped them into four categories.[28] These include: (1) screening tests that detect cognitive impairment, such as the Mini-Mental Status Exam[29] and the Blessed Orientation-Memory-Concentration Test[30]; (2) diagnostic instruments based on DSM criteria, such as the Confusion Assessment method[31]; (3) rating scales for delirium, such as the Delirium Rating Scale (DRS)[32]; and (4) physiological correlates of delirium that use laboratory or para-clinical exams, such as EEG or brain imaging studies.

Evaluation instruments in the first three categories can be incorporated with relative ease into patient assessment. It should be noted, however, that instruments that assess cognition alone, such as the Mini-Mental Status Exam,

Table 1.1. Research assessment methods for delirium in cancer patients

---

Diagnostic classification systems
  DSM-III, DSM-III-R, DSM-IV
  ICD-9, ICD-10

Diagnostic interviews/instruments
  Delirium Symptom Interview (DSI)
  Confusion Assessment Method (CAM)

Delirium rating scales
  Delirium Rating Scale (DRS)
  Confusion Rating Scale (CRS)
  Saskatoon Delirium Checklist (SDC)

Cognitive impairment screening instruments
  Mini-Mental State Exam (MMSE)
  Short Portable Mental Status Questionnaire (SPMSQ)
  Cognitive Capacity Screening Examination (CCSE)
  Blessed Orientation Memory Concentration Test (BOMC)

Laboratory examinations
  EEG, Brain Imaging
  Serum Anticholinergic Activity

---

can screen patients for impairment but do not provide enough information for the diagnosis of delirium. These instruments may provide a method for the monitoring of patients predisposed to delirium or those who are receiving treatment for this condition. Although no instrument has been validated as a measure of delirium severity, the use of a simple measure, such as the Mini-Mental Status Examination, may provide information that can facilitate diagnosis and therapeutic decision making.[33] Such information can also provide useful data for the study of delirium in advanced cancer.[12]

Differential Diagnosis

The differential diagnosis for delirium, because of the wide array of symptoms that may accompany it, encompasses a very broad spectrum of psychiatric disease.[34] The potential diagnoses in a patient with impaired cognition, for example, include delirium, dementias of various types, amnestic disorders, and drug-induced disorders. The DSM-IV categorizes this group as cognitive impairment disorders.[25]

Assessment of Etiology

Assessment of the etiology of delirium has been demonstrated to provide useful information even in extremely advanced disease.[35,36] In the cancer population, these etiologies include drugs, electrolyte imbalance, organ failure, nutritional deficiencies, vascular complications, and paraneoplastic syndromes.[37] The relative contributions of these disease-related and drug-related factors in cancer patients have not been assessed in any large prospective surveys. A recent survey of 94 delirious cancer patients referred initially for a neurology consultation demonstrated a multifactorial etiology in most.[35] Metabolic causes were found in 89% and were the primary cause in 44%. Medications were found to be contributory factors in 97%, but the primary cause in only 29%. Fifty percent of patients had fever and evidence of systemic infection, but bacteremia was documented in only 4%. Central nervous system metastases were found in 32% and were a major cause in all these patients. Disseminated intravascular coagulation was a contributing factor in 11%. The average number of contributing factors in each patient was four.

Approach to Clinical Assessment and Diagnostic Workup

Studies in patients with advanced cancer have demonstrated the utility of a thorough diagnostic assessment.[12,35] One study found that 68% of delirious cancer patients improved, despite a 30-day mortality of 31%.[35] Another found that one third of the episodes of cognitive failure improved following an evaluation that yielded a cause for these episodes in 43%.[12]

The extent of the diagnostic workup may be dictated by the goals of care but should generally include an assessment of potentially reversible causes of delirium. A physical examination should assess for evidence of sepsis, dehydration, or major organ failure. Medications that could contribute to delirium should be reviewed. A screen of laboratory parameters will allow assessment of the possible role of metabolic abnormalities, such as hypercalcemia, and other problems such as hypoxia or disseminated intravascular coagulation. Imaging studies of the brain and assessment of the cerebrospinal fluid may be appropriate in some instances.

Treatment

The appropriate approach in the management of delirium in the cancer patient includes interventions that are directed at both the underlying causes and the symptoms of delirium.[33,34,38] Except in cases where far advanced disease and particular goals of care may impose limitations, identification and correction of the underlying cause(s) of delirium must be undertaken while symptomatic and supportive therapies are being implemented.[34,39]

Reversible causes of delirium should be addressed. For example, in the cancer population, delirium is often associated with the use of an opioid. In such cases, simple interventions, such as dose reduction (if pain is controlled) or switching from one opioid to another, may resolve the delirium. Uncontrolled pain may require continued therapy at the same or a higher dose and occasionally, despite interventions, or while reversible causes are being addressed, the delirium will persist. The use of a concomitant neuroleptic drug (e.g., haloperidol) may be valuable in these settings.

Symptomatic treatment measures for delirium, regardless of cause, include support for and communication with the patient and family, reassurance, manipulation of the environment to provide a safe milieu, and the appropriate use of pharmacotherapies. To reduce anxiety and disorientation, measures should be implemented which increase structure and familiarity. Such measures may include encouraging the family to sit with the patient, and nursing the patient in a quiet, well-lit room with objects that assist in orientation such as a visible clock, calendar, or familiar objects from the patient's home. Often, these techniques alone are insufficient and treatment with neuroleptic or sedative medications is appropriate (Table 1.2). To prevent self-harm, particularly in the early stabilization phase of pharmacological treatment, the judicious use of physical restraints and one-to-one nursing observation may be appropriate.

Pharmacological Management of Delirium

Neuroleptic medications vary in their sedating properties and in their potential for producing orthostatic hypotension, neurologic side effects (acute dystonia, extrapyramidal symptoms), and anticholinergic effects. The acutely agitated patient may require a sedating medication; the patient with hypotension should be treated with the medication with the least effect on blood pressure; and the anti-psychotic medication with the fewest anticholinergic effects is preferred for use in the delirious post-operative patient who has an ileus or urinary retention.

To date, haloperidol remains the drug of choice for the treatment of delirium in the cancer patient. This neuroleptic agent is a potent dopamine blocker with useful sedating effects and low incidence of cardiovascular and anticholinergic effects. For the most part, relatively low doses of haloperidol (1–3 mg/day) are effective in targeting agitation, paranoia, and fear. Typically the initial dose may be in the range of 0.5–1.0 mg haloperidol (PO,IV,IM,SC), with repeat doses if necessary, titrated against symptoms at intervals of 45–60 minutes.[40] Although our experience has been that most patients respond to doses of less than 20 mg haloperidol in a 24-hour period, others have advocated high doses (up to 250 mg/24 h IV haloperidol) in selected cases.[34,40,41] Parenteral doses of haloperidol are roughly twice as potent as oral doses, and peak plasma concentrations are achieved in 2–4 hours after an oral dose, whereas measurable plasma concentrations of haloperidol occur 15–30 minutes after intramuscular administration. Although most delirious patients can

Table 1.2. Medications useful for managing delirium in adult cancer patients

Generic name	Approximate daily dosage range (mg)	Route
Neuroleptics		
Haloperidol	0.5–5 q2–12h	PO, IV, SC, IM
Thioridazine	10–75 q4–8h	PO
Chlorpromazine	12.5–50 q4–12h	PO, IV, IM
Methotrimeprazine	12.5–50 q4–8h	IV, SC, PO
Droperidol	0.5–5 q12h	IM, IV
Molindone	10–20 q4–6	PO
Benzodiazepines		
Lorazepam	0.5–2.0 q1–4h	PO, IV, IM
Midazolam	30–100 per 24h	IV, SC

PO = orally; IV = intravenously; SC = subcutaneously; IM = intramuscularly

In some cases, dose adjustments are prudent during parenteral use. Oral forms of medication are preferred. Intravenous bolus injections should be administered slowly. Intramuscular injections should be avoided if repeated use becomes necessary. Subcutaneous infusions are accepted modes of drug administration in the terminally ill.

be managed with oral haloperidol, the intravenous route facilitates rapid onset of medication effects, which may be preferable in very agitated or paranoid patients.[34,39–41] Although not yet approved by the Food and Drug Administration for intravenous use in the United States, haloperidol is commonly and safely administered by this route. If the clinical situation dictates the need for a prompt effect and intravenous access in unavailable, we suggest starting with intramuscular or subcutaneous administration and switching to the oral route when possible. The subcutaneous delivery of haloperidol is an approach commonly employed by palliative-care practitioners. Other neuroleptic medications, including thioridazine and chlorpromazine, may also be useful in the management of delirium. These medications have the potential to result in more sedation and orthostatic hypotension than haloperidol.

A drawback to the use of haloperidol, and other neuroleptic drugs, is the potential for causing extrapyramidal side effects and movement disorders. Acute dystonias and extrapyramidal side effects can generally be controlled by use of anti-parkinsonian medications (e.g., diphenhydramine, benztropine, trihexyphenidyl); akathisia responds to low doses of propranolol (e.g., 5 mg two to three times per day), lorazepam (0.5–1.0 mg two to three times per day), or benztropine (1–2 mg once to twice per day). The neuroleptic malignant syndrome is a rare complication of antipsychotics and must be recognized as a potential medical emergency. This syndrome may be fatal and is characterized by hyperthermia, increased mental confusion, leukocytosis, muscular rigidity, myoglobinuria, and high serum creatine phosphokinase. Although this syndrome may occur at any time during administration of this group of medications, it usually occurs after prolonged high-dose administration of neuroleptics or is precipitated by intercurrent illness. Treatment consists of discontinuing the neuroleptic, general supportive measures, treatment of precipitating factors, and the use of dantrolene sodium or bromocriptine mesylate.[42]

Methotrimeprazine (IV or SC) is often used to control confusion and agitation in delirium occurring in the setting of terminal disease.[43] Dosages range from 12.5 mg to 50 mg every 4–8 hours up to 300 mg/24 h. Hypotension and sedation are problematic limitations of this drug. The use of midazolam has been reported for the control of agitation related to delirium in the terminal stages of disease.[44,45] It has been given by subcutaneous or intravenous infusion in doses ranging from 30 mg to 100 mg/24 h. The goal of treatment with midazolam, and to some extent with methotrimeprazine, is to achieve quiet sedation. As opposed to neuroleptic drugs like haloperidol, benzodiazepines have not been shown to clear a delirious patient's sensorium or improve cognition. These clinical differences may be due to the underlying pathophysiology of delirium. For example, one hypothesis postulates that an imbalance of central cholinergic and adrenergic mechanisms underlies delirium, and so a dopamine-blocking drug may initiate a re-balancing of these systems.[46]

While in many cases neuroleptic drugs are most effective in diminishing agitation, clearing the sensorium, and improving cognition, these may not be attainable goals in the last days of life. Although delirium may still be reversible at this time of life, the processes causing delirium may, as death nears, be ongoing and irreversible. Ventafridda et al.[47] and Fainsinger and colleagues[48,49] have reported that a significant group (10%–20%) of terminally ill patients experience delirium that can only be controlled by sedation to the point of a significantly decreased level of consciousness. In such cases, and occasionally in the course of management of reversible delirium, a common strategy in the management of agitated delirium is to supplement the regimen of haloperidol with parenteral lorazepam.[40,41,43] Lorazepam 0.5 mg–1.0 mg every 1–2 h PO or IV, when administered with haloperidol, may result in more rapid sedation in the agitated delirious patient.

Despite these clinical observations suggesting lorazepam as an effective adjunct to antipsychotic medications, benzodiazepines alone have limited benefit in the treatment of delirium. In a double-blind, randomized trial comparing haloperidol with chlorpromazine and lorazepam, Breitbart and colleagues[50] demonstrated that lorazepam alone, in doses up to 8 mg in a 12-hour period, was ineffective in the treatment of delirium and in fact contributed to worsening delirium and cognitive impairment.[50] Both of the neuroleptic drugs studied, however, in low doses (approximately 2 mg haloperidol equivalent/ per 24 h) were highly effective in controlling the symptoms of delirium (dramatic improvement in DRS scores) and improving cognitive function (dramatic improvement in MMSE scores).

Conclusion

Delirium is a highly prevalent disorder in the population with advanced cancer. It is distressing for patients and their families and is often a management problem for staff. Frequently, delirium is reversible and, therefore, a management approach that incorporates a thorough diagnostic assessment is required so that specific treatment strategies may be implemented. Further research is needed to assess the nature of this condition and its appropriate treatment interventions.

Acknowledgments

This material was published previously, in part, in: Ingham J, Portenoy RK: The assessment of delirium in patients with cancer. *Quaderni di Cure Palliative* 2(2):121–125, 1994.

References

1. Lipowski ZJ. Delirium (acute confusional states). *JAMA* 1987; 258(13):1789–1792.
2. Rabins PV. Psychosocial and management aspects of delirium. *Int Psychogeriatr* 1991; 3:319–324.
3. Bruera E, Fainsinger RL, Miller MJ, and Kuehn N. The assessment of pain intensity in patients with cognitive failure: a preliminary report. *J Pain Symptom Manage* 1992; 7:267–270.
4. Trzepacz PT, Teague GB, Lipowski ZJ. Delirium and other organic mental disorders in a general hospital. *Gen Hosp Psychiatry* 1985; 7:101–106.
5. Johnson JC, Kerse NM, Gottlieb G, Wanich C, Sullivan E, Chen K. Prospective versus retrospective methods of identifying patients with delirium. *J Am Geriatr Soc* 1992; 40:316–319.
6. Lipowski ZJ. *Delirium: Acute Confusional States.* New York: Oxford University Press; 1990.
7. Levkoff SE, Evans DA, Liptzin B, Cleary PD, Lipsitz LA, Wetle TT, Reilly CH, Pilgrim DM, Schor J, Rowe J. Delirium: The occurrence and persistence of symptoms among elderly hospitalized patients. *Arch Intern Med* 1992; 152:334–340.
8. Derogatis LR, Morrow GR, Fetting J, Penman D, Piasetsky S, Schmale AM, Henrichs M, Carnicke CLM. The prevalence of psychiatric disorders among cancer patients. *JAMA* 1983; 249:751–757.

9. Levine PM, Silberfarb PM, Lipowski ZJ. Mental disorders in cancer patients: a study of 100 psychiatric referrals. *Cancer* 1978; 42:1385–1391.

10. Stiefel F, Fainsinger R, Bruera E. Acute confusional states in patients with advanced cancer. *J Pain Symptom Manage* 1992; 7:94–98.

11. Massie MJ, Holland J, and Glass E. Delirium in terminally ill cancer patients. *Am J Psychiatry* 1983; 140:1048–50.

12. Bruera E, Miller L, McCallion J, Macmillan K, Krefting L, Hanson J. Cognitive failure in patients with terminal cancer: a prospective study. *J Pain Symptom Manage* 1992; 7:192–195.

13. Inouye SK, Viscoli CM, Horwitz RI, Hurst LD, Tinetti ME. A predictive model for delirium in hospitalized elderly medical patients based on admission characteristics. *Ann Intern Med* 1993; 119:474–481.

14. Williams RP, Urquhart BL, Sharrock NE, Charlson ME. Post-operative delirium: predictors and prognosis in elderly orthopedic patients. *J Am Geriatr Soc* 1992; 40:759–767.

15. Marcantonio ER, Goldman L, Mangione CM, Ludwig LE, Muraca B, Haslauer CM, Donaldson MC, Whittemore AD, Sugarbaker DJ, Poss R, Haas S, Cook EF, Orav EJ, Lee TH. A clinical prediction rule for delirium after elective noncardiac surgery. *JAMA* 1994; 271:134–139.

16. Schor JD, Levkoff SE, Lipsitz LA, Reilly CH, Cleary PD, Rowe JW, Evans DA. Risk factors for delirium in hospitalized elderly. *JAMA* 1992; 267:827–831.

17. Tune LE, Bylsma FW. Benzodiazepine-induced and anticholinergic-induced delirium in the elderly. *Int Psychogeriatr* 1991; 3:397–408.

18. Portenoy RK, Thaler HT, Kornblith AB, McCarthy-Lepore J, Friedlander-Klar H, Coyle N, Smart-Curley T, Kemeny N, Norton L, Hoskins W, Scher H. Symptom prevalence, characteristics and distress in a cancer population. *Qual Life Res* 1994; 3:183–189.

19. Coyle N, Adelhardt J, Foley KM, Portenoy RK. Character of terminal illness in the advanced cancer patient: pain and other symptoms during the last four weeks of life. *J Pain Symptom Manage* 1990; 5:83–93.

20. Lichter I, Hunt E. The last 48 hours of life. *J Palliat Care* 1990; 6:7–15.

21. Lipowski ZJ. Delirium in the elderly patient. *N Engl J Med* 1989; 320:578–582.

22. Liptzin B, Levkoff SE. An empirical study of delirium subtypes. *Br J Psychiatry* 1992; 161:843–845.

23. Ross CA, Peyser CE, Shapiro I, Folstein MF. Delirium: phenomenologic and etiologic subtypes. *Int Psychogeriatr* 1991; 3:135–147.

24. Posner JB, Plum F. *Diagnosis of Stupor and Coma.* 3rd ed. Philadelphia: F.A. Davis; 1982.

25. American Psychiatric Association. *Diagnostic and Statistical Manual of Mental Disorders.* 4th ed. Washington, D.C.: American Psychiatric Association; 1994.

26. American Psychiatric Association. *Diagnostic and Statistical Manual of Mental Disorders.* 3rd, rev. ed. Washington, D.C.: American Psychiatric Association; 1987.

27. American Psychiatric Association, Task Force on DSM-IV. *Diagnostic and Statistical Manual of Mental Disorders–IV Draft Criteria.* Washington, D.C.: American Psychiatric Association; 1993.

28. Smith MJ, Breitbart WS, Platt MM. A critique of instruments and methods to detect, diagnose, and rate delirium. *J Pain Symptom Manage* 1994; 10:35–77.

29. Folstein MF, Folstein SE, McHugh PR. Mini-mental state. *J Psychiatr Res* 1975; 12:189–198.

30. Katzman R, Brown T, Fuld P, Peck A, Schechter R, Schimmel H. Validation of a short orientation-memory-concentration test of cognitive impairment. *Am J Psychiatry* 1983; 140:734–739.

31. Inouye SK, Van Dyck CH, Alessi CA, Balkin S, Siegal AP, Horwitz RI. Clarifying confusion: the confusion assessment method. *Ann Intern Med* 1990; 113:941–948.

32. Trzepacz PT, Baker RW, Greenhouse J. A symptom rating scale for delirium. *Psychiatry Res* 1988; 23:89–97.

33. Fainsinger RL, Tapper M, Bruera E. A perspective on the management of delirium in terminally ill patients on a palliative care unit. *J Palliat Care* 1993; 9:4–8.

34. Murray GB. Confusion, delirium, and dementia. In: Hackett TP, Cassem NH, eds. *Massachusetts General Hospital Handbook of General Hospital Psychiatry*. 2nd ed. Littleton, Mass: PSG; 1987:84–115.

35. Tuma R, DeAngelis L. Acute encephalopathy in patients with systemic cancer. *Ann Neurol* 1992; 32:288.

36. Leipzig RM, Goodman H, Gray G, Erle H, Reidenberg MM. Reversible, narcotic-associated mental status impairment in patients with metastatic cancer. *Pharmacology* 1987; 35:47–54.

37. Patchell RA, Posner JB. Cancer and the nervous system. In: Holland JC, Rowland JH, eds. *Handbook of Psychooncology*. New York: Oxford University Press; 1989:327–341.

38. Fleishman SB, Lesko LM, Breitbart W. Treatment of organic mental disorders in cancer patients. In: Breitbart W, Holland JC, eds. *Psychiatric Aspects of Symptom Management in Cancer Patients*. Washington, D.C.: American Psychiatric Press; 1993:23–47.

39. Fleishman S, Lesko LM. Delirium and dementia. In: Holland JC, Rowland JH, eds. *Handbook of Psychooncology*. New York: Oxford University Press; 1989: 342–355.

40. Adams F, Fernandez F, Andersson BS. Emergency pharmacotherapy of delirium in the critically ill cancer patient. *Psychosomatics* 1986; 27:33–37.

41. Fernandez F, Levy JK, Mansell PWA. Management of delirium in terminally ill AIDS patients. *Int J Psychiatry Med* 1989; 19:165–172.

42. Cooper PE. Disorders of the hypothalamus and pituitary gland. In: Joynt RJ, ed. *Clinical Neurology*. Vol. 3. Philadelphia: J.B. Lippincott; 1994:31–32.

43. Oliver DJ. The use of methotrimeprazine in terminal care. *Br J Clin Pract* 1985; 39:339–340.

44. Bottomley DM, Hanks GW. Subcutaneous midazolam infusion in palliative care. *J Pain Symptom Manage* 1990; 5:259–261.

45. De Sousa E, Jepson A. Midazolam in terminal care. *Lancet* 1988; 67–68.

46. Itil T, Fink M. Anticholinergic drug-induced delirium: experimental modification, quantitative EEG and behavioral correlations. *J Nerv Ment Dis* 1966; 143:492–507.

47. Ventafridda V, Ripamonti C, DeConno F, et al. Symptom prevalence and control during cancer patients' last days of life. *J Palliat Care* 1990; 6:7–11.

48. Fainsinger R, Bruera E. Treatment of delirium in a terminally ill patient. *J Pain Symptom Manage* 1992; 7:54–56.
49. Fainsinger R, MacEachern T, Hanson J, et al. Symptom control during the last week of life in a palliative care unit. *J Palliat Care* 1991; 7:5–11.
50. Breitbart W, Marotta R, Platt MM, et al. A double-blind trial of haloperidol, chlorpromazine and lorazepam in the treatment of delirium in hospitalized AIDS patients. *Am J Psychiatry* 1996; 153:231–237.

2

Assessment and Management of Reversible Delirium

NOÉMI D. DE STOUTZ AND FRITZ STIEFEL

Delirium (acute confusional states) is a common psychiatric complication in patients with cancer.[1–5] It is a neglected syndrome, partly because it is seen by nonpsychiatric physicians.[6] Since Engel and Romano's studies nearly 40 years ago,[7] there has been a lack of research compared to other psychiatric morbidity associated with cancer or its treatment.[8,9] For example, delirium has not been investigated until recently with newly developed techniques like computed tomography (CT) and magnetic resonance imaging (MRI). According to Lipowski,[9,10] who devoted extensive work to this syndrome and wrote the most comprehensive book on this subject: "My object in approaching so acknowledged a terra incognita is not, I regret to say, that I have any fresh contribution towards its elucidation to bring into the field, but rather to awaken a more lively inquiry amongst the profession as to its real nature and causes."

In this chapter, we review the most important elements a physician could need when confronted with a delirious cancer patient. Specifically, we concentrate on the etiology and pathogenesis of delirium in cancer patients, the usefulness of screening and assessment instruments, the possibilities and limitations of the medical workup, nonpharmacological management, and the approach to the patient.

Etiology and Pathogenesis

A variety of factors are known to cause delirium in patients with cancer. Posner[11] has distinguished two major types: direct effects on the brain by primary brain tumor or metastatic spread, and indirect effects (far more fre-

quent) due to infections, vascular complications, toxic or metabolic abnormalities, hematologic complications, treatment side effects, and paraneoplastic syndromes (Table 2.1). The following are the most frequently observed
causes[12]: (1) metabolic abnormalities (organ failure, electrolyte imbalance), (2)
infections (pneumonia, sepsis), (3) metastatic brain disease, (4) treatment side
effects (corticosteroids, chemotherapeutics, opioids, and medications with anticholinergic properties, such as some of the antidepressants), (5) vascular
complications (thromboembolic cerebral infarction), and (6) withdrawal from
alcohol or benzodiazepines. Patients with cancer who have advanced disease
have a relatively high risk of delirium, which is usually associated with multiple causes.[13] In a small study of patients with advanced disease, 10 of the 11
confusional states were attributed to multiple factors.[3] Because extensive clinical workup is rarely appropriate in patients with advanced disease, the processes causing delirium are rarely detected. In a retrospective study involving
patients of a highly specialized palliative care unit, the reason for delirium
remained unknown in 75% of the cases (Table 2.2).[14]

Different hypotheses have been elaborated to explain the pathogenesis of
delirium. It may be that different mechanisms contribute simultaneously to a
delirious state, or that the pathophysiology differs depending on the underlying etiology. The following hypotheses have been posited:[8]

1. Any state of (relatively) reduced oxidative metabolism of cerebral neuron. Engel and Romano[7] observed in their classical studies that the
   level of consciousness in delirium correlated with the slowing of electro-
   encephalogram (EEG) background activity, which parallels changes in
   the functional metabolism of cerebral neurons; since then, many other
   reports support this hypothesis.
2. Imbalance between acetylcholine and dopamine caused by drugs or
   other reasons.
3. Hypercortisolism caused by stress or medication.[15,16]
4. Structural damage to neurons by tumor growth.
5. Changes in endorphin levels.

These hypotheses and others indicate that any condition with increased cerebral energy requirements (fever), increased cerebral functional activity (stress,
anxiety), decreased energy supply (hypoxia) or anticholinergic imbalance
should be treated to support recovery. Recently, investigations using computed tomography and brain magnetic resonance imaging suggest that the
underlying pathophysiology of delirium may lie, at least in part, at the subcortical level.[17,18] Structural or functional changes in the basal ganglia or white
matter could disrupt afferent projections from association cortices, resulting in
an increased vulnerability to disturbance of attention, which is a cardinal
feature that may lead to other symptoms, such as perceptual misinterpreta-
tion, decreased awareness of self and surroundings, impaired directed thinking, difficulties in memory retrieval, spatiotemporal disorientation, hypoac-

Table 2.1. Causes of delirium in cancer patients

Direct effects

Primary tumor
Metastatic lesions by local extension, hematogenous or lymphatic routes

Indirect effects

Metabolic problems (organ failure and electrolyte imbalance)
Treatment effects (chemotherapeutic agents, radiation, medications)
Infections (pneumonia) and systemic infections
Withdrawal (alcohol, benzodiazepines)
Vascular complications (thromboembolic cerebral infarction, intracranial hemorrhage)
Hematologic abnormalities (anemias, coagulopathies)
Nutritional deficits (general malnutrition and vitamin deficits)
Paraneoplastic syndromes

Source: Modified from Posner.[72]

Table 2.2. Retrospective analysis of the treatment of 39 delirious patients with advanced cancer

Mean age/range (yr)	62.5/28–84
Sex (female/male)	18/21
Main cancer diagnosis (n)	
Lung	8
Colon	5
Gastric	3
Unknown	3
Others	20
Psychotropic drug treatment (n)	
Haloperidol	8
Lorazepam	5
Lorazepam and/or haloperidol	10
Midazolam	9
Established reason for delirium (n)	
Unknown	29
Brain metastases	5
Liver failure	4
Hypoxia	1

tive psychomotor behavior, cognitive impairment, and disorder in sleep–wake cycle.[19]

This proposed pathophysiology does not account for the observation that some patients develop a hyperactive, hyperalert delirium from the same metabolic disturbance that causes others to develop a hypoactive, hypoalert delirium. Individual differences in anatomy and membrane function may be the reason, but it is also possible that each type of clinical presentation is determined by an unique combination of factors, with the most obvious cause of the illness being only one.[20,21] From a clinical point of view, the onset of delirium always represents a state of fragility and is a serious sign of an underlying somatic process. It is, therefore, not surprising that delirium is a predictor of shortened survival.[22]

Early Detection, Assessment, and Screening

Because delirium is a frequent prelude to serious somatic complications, prolonged psychiatric morbidity, or death, prompt recognition and diagnosis is essential for patient safety, survival, and quality of life.[23] Generally, however, delirium is unrecognized and is likely to be misdiagnosed as "depression," "coping difficulties," "hysteria," and other nonspecific terms. When delirium is recognized in patients with advanced cancer it is often seen as heralding the terminal phase of the illness[3] and it may be too easily accepted as an unavoidable and irreversible part of the dying process, and thus not worthy of investigation.[24]

Delirium is reversible in an unknown proportion of cases, particularly when it is detected and treated early. Delirium can be the first symptom of a life-threatening complication, such as infection, that needs to be treated vigorously. Several groups have shown a benefit of early detection of delirium, even in terminally ill cancer patients.[25,26]

Early detection of delirium presupposes a high awareness of its often elusive clinical presentation. An accurate assessment must be applied repeatedly in all cancer patients.[27] Observation of cognitive functioning should be routine, not only on admission, but in daily contacts and by all the caregivers involved. Interspersing mental status questions with a discussion of personal history is useful. Orientation can be intact for a long time and should not be the only function tested. Confabulation and/or a nervous chuckle are common reactions in patients who recognize that they have some confusion.[28] Because of the variability of symptoms, observers may give strikingly divergent reports. The night staff should be particularly proficient at assessing the early signs of acute confusion.[29]

The following key features may be of help for the clinical assessment of delirium (Tables 2.3 and 2.4):

Table 2.3. DSM-III-R Criteria for Delirium (according to the American Psychiatric Association, 1987)

A.	Reduced ability to maintain attention to external stimuli (e.g., questions must be repeated because attention wanders) and to appropriately shift attention to new external stimuli (e.g., perseverates answer to a previous question).
B.	Disorganized thinking, as indicated by rambling, irrelevant, or incoherent speech.
C.	At least two of the following: 1. reduced level of consciousness, e.g., difficulty keeping awake during examination 2. perceptual disturbances: misinterpretations, illusions, or hallucinations 3. disturbance of sleep–wake cycle with insomnia or daytime sleepiness 4. increased or decreased psychomotor activity 5. disorientation to time, place, or person 6. memory impairment, e.g., inability to learn new material, such as the names of several unrelated objects, after 5 minutes, or to remember past events, such as history of current episode of illness
D.	Clinical features develop over a short period of time (usually hours to days) and tend to fluctuate over the course of a day.
E.	Either (1) or (2): 1. evidence from the history, physical examination, or laboratory tests of a specific organic factor (or factors) judged to be etiologically related to the disturbance 2. in the absence of such evidence, an etiologic organic factor can be presumed if the disturbance cannot be accounted for by any nonorganic mental disorder, e.g., manic episode accounting for agitation and sleep disturbance.

DSM-III-R = *Diagnostic and Statistical Manual of Mental Disorders*, 3rd ed., revised.

Table 2.4. DSM-IV Criteria for Delirium (according to the American Psychiatric Association, 1995) and their relation to DSM-III-R Criteria

A.	Disturbance of consciousness (i.e., reduced clarity of awareness of the environment) with reduced ability to focus, sustain, or shift attention. (= A + C1 in DSM-III-R)
B.	A change in cognition (such as memory deficit, disorientation, language disturbance) or the development of a perceptual disturbance that is not better accounted for by a preexisting, established, or evolving dementia. (= B + C2 + C5 + C6 in DSM-III-R)
C.	The disturbance develops over a short period of time (usually hours to days) and tends to fluctuate during the course of the day. (= D in DSM-III-R)
D.	There is evidence from the history, physical examination, or laboratory findings that the disturbance is caused by the direct physiological consequences of a general medical condition. (= E1 in DSM-III-R) Criteria C3, C4, and E2 in DSM-III-R have been omitted in DSM-IV.

DSM-IV = *Diagnostic and Statistical Manual of Mental Disorders*, 4th ed.

1. Cognition (perception, thinking, and memory) is always disturbed to some extent. Perceptions cannot be integrated meaningfully with previously acquired knowledge, and hallucinations, dreams, and illusions cannot be discriminated anymore. Thinking is disorganized, ranging from mild concentration difficulties to complete incoherence of thought, with emergence of unconscious conflictual material. Memory is impaired in all its key aspects—registration, retention, and recall—and there tends to be some degree of amnesia. Disorientation is just one consequence of this general inability to process information.[13]
2. Attention is invariably disordered in delirium, manifesting as either decreased or increased readiness to respond to stimuli. Focusing, directing, and shifting attention at will is always impossible.
3. Verbal and nonverbal psychomotor behavior is disturbed. Attention and behavior abnormalities exist in three forms: hypoalert–hypoactive, hyperalert–hyperactive, and a mixed form in which both extremes alternate.[10,19]
4. The sleep–wake cycle also is disturbed. Napping tends to be frequent during the day and adds dream fragments to the misperceptions of waking periods, further confusing the patient. Night sleep is usually short and fragmented, and periods of agitation occur mostly during the night.
5. Additional symptoms exist, which are neither constant nor essential for diagnosis. Intense emotions are experienced by many patients and are accompanied by sympathetic nervous system hyperarousal. Fear, apathy, and aggressiveness are commonly seen. Involuntary movements may be present, especially in substance-induced delirium.[13,30]

The patient himself should be asked about prodromal symptoms, such as disturbing dreams and transient hallucinations, and about difficulties in discriminating perceptions, images, dreams, and hallucinations.[30] A patient may remember what happened during his delirium and may appreciate talking things over once the syndrome has subsided.[31]

The clinical interview is generally used to detect delirium in research studies. Only exceptionally do these studies document how the criteria for the diagnosis of delirium are translated into practical procedures.[32] Standard nursing assessments have been developed at some centers[33] in an effort to systematize observations for diagnostic purposes. Such assessments take into account all the criteria defining delirium according to the *Diagnostic and Statistical Manual of Mental Disorder,* third edition, revised (DSM-III-R).[34] However, even if such a standard of nursing practice increases the nurses' awareness of the possible significance of patient behaviors, it is difficult to imagine the routine application of all its parts.

Family members are a very important source of information about the patient's prior level of mental functioning. They should also get involved in the early detection of delirium. Their observations need to be taken into account, but teaching is necessary to help them in recognizing relevant findings and to reduce their anxiety with regard to personality changes in a loved one. Early, mild symptoms worth noting include a change in sleep pattern with restlessness and occasional disorientation, increased irritability, withdrawal, and unusual forgetfulness.[13] The family's recognition might help to prevent disruptive behaviors that occur in more severe delirium.

In daily clinical work, where time for a more comprehensive assessment often is very limited, a useful first question may be to ask the patient what time he thinks it is. Patients with delirium often fail to answer this question correctly, and further assessment becomes warranted. So many environmental clues have to be perceived and processed to guess the approximate time of day that this would be an interesting screening tool to examine.

Serial screening is recommended by many authors. The ideal screening instrument would be short and easy to administer; independent of the patient's physical handicaps, education, and language; sensitive despite fluctuation of symptoms; and able to test for all the criteria of delirium as defined in DSM-III-R. Levkoff and colleagues published a review of existing instruments[35] and conclude that "further research is needed to refine these instruments and to compare their reliability and validity in the detection of this important syndrome."

In these screening tests, global scores have advantages over the tests that examine individual functions. They assess different areas independently, which increases their sensitivity, and as they quantify the impairments, they provide a means for longitudinal observation of patients. Deciding about cutoff points is crucial, as they have a marked impact on sensitivity and specificity of the tests. For patients with preexisting mental status impairment, changes in mental scores is more important in the detection of delirious episodes than a cutoff.

The following screening instruments have been used for clinical and scientific investigation (Table 2.5):

1. Both the left and right cerebral hemispheres are involved in the complex process of writing,[36] and having the patient write a sentence is sensitive to even subtle cerebral changes.[37] In Aakerlund and Rosenberg's study,[36] writing had a high positive predictive value, and, in one case, disturbances occurred before all DSM-III-R criteria for delirium were detectable. Larger studies are needed to confirm this finding and to standardize the criteria used for judging writing ability. The use of handwriting as a screening instrument for delirium cannot be used with aphasic patients, patients speaking foreign languages, and those whose baseline writing ability is limited by preexisting handicaps.

Table 2.5. Screening and assessment instruments for delirium

---

1. Clinical observation by
   Health care professionals
   Family
   Patient

2. Tests addressing complex cerebral processes
   Guessing the hour
   Handwriting

3. Tests addressing isolated DSM-III-R criteria for delirium
   Attention: Hand Held Tachistoscope, Trail Making Test
   Consciousness/attention: Global Accessibility Rating
   Orientation: Organic Brain Syndrome Scale

4. Scores quantifying cognitive functions
   Mini-Mental State Questionnaire
   Short Portable Mental State Questionnaire
   Cognitive Capacity Screening Examination

5. Scores operationalizing the DSM-III-R criteria
   Confusion Rating Scale
   NEECHAM Confusion Scale
   Delirium Rating Scale
   Delirium Symptom Interview

DSM-III-R = *Diagnostic and Statistical Manual of Mental Disorders*, 3rd ed., revised.

2. One of the core features of delirium is attention. Psychomotor tests for attention such as Hand-Held Tachistoscope[38] and the Trail-Making Test[39] have been used in research on delirium. Unfortunately both rely heavily on patient cooperation, and on physical and sensory functioning. Their usefulness is therefore limited in delirious patients, and especially in the physically ill such as cancer patients.

3. The Global Accessibility Rating[40] tests for clouding of consciousness or attention. Because the rating is done by a trained observer interacting with the patient, there is no need for patient cooperation. It has been used for diagnosis of delirium in one study only and does not cover all the DSM-III-R criteria.

4. The Organic Brain Syndrome scale (OBS-scale) is not aimed specifically at delirium and tests orientation to time, person, and present situation only.[41]

5. The Mini-Mental State Questionnaire (MMSQ) has been proposed by Folstein and colleagues "as a practical method for grading the cognitive state of patients for the clinician."[42] It is a short series of questions that requires 10 minutes to complete and tests orientation, registration, attention and calculation, recall, and language. Although valida-

tion studies have shown good sensitivity for cognitive impairment, specificity is low and the MMSQ does not differentiate delirium from dementia in a single examination.[35] The clinical value of some of the tasks included in the MMSQ is also controversial.[37,43] Noncognitive aspects are not tested, and there is no means to account for rapidity of onset and fluctuation of symptoms. This scale may therefore not be sensitive enough to detect mild forms of delirium. However, when the MMSQ is administered repeatedly, changes in a patient's score can be an early indication of delirium.[26,44]

6. The Short Portable Mental State Questionnaire[45] and the Cognitive Capacity Screening Examination[46] have similar limitations as the MMSQ. All were designed before the DSM-III criteria for delirium were established. They focus on cognitive function, rely on the patient's verbal response, and were designed to diagnose organic cognitive impairments, without distinction between acute and chronic impairments.

7. The Confusion Rating Scale[47] is a rating of confusional behavior over an 8-hour shift, administered by nurses. It was designed for diagnosis of postoperative delirium on an orthopedic ward, and is short enough to be used as a screening instrument. It does not cover all aspects of the DSM-III-R definition of delirium and has not been tested outside that surgical context.

8. The NEECHAM Confusion Scale[48] is a test scored by nurses at the bedside. It utilizes information on the patient's performance in activities of daily living and physiological data, but places a minimal response burden on the patient. It was designed to assess changes in information processing and to document acute confusional behavior, including delirium. It was not specifically designed to detect delirium as defined by DSM-III or DSM-III-R, but showed strong associations with those criteria. It has not been used by other investigators.

9. The Confusion Assessment Method (CAM) is a diagnostic algorithm based on those DSM-III-R criteria that can be observed at the bedside. It was shown to be sensitive and reliable for diagnosis of delirium when used by geriatricians and psychiatrists after structured interviews of the patients. It is probably reliable when used by nurses after routine daily care, and may be a candidate instrument for daily use.[49]

10. The Delirium Rating Scale (DRS) is rated by a clinician using whatever information is available from medical examination, nursing and family observations, laboratory tests, and so on. It is based on the DSM-III criteria and covers all the domains defined therein. Fluctuation of symptoms is accounted for by basing the scores on 24-hour periods.[50] The interrater reliability is high among raters familiar with the use of

the score, but standardization of the clinical judgment used to generate a score is difficult. This scale may therefore be more appropriate for scientific than clinical investigations.

11. The Delirium Symptom Interview (DSI) was designed for use in the Commonwealth-Harvard Study to circumvent the limitations of earlier instruments. It is a symptom checklist, with questions for patients and parallel questions for nurses. After adequate training, nonclinical research assistants can administer this instrument, and it has high specificity and sensitivity.[35] Its use as a screening method for delirium in routine clinical practice has yet to be attempted and the training seems to be rather complex, with a 37-page instruction manual.

The DSM-III-R criteria themselves have been questioned and recent literature has included proposals for improving the definition of delirium in DSM-IV. Thus, Lipowski has criticized the fact that memory impairment and perceptual disturbances are not considered an integral part of the syndrome.[30] Spitzer and colleagues have suggested a whole new classification that would no longer rely on a mind/body duality and would therefore drop the term "organic mental disorders." They propose to reorganize the classification to include a section called "cognitive mental disorders," comprising delirium, dementia, and amnestic disorders, and to distinguish "secondary" and "substance-induced" disorders as those with medical and chemical causes of delirium.[51] The classification in DSM-IV has been changed accordingly, and criteria for delirium have been reorganized to include only four elements: (A) consciousness and attention, (B) cognition or perception, (C) time course of symptoms, and (D) organic cause (Table 2.3).[52]

It is safe to say that neither the screening instruments nor the concepts for the clinical assessment are yet comprehensive enough to allow general acceptance of a "gold standard" for early detection and diagnosis of delirium.

The diagnosis of delirium is easy once the symptoms disturb the normal functioning of an oncology ward. But disruptive behavior may not occur, and hypoalert–hypoactive delirium is just as important to detect as hyperactive delirium. Some of the assessment instruments are not adequate for routine repeated screening, but rather qualify as research instruments. The mainstay of systematic early detection of delirium is a high level of suspicion, awareness of the frequency of the syndrome and its risk factors, knowledge of the diagnostic criteria, and familiarity with the subtle manifestations that could otherwise give rise to wild interpretations. Educating health care providers to this awareness is essential.

Systematic observation combined with routine use of even suboptimal screening instruments allows for further assessment of patients suspected of delirium. Implementation of such measures may be more realistic than designing the perfect instrument and lacking funds to administer it universally.

Differential Diagnosis

One of the challenges in diagnosing delirium is to distinguish it from acute stress reactions, depression, mania, schizophreniform disorders, and dementia. Often, an agitated patient is first thought to have an understandable stress reaction to the bad news of having cancer. Anxiety and anger may be interpreted in this way, especially by health care providers who misinterpret the writings of Kübler-Ross.[53] These writings describe different phases of adaptation to cancer, some of which may present with a picture similar to the symptomatology of early delirium. This may be one of the many reasons for the undertreatment of delirium.[54] Close monitoring of the disturbances mentioned above (Table 2.4) will clarify the differential diagnosis.

Delirium is also often misdiagnosed as depression. It is common for psychiatric consultation requests for "depression" to turn out to be a "delirium."[6] Although withdrawal and refusal to communicate, cognitive deficits, and depressive or anxious feelings may be present in both delirium and depression,[55,56] other symptoms, such as reduced level of consciousness, disorientation, or incoherent speech, are not seen in depression. In addition, the patient's psychiatric history and the family history for psychiatric morbidity may be helpful in diagnosing depression.

Manic states are often associated with disruptive behavior, aggression, and elevated mood, with ideation of grandiosity. It may be difficult in the acute situation to distinguish a manic episode from delirium. In such a situation, a psychiatric consultation becomes necessary to make the differential diagnosis and start adequate treatment. This also holds true for patients with hallucinations and delusions, who may be similar to patients with schizophreniform disorders. The diagnosis in this case is also possible from clinical examination, history, and the course of the disease. In the cancer population, it is far more likely that delusions, hallucinations and aggressive behavior reflect delirium than a manic episode or schizophreniform disorder.

The most difficult differential diagnosis is dementia. Delirium and dementia have many symptoms in common. The characteristics that most clearly distinguish delirium are its acute onset and rapid progression,[33] fluctuation over the course of a day, clouding of consciousness, and major attention disturbances.[57] Lipowski has proposed criteria for differentiating among delirium, dementia, and depression that are based essentially on systematic clinical observation over several days.[58] Selbst stresses that history is the most important diagnostic tool.[59]

Delirium and dementia can occur simultaneously or separately. Untreated delirium, or delirium caused by irreversible organic factors, is thought by some authors to be a risk factor for developing dementia[37] although prospective confirmatory studies are lacking.[30] More important, patients with preexisting dementia are more sensitive to the factors that can induce delirium. The presence of an underlying dementia in a newly admitted, delirious patient should be elicited by asking relatives about baseline functioning.[27] Incomplete recovery from a delirious episode can be due to preexisting dementia.

Tests for cognitive function do not discriminate sufficiently between delirium and dementia. A clinical workup, as described below, may reveal factors contributing to delirium that are potentially reversible. Treating them aggressively can restore the patient's baseline functioning.

Although the diagnosis of delirium may sometimes be difficult and time consuming, correct diagnosis is critical for therapy. Diagnosis is also important for discharge planning and placement, evaluation of rehabilitative interventions, and development of a strategy to optimize quality of life.[60]

Clinical Workup: Seeking and Managing Reversible Causes

There is a consensus that delirium is a manifestation of generalized cerebral insufficiency with widespread dysregulation of neurotransmitter systems; however, there are no appropriate laboratory tests to measure the internal milieu of the living brain.[37] The clinical workup essentially needs to identify those potential causes of delirium that can be corrected by adequate medical interventions. Delirium is usually caused by multiple factors[3,24] that should be addressed simultaneously.

Predisposing and facilitating factors for delirium are advanced age, chronic brain disease and brain damage, and, especially, dementia.[30] The etiologic role of psychosocial stress, sleep deprivation, sensory deprivation or sensory overload, and immobilization is unclear, but they certainly act as facilitating factors. Untreated pain seems to play some part in generating delirium, although little is known about its effect.[61] A hypothesis is that endorphins and other neurotransmitters are involved. The most dramatic problem is that pain assessment is unreliable during delirium, and pain medications tend to be given arbitrarily.[62]

Postoperative situations constitute a risk period for the development of delirium. The drugs used for anesthesia and the metabolic disturbances of the surgical procedure itself act synergistically to produce increased oxygen demand and decreased oxygen supply.[36]

Clinical examination

The workup starts with a thorough clinical examination. The first impression can reveal features that point to a cause of delirium.[13] Observation of skin color and temperature, and the amount of sweating can raise suspicion of a metabolic or pharmacologic origin of delirium. The deep and rapid breathing pattern associated with acidosis needs to be recognized. The level of consciousness can fluctuate rapidly in parallel with a Cheyne-Stokes breathing pattern.

Unstable vital signs may accompany sepsis or hemorrhage. Any sign of organ failure will be noted because each has metabolic consequences that will affect the brain. Cachexia is to be evaluated as renal failure and may be missed by laboratory tests when creatinine levels are low as the result of the decreased muscle mass. The neurological examination will help to exclude focal deficits due to a cerebrovascular accident or intracranial tumor growth. The size of the pupils point to opioid or anticholinergic toxicity. Ophthalmoscopy can reveal signs of intracranial hypertension or a hyperviscosity syndrome. Particular attention should be paid to possible infectious foci, for delirium can be the first sign of an infection.

Pertinent history

A thorough review of past and current medications is mandatory. Many patients use over-the-counter drugs, which also can interact with prescribed drugs.[27] Information about prior drug reactions can be obtained from relatives and from old hospital records. Changes in absorption, distribution, metabolism, and excretion may be important, especially in the elderly.[29] The cancer or anticancer treatment can also change pharmacokinetics. Polypharmacy should be avoided as much as possible.

Some antineoplastic agents have neurotoxic effects. Delirium has been described with 5-fluorouracil, high-dose methotrexate given intravenously or intrathecally, cytosine-arabinoside, ifosfamide, vinca alkaloids, bleomycin, cisplatin, L-asparaginase, procarbazine,[63] etoposide, carmustine,[27] and caracemide.[37] After treatment with hexamethylmelamine, the occurrence of delirium is delayed by days or weeks and is followed by spontaneous recovery.[64] Interferon and interleukin are increasingly included in treatment protocols and can cause delirium in some cases.[37] Delirium induced by all these agents is self-limited and subsides after discontinuation of the offending drug.

Some of the antineoplastic agents produce alterations in vital organs, which can enhance the patient's susceptibility to multicausal delirium. Thus, the lung fibrosis following bleomycin treatment and the myocardial damage after anthracycline therapy can induce hypoxia, and impaired renal function after platinum compounds or methotrexate can reduce clearance of drugs and their metabolites, even in the absence of uremic syndromes.

Corticosteroids are used as antitumor therapy and as a treatment for nausea or edema associated with brain and spinal cord lesions. They are known to cause mild nervous system disturbances, such as restlessness, hyperactivity, and insomnia.[65] In a prospective comparison study, Breitbart and colleagues found a tendency for a greater incidence of delirium in the corticosteroid group.[15] When corticosteroids are essential, they should be used at the lowest possible dose and psychotropic drugs should be added preventively for those patients who already have steroid-induced delirium.

During treatment with corticosteroids, close monitoring of blood sugar and insulin therapy, if necessary, will prevent hyperglycemic delirium. Steroids can mask the clinical manifestations of an infection, which itself may induce delirium.[13]

Other drugs that are often used in anticancer therapy and that can cause delirium include amphotericin B, acyclovir, and cimetidine.[13] The incidence of delirium associated with anticancer chemotherapy has not been systematically studied.[13] There are also no studies on the effect of delirium on cancer treatment outcomes and prognosis.[27] If a patient who has suffered from treatment-induced delirium is to undergo more cycles of the same therapy, psychotropic agents such as haloperidol should be considered as a preventive measure and the patient should be closely monitored. The patient and his family should be thoroughly informed about the reversible nature of drug-induced delirium.

Unwanted effects of cranial irradiation present either as an immediate somnolence syndrome and cognitive loss, or as a late dementia months or years after the treatment. Late adverse effects are most likely when irradiation is given in large fractions or combined with high-dose chemotherapy.[66] The immediate reaction can have all the characteristics of delirium, but as it is due to acute cerebral edema, other signs of intracranial hypertension are often associated.[67] The specific treatment is corticosteroids, whereas psychotropic drugs are not usually needed.

The opioid analgesics and their metabolites can induce all the disturbances described in the DSM-III-R criteria for delirium. The smallest dose of opioids that ensures good pain control should be prescribed. When delirium has been diagnosed, switching to a different pure μ-receptor agonist (for instance, from morphine to hydromorphone, or vice versa) may improve mental status while maintaining good pain control.[26,46,68]

A large group of drugs frequently used in oncology have anticholinergic properties and may induce delirium, presumably by disturbing the neurotransmitter balance.[30] They include antiemetics, antihistamines, antiparkinsonian drugs, atropine, scopolamine, antispasmodics, antipsychotics (especially the phenothiazine type), and tricyclic antidepressants.[13] It is not unusual to combine several of these drugs in palliative care, which enhances their potential to induce delirium.

Anticholinergic drugs should be discontinued in delirious patients whenever possible. They should be replaced by less anticholinergic medication, if necessary, at the lowest effective dose. In cases of life-threatening anticholinergic toxicity with hyperpyrexia, mydriasis, dehydration, vasodilatation, tachycardia, and urinary retention, the antidote physostigmine can be given, provided resuscitation equipment is available. However, supportive measures and constant observation are often sufficient until the offending drugs are metabolized.[13]

Hypnotic drugs are frequently given to cancer patients for anxiety or insomnia, and they can contribute to delirium. Sedative drugs given for acute agitation, often without evaluating the delirium, enhance the syndrome.[27] Many patients who are thought to be anxious become clearly delirious after receiving a benzodiazepine.[33] Agitated delirium is a rare paradoxical reaction to benzodiazepines.[69] Some degree of confusion, amnesia, disorganized thought, and impairment of mental and psychomotor functions is present at peak plasma concentrations of all benzodiazepines, with long-lasting residual effects after some of them.[70] Benzodiazepines are best avoided in patients predisposed to delirium, and should be discontinued when delirium occurs. If marked sedation is necessary in the management of a delirious patient, a short-acting benzodiazepine, such as midazolam, should be chosen. After discontinuation of the drug, an assessment of the improvement of the patient's delirium becomes rapidly possible, in contrast with longer-acting sedative drugs.[46]

Delirium may be the result of withdrawal in substance abusers. In hospitalized patients, withdrawal from alcohol and benzodiazepines is most common. Inadvertent discontinuation of prescribed medications, such as steroids, thyroid hormone substitution, and opioids, also can precipitate a delirium.[13]

A nutritional history should be obtained from the patient or from caregivers and family. This should assess the potential for deficiencies and for substance abuse. Nutritional status is compromised because of the anorexia of cancer patients or to treatment side effects such as mucositis or short bowel syndrome. Vitamin deficiencies have been linked to increased risk of delirium, especially thiamine, B_{12}, and folate deficiencies.[71]

Laboratory investigations

In the case of a life-threatening metabolic crisis, the following emergency tests need to be obtained: glucose, sodium, calcium, blood urea nitrogen, pH, Pco_2, Po_2. A lumbar puncture will help to exclude bacterial meningitis and subdural hemorrhage.[72] Determination of hemogram, coagulation tests, and liver and kidney function parameters as well as thyroid function studies can reveal additional causes of delirium.[37]

Some electrolyte disturbances may manifest as delirium and will be discussed briefly. Severe hyponatremia occurs in the presence of inappropriate secretion of antidiuretic hormone. This paraneoplastic syndrome is associated mostly with small-cell lung cancer and subsides when the tumor load can be reduced. Supportive treatment, such as restriction of fluid intake, sodium supplementation combined with furosemide, and demeclocycline, may be needed until a remission of the tumor is achieved.[73]

Hypercalcemia is a frequent cause of delirium in cancer patients. It can be a consequence of calcium release from extensive bone metastasis, or of paraneoplastic secretion of parathormone-like peptides.[74] In both cases, the treatment of choice is fluid repletion and intravenous bisphosphonates.[75–77] Rarely, hyperparathyroidism occurs in multiple endocrine neoplasia type II (MEN II;

Sipples syndrome), and hypercalcemia with delirium can be the first manifestation of the disease.[78]

Organ failure also has metabolic consequences that contribute to delirium. Cardiac failure and respiratory insufficiency induce tissue hypoxia, which has an impact on biosynthesis of neurotransmitters.[58] In global respiratory failure, hypercapnia is also possible and directly leads to "CO_2 narcosis," with delirium followed by intracranial hypertension and coma.[79] Pulse oximetry can be sufficient to diagnose hypoxia in cases where there is no suspicion of carbon dioxide retention and where capillary blood flow in the extremities is intact. Otherwise, blood gas analyses are warranted.

Renal function parameters must be evaluated in terms of the nutritional status of a cancer patient. In cachectic patients, serum creatinine can be normal despite very low creatinine clearance. Blood urea nitrogen depends not only on renal function, but also on protein intake. Therefore, creatinine clearance must be estimated on the basis of body weight, or determined using 24-hour urine, to diagnose renal failure. Delirium associated with renal failure is a consequence either of uremia or of accumulation of drugs and their metabolites. It is reversible only if the cause of renal impairment can be corrected, as is the case in prerenal failure due to nonsteroidal anti-inflammatory drugs, angiotensin-converting enzyme inhibitors, or dehydration.[24,80–82] Liver failure due to extensive hepatic metastases is seldom reversible. Reversible liver failure due to hepatotoxic agents, such as acetaminophen or anesthetic gases, is rare. Hepatic function tests include not only liver enzymes and bilirubin, but also parameters of hepatic synthesis such as albumin and coagulation tests.[37]

Hematologic tests can reveal many factors contributing to delirium. Anemia is directly responsible for tissue hypoxia. Leukocytosis with a left shift in the differential blood count, or severe neutropenia, must raise suspicion that delirium is caused by an infection. Culture of all body fluids must be obtained if an infection is suspected, and antibiotic therapy started before the results are known, if the situation warrants it. Thrombocytopenia and impaired coagulation puts the patient at risk for bleeding. An intracranial hemorrhage can be the cause of the delirium. Agitated behavior is particularly dangerous in patients at high risk of bleeding, and sedating medications should be readily given in these cases. Disseminated intravascular coagulation is usually a sign of infection, more rarely of tumor progression, and is associated with bleeding risks as described above.

Delirium can also be the consequence of endocrine disturbances. The most common problem is preexisting or iatrogenic diabetes mellitus. Hypothyroidism is occasionally the cause of a delirium. It can be seen following radiotherapy of head and neck cancer, with a delay of several months or years.[37] Carcinoid tumors are the most common endocrine malignancy to cause psychiatric symptomatology. Depression is the usual manifestation, but anxiety and confusion have also been observed.[83] No routine laboratory tests are available for this condition, in which peptide hormones are involved. Paraneoplastic hallucinosis has been described as the first symptom of pancreatic carcinoma.[60]

Imaging techniques

The direct effects of cancer that cause delirium are often treatable. Therefore, an aggressive search for disorders such as leptomeningeal spread, treatment-induced leukoencephalopathy, central nervous system leukemia, and solitary or multiple brain metastases is warranted.[37] CT scans and MRI are useful to rule out brain metastasis, and MRI and lumbar puncture are indicated when leptomeningeal spread is suspected.

Although the EEG is not routinely needed, it can confirm an encephalopathy or reveal an unsuspected disorder such as complex partial seizures.[23] In most cases, there is slowing of the EEG background activity, but in delirium due to withdrawal of alcohol and sedative–hypnotic drugs, there usually is low-voltage fast activity.[30]

Positron emission tomography may be useful to localize the distribution of abnormal brain metabolism. It is still experimental, but seems a promising tool for diagnosis of delirium and its mechanisms.[30]

Other evaluations can be obtained according to the suspected cause of delirium. In cases of electrolyte disturbances, arrhythmias, and suspected cerebral thromboembolism, an ECG and, if necessary, an echocardiogram will clarify the picture. Radiographs and sonograms can help in the search for infectious processes.

Decisions concerning investigations should depend on the therapeutic interventions that would be made if tests are positive. Sound clinical reasoning is essential in the search for reversible causes of delirium. A rational approach with a minimum of tests is possible, regardless of prognosis, and will be most beneficial to patients.[24,46]

Nonpharmacological management

General supportive treatments, such as measures to counteract sleep deprivation, constipation, and psychosocial stress,[58] and environmental manipulation (e.g., clock at the bedside) to help the patient's orientation may be helpful.[84] However, the most efficient treatment is to remove the underlying causative agent. If this is not possible, pharmacological symptomatic treatment is necessary, at least in patients with hallucinations, delusions, anxiety, agitation, and disruptive behavior. Such treatment should also be provided during the search for underlying causes. Early diagnosis and treatment may also ameliorate other conditions due to delirium, such as pain.[25]

An important, albeit rarely discussed, element in the management of delirium is the personal approach to the delirious patient. From clinical experience, three major points seem to be crucial:

First, in an emergency situation in which the patient exhibits disruptive behavior, agitation, and danger to self or others, the treating physician or the consulting psychiatrist should lead the action (most often ending with a treatment against the will of the patient). Any ambivalence in the situation or an absence of a plan (known to all staff members) will prolong or even worsen the situation. While the outcome of drug therapy cannot be known in advance and it is true that a "psychotropic straitjacket" will probably take away the opportunity to express strong emotions, it is also evident that severely agitated patients have to be treated for the security of themselves and others. There are many patients who clearly benefit from pharmacological treatment, from both a subjective and observer's point of view. It should not be forgotten that delusions and hallucinations due to organic brain disease are most often associated with a great deal of anxiety and suffering, and that this can be alleviated by pharmacological treatments. If doubts exist about treatment, it may well be possible to treat the patient and closely monitor his or her reports and cognitive state.[85]

Second, an open dialogue should be possible with patients who are able to communicate, at least during the periods of lucidity. When communicating, most of the patients experience relief from an experience of personal disorganization. Patients should be told that these states occur fairly frequently in patients with cancer, that they are usually reversible, and that they are not "going to lose their minds." The same holds true for the families of the patients, who have to be informed about our reflections.

Third, there is often concern from medical and nursing staff about the possibility of missed psychogenic reasons for the onset of delirium. While it is true that the contents of delusions and hallucinations may be directly related to prior experiences (conscious and unconscious) of the patient and that impulse control is diminished during these states (e.g., there may be thoughts and acts with aggressive and sexual contents), it is simply not possible that conflicts or other kinds of psychiatric morbidity explain the onset of delirium, except in very rare circumstances where severe anxiety or stress may cause delirium. However, anger or anxiety associated with delirium is often misinterpreted by the staff as a stress reaction or depression, and, occasionally, this delays early diagnostic and therapeutic action.[33] The liaison work of the psychiatric consultant becomes the most important tool to increase knowledge about this syndrome among the medical staff. In the verbal approach to the patient, a repeated and calm orientation to time, place, reason for admission, and actual treatment of the condition seems more appropriate than trying to interpret some of the communication or to "enter the unreal world" of the delirious patient. Too often, health personnel fail to realize that it is unrealistic to reason, apply logic, or argue with a delirious patient, except during a lucid interval.[27] Once again, repeated case conferences or other teaching methods are an appropriate tool to ameliorate the understanding of the situation among the staff.

Conclusion

The management of delirium is a very important task of each health care professional working in oncology. It is very unfortunate that research on delirium has lagged behind research in other psychiatric morbidity. Nonetheless, there is considerable knowledge about some aspects of delirium (such as etiology) and tools for the assessment, clinical workup, and treatment have been developed. These can all be used to ameliorate this distressing condition. As with other important areas of patient care, such as pain management, teaching of the health care professionals remains the key for the improved management of delirious cancer patients.

References

1. Breitbart W. Identifying patients at risk for, and treatment of major psychiatric complications of cancer. *Support Care Cancer* 1995; 3:45–60.
2. Bruera E, Chadwick S, Weinlick A et al. Delirium and severe sedation in patients with terminal cancer (letter). *Cancer Treat Rep* 1987; 71:787–788.
3. Massie MJ, Holland J, Glass E. Delirium in terminally ill cancer patients. *Am J Psychiatry* 1983; 140:1048–1050.
4. Leipzig RM, Goodman H, Gray G, et al. Reversible, narcotic associated mental status impairment in patients with metastatic cancer. *Pharmacology* 1987; 35:47–54.
5. Stiefel F, Razavi D. Common psychiatric disorders in cancer patients. II Anxiety and acute confusional states. *Support Care Cancer* 1994; 2:233–237.
6. Levine PM, Silberfarb PM, Lipowski ZJ. Mental disorders in cancer patients: a study of 100 psychiatric referrals. *Cancer* 1978; 42:1385–1391.
7. Engel GL, Romano G. Delirium, a syndrome of cerebral insufficiency. *J Chronic Dis* 1959; 9:260–277.
8. Stiefel F. Age and the syndrome of delirium—a workshop of the National Institute of Mental Health, Washington, DC, June 1989. *Schweiz Rundsch Med Prax* 1989; 78:1329.
9. Lipowski ZJ. *Delirium: Acute Brain Failure in Man.* Springfield, Ill: Charles C Thomas; 1980.
10. Lipowski ZJ. *Delirium: Acute Confusional States.* New York: Oxford University Press; 1990.
11. Posner JB. Neurologic complications of systemic cancer. *Dis Mon* 1978; 25:1–60.
12. Stiefel F, Holland J. Delirium in cancer patients. *Int Psychogeriatr* 1991; 3:333–336.
13. Fleishman S, Lesko LM. Delirium and dementia. In: Holland JC, Rowland RH,

eds. *Handbook of Psychooncology*. New York: Oxford University Press; 1989:342–355.

14. Stiefel F, Fainsinger R, Bruera E. Acute confusional states in patients with advanced cancer. *J Pain Symptom Manage* 1992; 7:25–29.

15. Breitbart W, Stiefel F, Kornblith AB, Panullo S. Neuropsychiatric disturbance in cancer patients with epidural spinal cord compression receiving high dose corticosteroids: a prospective comparison study. *Psycho-Oncology* 1993; 2:233–245.

16. Stiefel F, Breitbart W, Holland J. Corticosteroids in cancer: neuropsychiatric complications. *Cancer Invest* 1989; 7:479–491.

17. Trzepacz PT, Sclabassi RJ, Van Thiel DH. Delirium: a subcortical phenomenon? *J Neuropsychiatry* 1989; 1(3):283–290.

18. Figiel GS, Krishnan RK, Doraisamy M. Subcortical structural changes in ECT-induced delirium. *J Geriatr Psychiatry Neurol* 1990; 3:172–176.

19. Stiefel F, Bruera E. Psychostimulants for hypoactive-hypoalert delirium? *J Palliat Care* 1991; 7(3):25–26.

20. Strub RL, Black FW (eds). Aute confusional states (Delirium). In: *Neurobehavioral Disorders*. Philadelphia: F.A. Davis Co.; 1988:107–139.

21. Hales RE, Polly S, Orman D. An evaluation of patients who received an organic mental disorder diagnosis on a psychiatric consultation-liaison service. *Gen Hosp Psychiatry* 1988; 11:88–94.

22. Bruera E, Miller MJ, Kuehn N, MacEachern T, Hanson J. Estimate of survival of patients admitted to a palliative care unit: a prospective study. *J Pain Symptom Manage* 1992; 7:82–86.

23. Adams F. Neuropsychiatric evaluation and treatment of delirium in the critically ill cancer patient. *Cancer Bull* 1984; 36:156–160.

24. de Stoutz N, Tapper M, Fainsinger RL. Reversible delirium in terminally ill patients. *J Pain Symptom Manage* 1995; 10(3):249–253.

25. Coyle N, Breitbart W, Weaver S, Portenoy R. Delirium as a contributing factor of "crescendo" pain. *J Pain Symptom Manage* 1994; 9(1):44–47.

26. Bruera E, Franco JJ, Maltoni M, Watanabe S, Suarez-Almazor M. Changing pattern of agitated impaired mental status in patients with advanced cancer: association with cognitive monitoring, hydration and opiate rotation. *J Pain Symptom Manage* 1995; 10(4):287–291.

27. Weinrich S, Sarna L. Delirium in the older person with cancer. *Cancer* 1994; 74:2079–2091.

28. Drachman D, Friedland RP, Larson EB, Williams M. Making sure it's really Alzheimer's. *Patient Care* 1991; 26:13–28.

29. Welch-McCaffrey D, Dodge J. Acute confusional states in elderly cancer patients. *Semin Oncol Nurs* 1988; 4(3):208–216.

30. Lipowski ZJ. Update on delirium. *Psychiatr Clin North Am* 1992; 15(2):335–346.

31. Andersson EM, Knutsson IK, Hallberg IR, Norberg A. The experience of being confused: a case study. *Geriatr Nurs* 1993; 14:242–247.

32. Gottlieb GL. Delirium in the medically ill elderly: Operationalizing the DSM-III-R criteria. *Int Psychogeriatr* 1991; 3:181–186.

33. Zimberg M, Berenson S. Delirium in patients with cancer: nursing assessment and intervention. *Oncol Nurs Forum* 1990; 17(4):529–538.

34. American Psychiatric Association. *Diagnostic and Statistical Manual of Mental*

Disorders. 3rd ed rev. Washington, D.C.: American Psychiatric Association; 1987.

35. Levkoff S, Liptzin B, Cleary P, Reilly CH, Evans D. Review of research instruments and techniques used to detect delirium. *Int Psychogeriatr* 1991; 3(2):253–271.

36. Aakerlund LP, Rosenberg J. Writing disturbances: an indicator for postoperative delirium. *Int J Psychiatry Med* 1994; 24(3):245–257.

37. Adams F. Neuropsychiatric evaluation and treatment of delirium in cancer patients. *Adv Psychosom Med* 1988; 18:26–36.

38. Pauker NE, Folstein MF, Moran TH. The clinical utility of the hand-held tachistoscope. *J Nerv Ment Dis* 1978; 166:126–129.

39. Reitan R. Validity of the trail-making test as an indicator of organic brain damage. *Percept Mot Skills* 1958; 8:271–276.

40. Anthony JC, le Resche L, Niaz U, Vonkorff MR, Folstein MF. Limits of the "Mini-Mental State" as a screening test for dementia and delirium among hospital patients. *Psychol Med* 1982; 12:397–408.

41. Gustafsson L, Lindgren M, Westling B. The OBS-scale: a new rating scale for evaluation of confusional states and other organic brain syndromes. Presented at the 2nd International Congress on Psychogeriatric Medicine; 1985, Umea, Sweden.

42. Folstein MF, Folstein S, McHugh PR. "Mini-mental state": a practical method for grading the cognitive state of patients for the clinician. *J Psychiatr Res* 1975; 12:189–198.

43. Tsai L, Tsuang MT. The mini-mental state test and computerized tomography. *Am J Psychiatry* 1979; 136(4A):436–439.

44. Fainsinger RL, Tapper M, Bruera E. A perspective on the management of delirium in terminally ill patients on a palliative care unit. *J Palliat Care* 1993; 9(3):4–8.

45. Pfeiffer E. A short portable mental status questionnaire for the assessment of organic brain deficit in elderly patients. *J Am Geriatr Soc* 1975; 23:433–441.

46. Jacobs JW, Bernhard MR, Delgado A, Strain JJ. Screening for organic mental syndromes in the medically ill. *Ann Intern Med* 1977; 86:40–46.

47. Williams MA, Ward SE, Campbell EB. Confusion: testing versus observation. *J Gerontol Nurs* 1986; 14(1):25–30.

48. Champagne MT, Neelon VJ, McConnell ES, Funk S. The NEECHAM confusion scale: assessing acute confusion in the hospitalized and nursing home elderly. *Gerontologist* 1987; 27:4A.

49. Inouye SK, van Dyck CH, Alessi CA, Balkin S, Siegal AP, Horwitz RI. Clarifying confusion: the confusion assessment method. *Ann Intern Med* 1990; 113:941–948.

50. Trzepacz PT, Baker RW, Greenhouse J. A symptom rating scale for delirium. *Psychiatry Res* 1988; 23:89–97.

51. Spitzer RL, First MB, Williams JBW, Kendler K, Pincus HA, Tucker G. Now is the time to retire the term "organic mental disorders." *Am J Psychiatry* 1992; 149(2):240–244.

52. American Psychiatric Association. *Diagnostic and Statistical Manual of Mental Disorders.* 4th ed. Washington, D.C.: American Psychiatric Association; 1995.

53. Kübler-Ross E. Interviews mit Sterbenden. Stuttgart: Kreuz-Verlag; 1980.

54. Stiefel FC, Kornblith AB, Holland JC. Changes in the prescription patterns of psychotropic drugs for cancer patients during a 10-year period. *Cancer* 1990; 65:1048–1053.
55. Cassens G, Wolfe L, Zola M. The neuropsychology of depressions. *J Neuropsychiatry Clin Neurosci* 1990; 2:202–213.
56. Raskin A. Partialing out the effects of depression and age on cognitive functions: experimental data and methodological issues. In: Poon L, ed. *Handbook for Memory Assessment of Older Adults.* Washington, D.C.: American Psychological Association; 1986:244–256.
57. Liston EH. Diagnosis and management of delirium in the elderly patient. *Psychiatr Ann* 1984; 14:109–118.
58. Lipowski ZJ. Delirium (acute confusional states). *JAMA* 1987; 258(13):1789–1792.
59. Selbst RA. Evaluating the "confused" patient. *Consultant* 1984; 4:209–221.
60. Schölzel-Dorenbos CJM. Casuistische mededelingen; Verwaardheid: meer dan dementie alleen. *Tijdschr Gerontol Geriatr* 1994; 25:117–119.
61. Marzinski LR. The tragedy of dementia: clinically assessing pain in the confused, non-verbal elderly. *J Gerontol Nurs* 1991; 17(6):25–28.
62. Bruera E, Fainsinger R, Miller MJ, Kuehn N. The assessment of pain intensity in patients with cognitive failure: a preliminary report. *J Pain Symptom Manage* 1992; 7:267–270.
63. Young DF, Posner JB. Nervous system toxicity of the chemotherapeutic agents. *Handbook of Clinical Neurology.* Amsterdam: North-Holland; 1980:91–129.
64. Peterson LG, Popkin MK. Neuropsychiatric effects of chemotherapeutic agents for cancer. *Psychosomatics* 1980; 21:141–153.
65. Stiefel F, Breitbart W, Holland J. Corticosteroids in cancer: neuropsychiatric complications. *Cancer Invest* 1989; 7(5):479–491.
66. Johnson BE, Becker B, Goff WB, Petronas N, Krehbiel MA, Mukuch RW, McKenna G, Glatstein E, Ihde DC. Neurologic, neuropsychiatric and computed tomography scan abnormalities in 2- to 10-year survival of small cell lung cancer. *J Clin Oncol* 1985; 3:1659–1667.
67. Levin VA, Gutin PH, Leibel S. Neoplasms of the central nervous system. In: de Vita VT, Hellman S, Rosenberg SA, eds. *Cancer: Principles and Practice of Oncology.* 4th ed. Philadelphia: J.B. Lippincott Co; 1993:1679–1737.
68. de Stoutz ND, Bruera E, Suarez-Almazor M. Opioid rotation for toxicity reduction in terminal cancer patients. *J Pain Symptom Manage* 1995; 10(5):378–384.
69. Hall RC, Zisook S. Paradoxical reactions to benzodiazepines. *Br J Clin Pharmacol* 1981; 11 (suppl 1):99–104.
70. Rall TW. Hypnotics and sedatives; ethanol. In: Gilman AG, Rall TW, Nies AS, Taylor P, eds. *The Pharmacological Basis of Therapeutics.* 8th ed. New York: Pergamon Press; 1990:345–382.
71. Tchekmedyan NS, Zahyna D, Halpert C, Heber D. Assessment and maintenance of nutrition in older cancer patients. *Oncology Suppl* 1992; 6:105–111.
72. Posner JB. Delirium and exogenous metabolic brain disease. In: Beeson PB, McDermott W, Wyngaarden JB, eds. *Cecil Textbook of Medicine.* Philadelphia: W.B. Saunders; 1979:644–651.
73. Bunn PA, Ridgway EC. Paraneoplastic syndromes. In: de Vita VT, Hellman S, Rosenberg SA, eds. *Cancer: Principles and Practice of Oncology.* 4th ed. Philadelphia: J.B. Lippincott Co; 1993:2026–2071.

74. Pfeilschifter J. Cytokines as mediators of hypercalcemia of malignancy. In: Raue F, ed. *Recent Results in Cancer Research*. Vol 137. *Hypercalcemia of Malignancy*. Berlin: Springer-Verlag; 1994:1–19.

75. Warrell RP. Metabolic emergencies. In: de Vita VT, Hellman S, Rosenberg SA, eds. *Cancer: Principles and Practice of Oncology*. 4th ed. Philadelphia: J.B. Lippincott Co; 1993:2128–2134.

76. O'Rourke NP, McCloskey EV, Vasikaran S, Eyres K, Fern D, Kanis JA. Effective treatment of malignant hypercalcemia with a single intravenous infusion of clodronate. *Br J Cancer* 1994; 67:560–563.

77. Thürlimann B, Waldburger R, Senn HJ, Thiébaud D. Plicamycin and pamidronate in symptomatic tumor-related hypercalcemia: a prospective randomized cross-over trial. *Ann Oncol* 1992; 3:619–622.

78. Billy C, Rivasseau-Jonveaux T, Gil R. Faits cliniques et lettres: Syndrome confu-sionnel isolé à rechutes révélateur d'une polyadénomatose de type IIa (syn-drome de Sipple). *Ann Med Interne (Paris)* 1991; 142(1):69–71.

79. Victor M, Adams RD. Metabolic diseases of the nervous system. In: Isselbacher KJ, Adams RD, Braunwald E, Petersdorf RG, Wilson JD, eds. *Harrison's Principles of Internal Medicine*. 9th ed. New York: McGraw-Hill Book Co; 1980:1977–1985.

80. Fainsinger RL, Miller MJ, Bruera E. Morphine intoxication during acute revers-ible renal insufficiency. *J Palliat Care* 1990; 8(2):52–53.

81. Stiefel F, Morant R. Morphine intoxication during acute reversible renal insuffi-ciency. *J Palliat Care* 1991; 7(4):45–47.

82. Fainsinger RL, Schoeller T, Boiskin M, Bruera E. Palliative care round: cognitive failure (CF) and coma after renal failure in a patient recieving captopril and hydromorphone. *J Palliat Care* 1993; 9(1):53–55.

83. Peterson LG, Perl M. Psychiatric presentations of cancer. *Psychosomatics* 1982; 23:601–604.

84. Rabins PV. Psychosocial and management aspects of delirium. *Int Psychogeriatr* 1991; 3(2):319–324.

85. Murray GB. Confusion, delirium, and dementia. In: Cassem NH, ed. *Massa-chusetts General Hospital Handbook of General Hospital Psychiatry*. 1987:89–120.

3

Counseling the Confused
Patient and the Family

CLAUDIA BORREANI, AUGUSTO CARACENI,
AND MARCELLO TAMBURINI

Delirium is frequent in progressive diseases such as cancer and AIDS. At times it can be reversible, but often it characterizes the terminal evolution of the disease. In many cases, therefore, delirium not only heralds death but also, as popular wisdom has it, is a way of dying.[1,2] This chapter will focus on the role and content of counseling in cases of cognitive impairment or delirium occurring in the course of advanced cancer. Communication with the patient and the family in this clinical circumstance is not easy and is very much influenced by psychological and organic factors: cognitive failure, coping abilities, perception and knowledge of the disease, perception and knowledge of terminality, fluctuation of symptoms, and reversibility or irreversibility of consciousness impairment.

Counseling

Definition and application in medicine

The scope of counseling is an action to support decision making.[3,4] Counseling should help to build up decisional autonomy through the awareness of the conscious and unconscious factors and feelings that are implicated in decision making. A realistic appreciation of self and of social environment and a reduction of conflicts arising from subjective variables are encouraged to ease choices.

Counseling has elective application in situations requiring the communication of information with strong emotional content, when decision making is implied, or when a change in the subject's behavior is deemed useful.

Counseling in medicine is an integral part of the patient–caregiver relationship. A formal analysis and theory of the content and structure of this relationship has been described mainly in the following situations:

HIV infection: in communicating positive serodiagnosis or AIDS diagnosis and in different phases of the disease.[5,6]

Cancer: especially in supporting patients and family in the many critical moments of the disease from diagnosis to the terminal phase.[7–10]

Genetics: in communicating the risks of genetically determined disease. This specific application now has examples also in oncology.[11–13]

Counseling techniques

Although counseling should be mainly a type of aid relationship, in the specific case of medical counseling between caregiver and patient or family, it uses techniques developed to fit different clinical situations.[14–16]

Informative counseling is aimed at giving information to help patients in decision making. This is done through creating a relationship that leaves wide opportunities for expressing doubts, perplexities, and requests of explanations by the patients. The aim of this intervention is the rational understanding of the situation.

Confrontational counseling is a second level in counseling with the scope of modifying dysfunctional thoughts and inefficacious coping strategies that prevent confronting the disease. It is again a cognitive intervention that uses feedback to make the patient acknowledge his or her maladaptive behavior and allows progressive adaptation to take place.

Cathartic counseling works at a more profound level. After creating an empathic context, it allows the patient to express his or her anxieties, fears, and most hidden thoughts; as emotional tension is released, a more realistic appreciation of the situation may be achieved.

Catalytic counseling is a further phase. After the patient understands the situation, he or she is encouraged to define realistic aims of change and to use his or her resources in achieving these aims, finally reaching a better sense of control during stressful events.

Supportive counseling, a fundamental component of every counseling intervention in medicine, is especially important when it is difficult to intervene in the patient's cognitive functions because of the presence of acute anxiety, cognitive failure, or very advanced disease and physical debility. The aim of this intervention, therefore, is to convey understanding and acceptance of the patient's needs and fears while focusing more on the existence of the relationship than on therapy goals.

Oncological counseling has a specific role. Listening to the patient, and helping him or her to understand individual reactions and difficult situations caused by the disease or unrelated life events, is considered the first step in this process. The patient can then be encouraged to take appropriate steps when action is possible.

Different counseling components will be emphasized if patients' cognitive functions are preserved and when dealing with family members. The case of the confused patient is unique because cognitive function, which is a mainstay of counseling possibilities, is impaired. In this situation emotional support will be used to help communicate with patients who have mild confusion. In cases of severe delirium, counseling interventions will focus on the family and on the personnel involved in the care of the patient.

Advanced cancer and counseling

Any psychological intervention in oncology is primarily supportive. Information, personal relationships, and support are the three pillars of psychological help. Educating the patient and the family about the disease and its treatment is fundamental to reassure them, to help normalize their reactions, and to prepare them to face the evolution of the disease.

Advanced progressive disease imposes a difficult psychological adaptation process on the patient and the family. Family has an important role in offering practical and psychological support; this implies a heavy emotional burden on the family members.[17-19] The emotional distress of family members of patients with severe illness is indeed comparable to the patient's own psychological distress. In the terminal phase of the patient's illness, anxiety, mood, and mental health disturbances are even more acute.[20]

Counseling interventions should therefore be planned earlier in the history of incurable illness, to help the patient and the family adapt to the disease with a free communication of emotion, elaboration of deep feelings, and a progressive resetting of family relationships.

Counseling should be used to focus on emergent and specific problems: information will be given to help in understanding diagnostic and therapeutic procedures; cognitive skills or techniques will be suggested to favor better coping strategies; cathartic aspects will be underlined in expressing thoughts, fears, and feelings with empathy and acceptance; and emotional support will be given in crisis situations.[16] A flexible approach enables us to choose or integrate one or more aspects of diverse counseling components.

Counseling the Confused Patient

General aspects

In counseling the patient with delirium and the family, the specificity of each condition is to be carefully considered: the degree of the cognitive impairment should guide patient communication and the extent of the family's understanding of the patient's condition should be taken into account as well when giving an explanation to family members.

The need for psychological support in cases of delirium is suggested by clinical experience. Fainsinger and coworkers[21] and Cherny and coworkers[22] independently described the destructive triangle created by a delirious agitated patient, high family distress, and a caring staff overwhelmed by the family requests for help. Strong emotional pressure can result in sedating the patient to relieve the family and perhaps the staff. This should be clarified with the family in a supportive and informative, but also directive, counseling setting. Although sedating the patient can be rewarding in terms of family gratitude, it is not always necessary; talking with the family about therapeutic decisions can facilitate optimal care, which in turn can, in many cases, avoid unnecessary psychotropic medication.[21–23]

Orientation to time and space is of uppermost importance; therefore, environment and behavior interventions can be very helpful: for example, keeping the room quiet and well lit, with some light also during the nighttime, and using objects that are familiar to the patient. Company should always be provided by family members or by somebody the patient knows well in an individualized and consistent care setting.[24–26]

When delirium is not severe the patient can be encouraged to walk, read, and participate in his own care, in an attempt to keep him in better touch with reality. This should be done carefully, paying attention not to confuse the patient even more through excessive sensory stimulation (sensory overload).

Delirium primarily affects communication, and this will generate anxiety in the family member who is trying to keep alive the personal relationship. It is therefore important to emphasize the emotional aspects of communication that can still be possible when the more rational bonds are lost.[26]

Slight to moderate delirium and hypoactive delirium should be differentiated from severe agitated delirium; in the latter, the previously mentioned issues may be compounded by medico-legal and ethical considerations such as in the case of a patient displaying aggressive behavior with potential danger for family members, caregivers, and the patient himself. When physical restraint is necessary, its use has to be explained to the family, and it should never be used as a substitute for accurate and compassionate pharmacological and psychological care.[25] In cases of severe delirium, the therapeutic and caring decisions will be more specific and will require more coordination of the members of the caring unit (professional and nonprofessional). Several risks are associated with the delirious conditions, including the possibility of suicidal acts due to disinhibition of a latent suicidal ideation or triggered by fearful hallucinations and persecutory delusions.[27]

In reviewing the literature on the concept of suffering in medicine, Cherny and colleagues emphasized the relevance of the interaction of medical, psychosocial, and practical aspects in the care of the patient with terminal illness.[22] Delirium exemplifies a physical and psychological symptom affecting quality of life and posing demanding burdens on family and staff. Interventions should therefore be planned on the basis of a rational review of all the different factors involved[22] in optimizing family and staff resources.

Specific patient interventions

The counseling strategies very briefly mentioned above can apply to the patient with delirium, depending on the level of psychological distress and cognitive and emotional resources still available on the side of patient and family. Several specific clinical situations may require a counseling intervention in the case of a patient with delirium.

When predictive factors of cognitive impairment are found, such as advanced aged, brain metastases, or metabolic failure, a "preventive" counseling intervention with the family and, at times, the patient (e.g., explicit questions about mode of disease progression) can be useful to make subsequent events less unexpected—in much the same way that drug side effects are explained before therapy changes.

The patient's awareness of his or her confusion is an obvious basic but sometimes overlooked question. "Do you feel confused?"; this simple question can be the key to the patient's insight into his own mental disturbance. Anosognosia is very frequent with delirium, but in early phases the patient perceives the internal change and suffers by losing control of his mind. Anxiety, perplexity, and depression are frequent emotional reactions. Few descriptions of delirious experiences are available, and they are often frightening. Unpleasant twilight states between sleep and wakefulness, horrible dreams, fear, and frightening experiences have been reported. Most often amnesia for the experienced sensations and thoughts follows.[2] Patients treated with opioids for cancer pain who recovered from delirium were found to have lower pain ratings and to request fewer opioid extra doses when back to their baseline mental condition, compared with the staff pain rating and consequent opioid dosing made when the patients were delirious and uncooperative. These patients did not recall their pain during the episode.[28]

Attention failure is one of the main manifestations of delirium and often results in short-term memory impairment. Reorientation and reassurance can help the patient; communication can still be effective using the relatively unaffected content of long-term memories. It is better not to challenge the patient with issues that are not recalled and not to leave them blocked on mistakes. Emotional lability is frequent and mood can be suddenly affected by excessive or inappropriate cognitive stimulation. Patients should be allowed to respond at their own time and pace, and nonverbal skills can be used to fill sudden communication gaps.

Emotion and prevailing feelings can be influenced, as mentioned, by the content of the pathological thought process, which may be affected by hallucinations and delusions; their evaluation is necessary to understand the patient experience. Attention should be paid to fears and worries, and to the presence of hallucinations or delusions. These symptoms should not be overemphasized or disregarded; on the contrary, the patient should be free to express his feelings within a protective, reassuring environment. A careful assessment of the previous psychological factors should be made to keep alive the therapeutic relationship with the patients as much as the severity of the delirium allows.

Specific family interventions

Family resources are very important when delirium is present. The meaning of this event for the family is especially important, for a change in mental function is indeed often perceived as related to the imminence of death. The family often needs more help than does the patient in accepting this situation and facing approaching death. Fear and feelings of loss can be present and evoke previous loss experiences that were not elaborated. Leaving an open door to the expression of such feelings is very important.

Table 3.1 highlights issues that can need a counseling intervention with the family. Family should be warned about the possibility of fluctuations of mental conditions and encouraged to talk and behave always as if the patient could understand. Relatives should be prepared for the onset of hallucinations and delusions and how to react appropriately to them. The patient's expression of paranoid fears and frightening visions should be quietly corrected while unharmful experiences, such as occupational delusions ("I need to go to the barn to milk the cow"), can be controlled with more indulgence ("We will go later this afternoon").

Family members have to know if the patient is suffering from pain or other symptoms and how to control them, and they should be involved in assessing the patient's awareness and perception.

Goals of care are listed as the last issue in Table 3.1 but indeed summarize most of the other issues already mentioned. The discussion with the family on goals of care has to be open and clear. It is very important that family realizes

Table 3.1. Critical issues in family counseling on delirium characteristics

Communication barrier
Patient's awareness of physical and psychological suffering
Reversibility
Short-term prognosis
Fluctuations of cognitive functions
Opioid therapy as the cause of delirium
Is it necessary to sedate patient?
Goals of care

that in cases when multiple factors are contributing to delirium (e.g., sepsis, metastases, metabolic derangement, drugs) it is difficult to find a single cause and eventually treat it, or that short-term prognosis can be difficult to establish and that it can change in a relatively short time. This implies that conservative treatment (e.g., antibiotics or hydration) can be appropriate when the condition is still believed to be reversible but can become inappropriate when the clinical conditions are deteriorating or when reversibility of some physiological functions would be achieved only at the price of enormous suffering and palliative care is the only goal of therapy.

Classification and explanation of etiology is also necessary because of the frequent tendency of family members to blame therapies (e.g., opioid analgesics) for cognitive failure. Clinical experience tells us that family members are often afraid of and can feel guilty about giving medications that they think are responsible for compromising cognitive functions. A discussion of the disease-related variables that are indeed responsible for the clinical course is usually helpful.

Major changes in attitudes, reactions, disinhibition of fears and conflicts, can develop in the course of delirium, leading to unusual behaviors (excessive complaints of minor symptoms, excessive unreasonable demands) or to a change in personality traits which can involve more or less profound levels (for instance, a patient awakening from an almost stuporous state of 24-hour duration: "Why are you starving me—I want to eat pizza," when she always hated pizza in her life). The family can have problems in adapting to these "personality" changes and may have unrealistic expectations of seeing their dear ones as they used to know them.

The decision to increase neuroleptic and/or benzodiazepine doses to the point of reducing the patient's consciousness, with the aim of controlling terminal agitated delirium[29,30] is a difficult one. Patients—even if delirious—can be part of this decision, expressing the desire to sleep, to rest, not to feel anymore what is happening to them, or can have expressed this wish before they were confused. The patient's wishes—or "living will"—about cardiopulmonary resuscitation (CPR) should be known at this time or should be discussed with the proxy. In general, CPR is considered futile when sedation has been chosen for symptom control.[31] Family involvement is important: family concerns often include the fear of accelerating death with sedation. These worries should be addressed. The family should know that the likelihood that clinical course is affected by treatment is low and ethical commitment to implement the most appropriate treatment balances the eventual risk of accelerating death when primacy is given to relieve suffering.[30,31]

Opposite pressures from the family to shorten the patient's life or to "put him or her to sleep" need as well to be identified and discussed openly. Experienced physicians are not afraid of admitting that although they "do not kill patients," at the same time they are not going to watch them suffer without appropriate treatment.[32] Shortening the patient's life is not among the goals of care,[32] and, more important for the purpose of counseling, is not usually necessary to achieve symptom control in most terminal patients with delirium. Family distress and emotional reactions in this situation need to be specifically addressed, as they influence the patient's care and may generate conflicts with the staff.

Conclusion

Counseling confused patients and families does not require specialized psychotherapy techniques. The intervention can be performed by medical and nursing staff involved in the care of the patient, provided the following conditions are satisfied:

- Complete knowledge of the clinical conditions, including a formal assessment of delirium and mental state.
- Assessment of the patient and family understanding of the clinical conditions, of their culture and family relationship.
- Empathic and good interpersonal relationship attitudes.
- Identification of maladaptive psychological reactions in the patient or the family.

It is evident from these considerations that well-developed professional skills are required of counselors in this difficult situation. It is also true that most professionals involved in the care of cancer patients have no formal training in counseling.[15]

Acknowledgments

This work has been partially funded by CNR grant ACRO n. 95.00495.PF39.

References

1. Massie MJ, Holland J, Glass E. Delirium in terminally ill cancer patients. *Am J Psychiatry* 1983; 140(8):1048–1050.
2. Lipowsky ZJ. *Delirium: Acute Confusional States*. New York: Oxford University Press; 1990:109–140.
3. May R. *The Art of Counselling*. New York: Gardner Press Inc; 1989.
4. Carkhuff RR. *The Art of Helping*. Amherst, Mass.: Human Resources Development Press; 1987.
5. Serpelloni G, Morgante S. HIV/AIDS counselling and screening—*Manuale Teorico Pratico Verano*. Leonard Edizioni Scientifiche; 1993:74–75.
6. Green J, McGreaner A. *Counselling in HIV Infection and AIDS*. London: Blackwell Scientific Publication; 1989.

7. Ferlic M, Goldman A, Kennedy BJ. Group counselling in adult patients with advanced cancer. *Cancer* 1979; 44:760–766.

8. Linn MW, Linn BS. Effects of counselling for late-stage cancer patients. *Cancer* 1982; 1048–1055.

9. Maguire GP, Tait A, Brooke M, Thomas C, Sellwood R. The effects of counselling on the psychiatric morbidity associated with mastectomy. *Br Med J* 1980; 28:1454–1456.

10. Watson H. Psychological intervention with cancer patients: a review. *Psychol Med* 1983; 13:839–846.

11. Learman C, Lustbader E, Rimer B, Daly M, Miller S, Sands C, Balshem A. Effects of individualized breast cancer risk counselling: a randomized trial. *J Natl Cancer Inst* 1995; 87:286–292.

12. Gardner M, St John J. Gene testing and genetic counselling in familial polyposis. *Med J Aust* 1995; 162:457.

13. Evans DRG, Blair R, Greenhalgh R, Hopwood P, Howell A. The impact of genetic counselling on risk perception in women with a family history of breast cancer. *Br J Cancer* 1994; 70:934–938.

14. Razavi D, Delvaux N. Les interventions psychologiques. In: Razavi D, Delvaux N, eds. *Psycho-oncologie*. Paris: Masson; 1994:165–194.

15. Roger CR. *On Becoming a Person*. Boston: Houghton Mifflin; 1961.

16. Fallowfield L. Counselling for patients with cancer. *Br Med J* 1988; 297:727–728.

17. Astudillo W, Mendinueta C, Astudilo E, Munoz A, Horcjada JP. How can relations be improved between the family and the support team during the care of terminally ill patients? *Support Care Cancer* 1995; 3:72–77.

18. Razavi D, Bredart A, Delvaux N, Hennaux P. Les reactions familiales. In: Razavi D, Delvaux N, eds. *Psycho-oncologie*. Paris: Masson; 1994:79–93.

19. Wellisch DK, Wolcott DL, Pasnau RO, Fawzy FI, Landsverkj L. An evaluation of the psychosocial problems of the homebound cancer patients: relationship of patient adjustment to family problems. *J Psychosoc Oncol* 1989; 7:55–76.

20. Cassileth BR, Lusk EJ, Strouse TB, et al. A psychological analysis of cancer patients and their next-of-kin. *Cancer* 1985; 1:72–76.

21. Fainsinger RL, Tapper M, Bruera E. A perspective on the management of delirium in terminally ill patients on a palliative care unit. *J Palliat Care* 1993; 9(3):4–8.

22. Cherny NI, Coyle N, Foley KM. Suffering in the advanced cancer patient: a definition and taxonomy. *J Palliat Care* 1994; 10(2):57–70.

23. Caraceni A, Martini C. Confusione mentale e sintomi neuropsichici nel paziente oncologico. In: S. Mercadante, ed. *Trattamento del Dolore e dei Sintomi nel Cancro Avanzato*. Padova: Piccin Editore; 1994:189–203.

24. Lesko LM, Fleishman S. Treatment and support in confusion states. In: *Recent Results in Cancer Research*. Berlin Heidelberg: Springer-Verlag; 1991:378–392.

25. Fainsinger R, Bruera E. Treatment of delirium in a terminally ill patient. *J Pain Symptom Manage* 1992; 7(1):54–56.

26. Weinrich S, Sarna L. Delirium in the older persons with cancer. *Cancer Supplement* 1994; 7(10):2079–2091.

27. Breitbart W. Cancer pain and suicide. In: Foley K, et al., eds. *Advances in Pain Research and Therapy*. New York: Raven Press; 1990:399–412.

28. Bruera E, Fainsinger RL, Miller MJ, Kuehn N. The assessment of pain intensity in

patients with cognitive failure: a preliminary report. *J Pain Symptom Manage* 1992; 7(5):267–270.

29. Burke AL, Diamond PL, Hulbert J, Yeatman J, Farr EA. Terminal restlessness— its management and the role of midazolam. *Med J Aust* 1991; 155:485–487.

30. Cherny NI, Portenoy RK. Sedation in the treatment of refractory symptoms: guidelines for evaluation and treatment. *J Palliat Care* 1994; 10(2):31–38.

31. Pius XII. Discorso sulle le varie questioni in relazione all'anestesia, 24 febbraio 1957, AAS 49:129–147.

32. Cherny NI, Coyle N, Foley KM. The treatment of suffering when patients request elective death. *J Palliat Care* 1994; 10(2):71–79.

II

GASTROINTESTINAL DISORDERS IN PATIENTS WITH ADVANCED CANCER

Introduction: A Call for Research to Elucidate Causes, Assessment, and Management of Common Gastrointestinal Symptoms

EDUARDO BRUERA

Chronic nausea and vomiting, anorexia, constipation, and malnutrition are among the most frequent and devastating complications in patients with advanced cancer.[1,2]

These different symptoms were initially studied in isolation from each other. However, there is growing evidence that there is a strong association among them. Anorexia, early satiety, chronic nausea, and constipation are all major manifestations of the cachexia syndrome.[1,2] These symptoms also occur in patients with autonomic failure due to cancer and other conditions.[3] Finally, these symptoms are also frequently observed in patients receiving opioids.[4]

The presence of common symptoms associated with cachexia, autonomic failure, and opioid therapy suggest that these three conditions produce similar pathophysiological abnormalities. The nature of the symptoms points toward abnormalities in gastrointestinal motility.

Abnormal gastrointestinal motility has been documented in association with opioid therapy and autonomic failure, as well as with some of the humoral mediators of cancer cachexia. Autonomic failure can occur as a paraneoplastic syndrome and can be aggravated by cachexia or by therapy with a number of drugs frequently used in cancer patients, such as opioids, tricyclic antidepressants, phenothiazines, or anticholinergic drugs. This syndrome can, in turn, aggravate malnutrition.

These recent findings suggest that a certain degree of gastrointestinal dismotility is likely present in the great majority of terminal cancer patients. These abnormalities are also likely in other conditions in which patients develop severe malnutrition and frequently receive opioids, tricyclics, or anti-cholinergics—for example, in advanced AIDS.

The recognition of functional abnormalities in gastrointestinal motility raises questions relating to both the assessment and the management of this problem.

In relation to assessment, it is important to establish that certain types and characteristics of symptom complaints are associated with specific patho-physiological changes and prognosis. In pain assessment, certain clinical de-scriptors such as those associated with neuropathic or incidental pain have therapeutic and prognostic implications. Do specific characteristics of nausea, vomiting, or anorexia have similar meaning?

Prospective studies that carefully assess the characteristics of these symp-toms would be required in order to address this question. It is also unclear if tests of gastrointestinal motility (e.g., radiological or radionuclide assessment of gastric emptying time) will be useful in order to characterize the severity of the disorder or the response to different treatments. Will simple, clinical bedside tests such as those used to assess cardiovascular autonomic failure be a useful alternative to more invasive tests in palliative care patients?

In the area of therapy, several questions remain unanswered. There are several drugs with documented effects on gastrointestinal motility, including metoclopramide, domperidone, and cisapride. The relative contribution of these agents to better symptom management needs to be established. Com-parative trials are also needed between these drugs and the more classical antiemetics such as prochlorperazine, haloperidol, dimenhydrinate, and on-dansetron.

In addition, other drugs such as corticosteroids and megestrol acetate have effects on symptoms that have been associated with gastrointestinal motility disorders. The possibility of effective drug combinations should be explored.

Mechanical bowel obstruction is another major cause of symptom distress in patients with intra-abdominal malignancies. These patients frequently present with partial syndromes with a complex clinical course, in which func-tional gastrointestinal motility disorders probably also play a major role. Until recent years, surgery or mechanical drainage of the gastrointestinal contents was considered the only possible approach. In recent years, a number of effective pharmacological interventions have emerged. The relative role of corticosteroids, pro-motility agents, anticholinergics, and octreotide will need to be established in prospective clinical trials.

Constipation is another complex, poorly understood, and poorly managed syndrome. It is one of the manifestations of autonomic failure, opioid therapy, and mechanical bowel obstruction. In addition, it is also associated with neuro-logical damage, decreased activity, poor oral intake, dehydration, hyper-calcemia, and treatment with a variety of drugs. This symptom continues to be poorly assessed and managed, even by palliative care groups.[5]

Very few clinical trials have been conducted comparing the effectiveness, toxicity, and patient compliance with common laxatives. In addition, in recent years, new agents such as naloxone or cisapride have been proposed for severe constipation. These agents might effectively potentiate common laxatives.

Finally, the spectrum of severe symptoms associated with constipation, including anorexia, nausea, emesis, abdominal pain, abdominal distention, and urinary retention should be characterized in prospective studies. One possible explanation for the poor management of constipation even among palliative care groups is that the "symptomatic price" of neglecting this problem has not been clearly established in prospective studies.

The following chapters address selected aspects of gastrointestinal motility. Two observations are common to all areas covered in this part: (1) these are common, everyday problems that cause a great amount of concern to palliative care patients and their families; (2) there is an alarming lack of clinical research on both the assessment and management of these problems. As a result, an evidence-based approach to this area is not possible at the present time.

The hoped-for outcome of this part is that research is stimulated in all aspects of this problem.

References

1. Bruera E, Fainsinger RL. Clinical management of cachexia and anorexia. In: Doyle D, Hanks G, MacDonald N, eds. *Oxford Textbook of Palliative Medicine*. Oxford: Oxford Medical Publications; 1993:330–337.
2. Alexander HR, Norton J. Pathophysiology of cancer cachexia. In: Doyle D, Hanks G, MacDonald N, eds. *Oxford Textbook of Palliative Medicine*. Oxford: Oxford Medical Publications; 1993:316–329.
3. Henrich W. Autonomic insufficiency. *Arch Intern Med* 1982; 142(2):339–344.
4. Manara L, Bianchetti A. The central and peripheral influence of opioids on gastrointestinal propulsion. *Annu Rev Pharmacol Toxicol* 1985; 75:249–273.
5. Bruera E, Suarez-Almazor M, Velasco A, Bertolino M, MacDonald SM, Hanson J. The assessment of constipation in terminal cancer patients admitted to a palliative care unit: a retrospective review. *J Pain Symptom Manage* 1994; 9(8):515–519.

4

Gastrointestinal Motility Disorders in Patients with Advanced Cancer

CARLA RIPAMONTI AND CARLOS RODRIGUEZ

Gastrointestinal (GI) motility disorders can be defined as abnormalities in smooth muscle contraction secondary to neural, humoral, and myogenic dysfunction.[1]

There are many symptoms associated with impaired GI motility. They include pyrosis, chest pain, dysphagia, regurgitation, nausea, vomiting, early satiety, dyspepsia, abdominal pain, bloating, abdominal distention, constipation, diarrhea, and halitosis. Among these symptoms, only a few are organ specific (i.e., dysphagia and fecal incontinence). Table 4.1 shows the frequency of some of the symptoms reported by patients with GI motility disorders.

In general, GI symptoms resulting from motility disorders are caused by delayed or accelerated transit, nonperistaltic contractions (often referred to as spasms), or alterations of the motility patterns at GI sphincter sites. There are many agents that can cause a delay in GI transit (Table 4.2).

Unfortunately, GI motility disorders are not classified in a uniform manner. Indeed, they are often reported or defined according to different criteria, such as radiographic, manometric, or pathological findings, or clinical syndrome. In the case of advanced cancer patients, recognized clinical syndromes include small or squashed stomach syndrome associated with hepatomegaly; cancer anorexia–cachexia syndrome; cancer-associated dyspepsia syndrome; autonomic failure; and narcotic bowel syndrome. In addition to these specific syndromes cancer patients can also suffer from GI motility disorders that are very common in the general population.

Table 4.1. Frequency, in percent, of GI symptoms in advanced cancer patients according to eight sources

Symptom	Grond et al.[174] (N=1635)	Twycross and Lack[175] (N=6677)	Reuben et al.[176] (N=1592)	Brescia et al.[177] (N=1103)	Seale[178] (N=168)	Ventafridda et al.[179] (N=115)	Curtis et al.[180] (N=100)	Coyle et al.[181] (N=90)
Loss of appetite (anorexia)	48	67	79	31	71	30	55	8
Dysphagia	22	23	43	22	38	9	9	3
Dyspepsia	11	—	—	—	—	—	17	—
Nausea	27	40	44	19	51	6	32	12
Vomiting	20	—	—	—	—	4	25	—
Constipation	33	47	54	—	47	23	40	4
Diarrhea	6	4	25	—	—	5	—	<5

Source: Adapted from Grond et al.[174]
—: not available.

Table 4.2. Agents that delay GI transit

Agent type	Specific examples	Effects
Agents that modify luminal contents	Fat, fiber	Modify the physical characteristics of GI contents or alter the balance of regulatory factors by interacting with the mucosa
Anticholinergic agents	Atropine, scopolamine, scopolamine hydro-bromide, and butylbromide	Promote peripheral effects on intestinal wall Central inhibitory effects on transit
Sympathomimetic agents	Clonidine, lidamidine	Interact with alpha 2 adrenoreceptors or presynaptic cholinergic neurons to inhibit ACh release
Calcium channel antagonist	Nifedipine, verapamil	Limits calcium entry through the smooth muscle cells May also alter neurotransmitter release
Opioids	Endogenous, exogenous	Delay GI transit due central or peripheral mechanisms
Peptides	Calcitonin, glucagon, neurotensin peptide YY, and cholecysto-kinin	Modify GI motility through different mechanisms

Pathophysiological Aspects of Motility Disorders

In general, GI motility has two components to phasic contractions (spatial and temporal). These patterns are controlled by three primary mechanisms: myogenic activity, intrinsic and extrinsic nervous system, and chemical or hormonal action. Each of these systems can be activated in response to sensory information mediated by mechanoreceptors or chemical receptors in the gut wall.[2–4]

Electrical control activity (ECA) is the basis of the myogenic control that coordinates the different phases of contraction. ECA comprises the resting membrane potential, the frequency and amplitude of periodic oscillations of membrane potential, and the phase relationships between oscillations in the adjacent groups of cells.[3] The ECA results in the following types of myogenic response:

1. Phasic contractions: Constant contractions with varying intensities and velocities that occur as part of basic GI function (alimentary mixing and propulsive movements).
2. Tonic contractions: Contractions mainly present at sphincteric levels or in regions, such as the gallbladder and the fundus of the stomach, that

minimize reflux and regulate the rate of transfer of food between adjacent organs.

3. Special situation contractions: Rapid unidirectional movements of intraluminal contents.[3,5,6]

Figure 4.1 shows the neurogenic control of the GI motility. The extrinsic nervous system includes central nervous system (CNS) and autonomic system (sympathetic and parasympathetic) structures. The sympathetic stimulation inhibits muscular contraction, whereas parasympathetic stimulation has two effects: the cholinergic excitatory and the noncholinergic nonadrenergic inhibition of the smooth muscle contraction. The intrinsic or enteric nervous system consists of the myenteric Auerbach's plexus, located between the circular and longitudinal muscle layers, and the submucosal Meissner's plexus, located between the submucosa and circular muscle layer. The axons from these neurons synapse with the muscle and glandular structures. The neurons develop the activity of pacemakers and have many fibers containing chemical substances important for neuromuscular transmission and the regulation of motility. The chemical control of GI motility occurs through the liberation of neurotransmitters that are generally classified as cholinergic agonists. These neurotransmitters include acetylcholine (ACh) and may also include serotonin, vasoactive intestinal polypeptide (VIP), or substance P. The neurokinins (substance P and substance K) may also be important and have demonstrated inotropic activity over muscle strips of the esophagus, small bowel, proximal and distal colon, and rectum.[2–4,6–10]

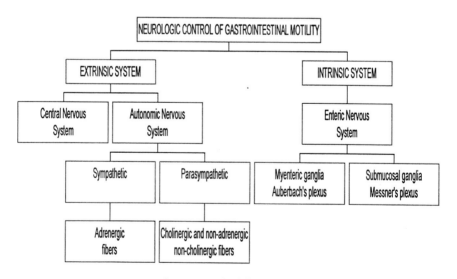

Figure 4.1. Neurologic control of the gastrointestinal motility.

Esophagus Motility Disorders

Normal esophageal function is a complex coordinated activity that allows transit of solids and liquids from the mouth to the stomach. This mechanism also prevents aspiration into the lung, nasal regurgitation, and reflux through the lower esophageal sphincter (LOS). Causes and symptoms of gastro-esophageal motility disorders are summarized in Table 4.3.

Dysphagia is the major symptom that signals an esophageal motility disorder. Dysphagia is defined as difficulty in swallowing and is a subjective sensation of some disturbance in the passage of a solid or liquid bolus from the mouth, down the esophagus, and into the stomach.

Not all patients who report dysphagia present real difficulty in swallowing solids and liquids.[11] Nonetheless, the presence of dysphagia almost always indicates a significant problem with the anatomy or motor function of the oral cavity, pharynx, esophagus, or cardia of the stomach.

Dysphagia has multiple causes in cancer patients (Table 4.4). Odynophagia (painful swallowing) is generally secondary to inflammatory processes such as reflux esophagitis or infection.

Whereas esophageal dysphagia usually results from esophageal disease, most cases of oropharyngeal dysphagia are the result of neurologic or muscular diseases, and oropharyngeal dysfunction is only a manifestation.[12] Perineural tumoral spread is associated with both cystic adenocarcinomas and squamous cell carcinomas. Sometimes the combination of motor neuropathy and local fibrosis causes severe functional dysphagia, which can simulate an organic obstruction.[13] Obstructive lesions initially provoke dysphagia for solids,

Table 4.3. Gastro-esophageal disorders

Causes	Symptoms
Obstruction of the esophagus by intrinsic or extrinsic tumor	Retching
Neurological damage to swallowing reflex	Dysphagia
	Chest pain
	Regurgitation
Gastric stasis due to:	Nausea
Drugs (e.g., morphine, anticholinergics)	Dyspepsia
Hepatomegaly, ascitis, pancreatic carcinoma, peptic ulceration	Early satiety
Gastric atony	Abdominal pain
Bowel obstruction	Large amounts of vomit
Severe constipation	
Gastric irritation due to:	Nausea
Drugs: NSAIDs, iron, antibiotics	Vomiting
Alcohol	Dyspepsia
Biliary reflux	Epigastric pain
Infection	
Blood in stomach	

Table 4.4. Causes of dysphagia in cancer patients

Cancer in oral cavity, pharynx, esophagus, cardia
Extrinsic esophageal compression: mediastinal mass, lung cancer
Infiltration of pharyngeal–esophageal wall
Perineural tumor spread: vagus, sympathetic
Cerebral metastatic disease (bulbar palsy)
Leptomeningeal infiltration
Cranial nerve damage (metastasis in base of skull)
Disorders of the neuromuscular transmission
Surgery in oral cavity
Post-radiation fibrosis
Dry mouth
Infections of the mouth, pharynx, or esophagus: Candida, herpes
Gastro-esophageal reflux disease (GERD)
Esophageal spasm
Generalized weakness
Neuromuscular-associated disease

whereas neuromuscular disorders first cause dysphagia for liquids and successively for solids as well. Radiotherapy of the esophagus and mediastinum can cause dysphagia as the result of fibrosis of the oropharyngeal musculature. Dysphagia can also be due to dry mouth following fibrosis of the submandibular or parotid glands. Central nervous system disorders may damage the swallowing center and cause uncoordinated swallowing. Cranial nerve damage, disorders of neuromuscular transmission, and myotonia can all reduce pharyngeal or esophageal contraction.

Gastro-esophageal reflux disease may cause dysphagia through a nonobstructive dysmotility characterized by failed esophageal peristalsis; hypotensive peristalsis; or nonperistaltic, simultaneous contractions.

Diagnosis of the anatomical region associated with dysphagia (buccal, pharyngeal, esophageal) and the cause of the dysphagia is based on a careful evaluation of the symptoms reported by the patient. Important points include the presence/absence of pain, location of pain (retrosternal, neck, between the shoulder blades), dysphagia to solids or liquids or both, nasal regurgitation or food retention in the mouth. The examination should include the assessment of the lower cranial nerves. If there is any doubt about the cause or severity of the dysphagia, diagnostic investigation can be completed with barium studies, endoscopy, and eventually videofluoroscopy.[14]

Spastic motility disorders

Esophageal motility disorders can be classified according to manometric criteria: achalasia, diffuse esophageal spasm, nutcracker esophagus, hypertensive lower esophageal sphincter (LOS), scleroderma esophagus, and nonspecific esophageal motor disorder. These groups have many characteristics in common, such as clinical presentation, poor knowledge of the pathological basis, treatment, and the fact that no specific outcome for any one subset is recognized.[15] Spastic motility disorders of the esophagus can appear at any age and are more frequent in women.

In diffuse esophageal spasm, manometric patterns are characterized by normal peristalsis that is intermittently interrupted by simultaneous contractions, high-amplitude or long-duration waves, or incomplete LOS relaxation.

The mechanism of dysphagia may involve intermittent simultaneous (nonpropulsive) contractions, which occur after 10% to 30% of swallows. Up to 30% of patients with diffuse esophageal spasm have high LOS pressure or impaired post-deglutition LOS relaxation. In patients with diffuse esophageal spasm, the barium study may reveal uncoordinated movement of the lower two thirds of the esophagus.

Gastro-esophageal reflux disease (GERD) is commonly associated with spastic motility disorders; it frequently presents with dysphagia and chest pain that may be taken for ischemic cardiac pain.[16] This is because the sensory innervation of the esophagus is similar to that of the heart. Dysphagia, which is present in 30% to 60% of patients, usually includes both liquids and solids but does not usually prevent the consumption of food completely. The chest pain is localized at the retrosternal level and radiates to the back, neck, jaw, and arms.

The spastic motility disorders associated with normal peristalsis (nutcracker esophagus, hypertensive LOS) are usually associated with normal barium esophagrams. Esophageal pH monitoring indicates the possible presence of abnormal acid reflux.[15]

The therapeutic approach to motility disorders is based on the treatment of gastro-esophageal reflux, if suspected, and reassuring the patient that symptoms are not cardiac in origin. In the treatment of the spastic esophageal motility disorders, various drugs have also been used, such as smooth muscle relaxants, anticholinergics, and calcium channel blockers, but no clinical studies have been carried out to assess their efficacy. In a double-blind, placebo-controlled study, low doses of the antidepressant trazodone hydrochloride produced global improvement and reduced stress from esophageal symptoms independently of any changes in manometric patterns.[17]

Gastro-esophageal reflux disease (GERD)

Chronic gastro-esophageal reflux is a very common clinical problem. The reflux of gastric contents into the esophagus through the LOS can cause esophageal mucosal damage ranging from inflammation to erosion and ulceration. GERD is primarily caused by a motility disorder of the esophagus and the stomach, rather than an excessive production of acid.[18] In fact, although there is a positive association between the severity of esophagitis and the duration of esophageal acid exposure, there is no association between the severity of esophagitis and the basal or maximal acid output.[19-21] There is a small group of patients with Zollinger-Ellison syndrome, whose excessive gastric acid secretion significantly contributes to the pathogenesis of esophagitis and presents a high incidence of GERD.[22,23] GERD may result from an incompetence of the LOS or impaired clearance of acid from the esophagus due to insufficient peristalsis or delayed gastric emptying.

Pathological reflux has also been shown to occur in conditions associated with diffuse GI dysmotility such as idiopathic intestinal pseudo-obstruction, irritable bowel syndrome, primary anorexia nervosa, and progressive systemic sclerosis.[24] Although some of these disorders, such as scleroderma, are characterized by a reduction of the resting LOS pressure, which could explain the gastro-esophageal reflux, most patients with GERD experience reflux because of spontaneous (transient or inappropriate) relaxation of the LOS independent of the normal swallowing sequence. The most frequent symptoms associated with GERD are regurgitation, pyrosis, dysphagia, and chest pain that mimics cardiac pain. Other manifestations include chronic hoarseness secondary to posterior laryngitis, bronchospastic conditions (asthma or chronic cough) precipitated by gastro-esophageal reflux, hiccup, loss of dental enamel, and night sweats.[18]

To reduce dyspeptic symptoms, antireflux measures are employed, such as the consumption of small quantities of food at a time and low-fat meals; reduced intake of acidic juices, coffee, and alcohol; and avoidance of recumbency immediately after eating and sitting as long as possible. It is also important to reduce or eliminate drugs that potentially lower the pressure of LOS such as anticholinergics, tranquilizers, tricyclic antidepressants, theophylline, and calcium channel blocking agents.[18]

Pharmacological therapy includes the use of an H2 blocking agent at full doses for long periods of time. However, recent studies indicate that approximately 50% of patients experience relapses even with continuous therapy.[25] Omeprazole has been shown to give an almost complete suppression of acid when administered in a single daily dose and moreover to give a high recovery percentage in patients with erosive esophagitis. Omeprazole was more effective than ranitidine in patients with grade I, II, and III reflux esophagitis.[26] Unfortunately most patients suffer a relapse within a short time after discontinuing omeprazole.[18] Patients who have an early relapse of esophagitis and in whom symptoms recur early, despite continuation of maintenance treatment with acid-inhibiting drugs, have been shown to have a lower LOS pressure than patients who can be maintained in remission for a long period of time.

Prokinetic drugs might offer a rational alternative to antisecretory therapy.

Stomach Motility Disorders

The control of stomach emptying is exerted at different levels: electromechanical, neurohormonal feedback, and brain.[3,6–8,10,27,28] Alterations occurring at any of these levels may cause gastric stasis and symptoms such as regurgitation, nausea, retching, vomiting, abdominal pain, and constipation.

Small or squashed stomach syndrome

Squashed stomach syndrome refers to dyspepsia caused by the inability of the stomach to distend normally because of hepatomegaly. Similar symptoms occur after partial gastrectomy (small stomach syndrome).[14] The frequency of this syndrome in advanced cancer patients is not known.

The symptoms associated with this syndrome include early satiety, epigastric fullness, epigastric pain, flatulence, hiccup, nausea, vomiting, and pyrosis. According to Twycross,[14] the treatment of squashed stomach syndrome is based on eating little and often, the use of defoaming antiflatulents after meals and at bedtime, and the use of prokinetic drugs.

Gastroparesis

Gastroparesis is a motility disorder caused by an alteration of the transit of the intraluminal content from the stomach to the duodenum in the absence of mechanical obstruction. Gastroparesis may be idiopathic or result from different conditions, such as severe chronic constipation, diabetes mellitus,[29] systemic sclerosis, myotonic dystrophy, progressive muscular dystrophy, vagotomy and pyloroplasty, or partial gastric resection. Acute gastroparesis may complicate gastroenteritis. The possible mechanisms of gastroparesis include impaired fundus tone, weak "antral pump," arrhythmia of the gastric pacemaker, or a lack of coordination between the antral peristaltic wave and the pyloric sphincter relaxation or proximal duodenal contractions.[30] Therapy is based on the use of prokinetic drugs. A single small study in cancer patients has shown that gastric stasis may be reversible with metoclopramide therapy.[31]

The cancer anorexia–cachexia syndrome (CACS)

This syndrome is a common problem in patients with advanced cancer.[32] Although many possible etiologies have been investigated, the cause has not yet been determined. Alteration in GI motility seems to be a primary factor in the pathogenesis of CACS.

In a review of the literature, Nelson and colleagues[33] reported that the prevalence of anorexia in cancer patients ranges from 15% to 40% at cancer diagnosis and goes up to 80% in the advanced stage. In addition to anorexia, weight loss is due to other factors, including nausea, vomiting, early satiety, pain, emotional distress, GI cancer, and the effects of radiation or chemotherapy. Furthermore, most cancer patients present oral cavity pathologies, such as mucositis, ulcerations, taste alteration, and dry mouth, which are often subsequent to anticancer therapy[34] and also greatly reduce food intake. Anorexia, early satiety, nausea, vomiting, bloating, and postprandial fullness are considered to be pathognomonic of delayed gastric emptying in diabetic patients.

Cancer-associated dyspepsia syndrome (CADS)

CADS was identified by Nelson and Walsh,[33] who highlighted the relationship between GI symptoms, particularly early satiety, and reduced upper GI motility in advanced cancer patients.[35] Because the GI symptoms are frequent and occur with or without anorexia, the authors named this symptom complex the "cancer-associated dyspepsia syndrome" (CADS). CADS appears to be a precursor of the cancer anorexia–cachexia syndrome. The causes of this syndrome may include central abnormalities (metabolic, biochemical, or humoral) or peripheral abnormalities (gastroparesis or direct tumor invasion). In a study carried out by the same authors, metoclopramide was found to significantly reduce many dyspeptic symptoms associated with anorexia, such as bloating, eructation, and nausea, and also produced an increase in appetite.[36]

Functional (non-ulcer) dyspepsia

Functional (non-ulcer) dyspepsia is a heterogeneous disorder characterized by recurrent or chronic abdominal pain or discomfort in the upper abdomen without evident lesions of the GI apparatus.[37] The prevalence of dyspepsia was about 40% in one community survey.[38] Other than pain, the symptoms reported by patients include early satiety, abdominal bloating, nausea, vomiting, pyrosis, and eructation. Usually, dyspeptic symptoms are chronic and exacerbated by food intake. The causes of these symptoms could be linked to abnormal upper GI motility, an altered visceral perception of pain, or increased sensitivity to gastric acid with or without inflammation of the mucosa.[39] In some cases, dyspepsia may be induced by drugs, such as nonsteroidal anti-inflammatory agents (NSAIDs), theophylline, digitalis, antibiotics, and potassium or iron supplements.

Subcategories have been proposed for functional dyspepsia and may be useful in clinical practice. In "ulcer-like dyspepsia," predominant symptoms include well-localized epigastric pain, with relief upon ingestion of food and antiacids. The patient has long periods without pain alternating with periods of intense pain that can occur also during the night, preventing sleep.[40] In "reflux-like dyspepsia," prominent symptoms include abdominal bloating, distention, early satiety, acid regurgitation, and pyrosis. In "dysmotility-like dyspepsia," the symptoms suggest gastric stasis or upper intestinal dysmotility, such as nausea and vomiting, abdominal bloating, anorexia or weight loss, and discomfort after meals.[40]

Some causes of functional dyspepsia are specific to the cancer population.

These include delayed gastric emptying due to administration of opioids, anticholinergics, or chemotherapeutics; gastritis due to irritant drugs, such as iron, metronidazole, NSAIDs, and corticosteroids; direct effects of gastric cancer; gastroparesis due to autonomic dysfunction; small stomach syndrome; and reflux esophagitis following surgery and/or radiotherapy.

Delayed gastric emptying and postprandial antral hypomotility were observed in 25% to 50% of the patients with functional dyspepsia.[41] Prokinetic drugs have been proposed as a rational treatment, particularly for patients with dysmotility-like symptoms. H2 antagonists are an alternative, and both cimetidine and ranitidine are modestly superior to placebo;[42,43] these drugs are more efficacious in patients with ulcer-like dyspepsia. The results of controlled clinical studies of sucralfate in the treatment of dyspepsia are still controversial.[44,45] Antacids are frequently used in patients with functional dyspepsia, but studies suggest their efficacy is no different from that of placebo.[46] The beneficial effect of antibiotic treatment of *Helicobacter pylori* infection for controlling dyspeptic symptoms has not yet been defined. Simethicone, a defoaming antiflatulent, is helpful for gas-related symptoms (fullness, distention, bloating).[47] Because patients often take multiple drugs, it is advisable to review therapy carefully and eliminate any nonessential drugs that could delay gastric emptying, stimulate gastric acid secretion, or physically irritate the gastric mucosa.

Intestinal Motility Disorders

Both the mixing of the chyme with the biliary, pancreatic, and intestinal secretions, and the propulsion of the chyme for intestinal absorption occur at the proximal bowel level. Absorption depends on the speed of contraction.[3,7,10] The control of the peristaltic circuit is determined by both neurogenic and chemical factors. This stimulation coordinates, in association with ECA, the actions of the circular and longitudinal muscle layer (direction and velocity of propagation, and the timing of contractions).[3,6,7,48,49] Colonic contractile activity may be grossly divided into segmental and propagated contractions.

Narcotic bowel syndrome

Opioid analgesics produce alterations of GI motility through more than one mechanism and at different points of the digestive tract[50–53] (Fig. 4.2). Both upper and lower level effects are probably mediated by the central nervous system and local mechanism in the walls of the stomach and intestine.[51,54] Numerous studies have shown that enkephalins and dynorphin may act as neurotransmitters in the GI tract by interacting with specific μ-, δ-, and κ-receptor subtypes.[52,55–58] The actions of opioids are either indirect, the

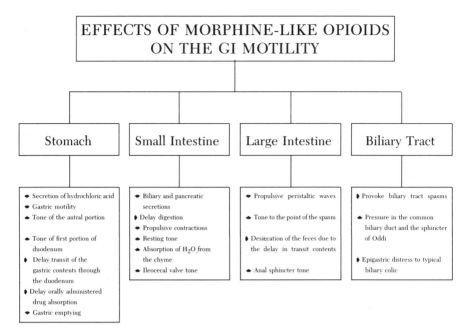

Figure 4.2. Effects of morphine-like opioids on the GI motility. [Adapted from Jaffe JH, and Martin W.[51]]

result of neural interaction through the inhibition of Ach or VIP, or direct, due to contraction of smooth muscle.[59–62]

Opioids reduce motility by increasing segmental motor contractility and preventing longitudinal peristalsis. Opioid administration can produce narcotic bowel syndrome (NBS), as described by Sandgren and coworkers[63] in five patients who were taking large doses of opioid analgesics to control abdominal pain. In one survey, NBS appeared in 4% of cancer patients treated with oral opioids.[64] This syndrome is characterized by nausea and vomiting, mild abdominal discomfort, constipation, gaseous abdominal distention, features of intestinal pseudo-obstruction, and weight loss. Rapid resolution of symptoms and signs of NBS can occur within days of complete withdrawal of opioids.[63] Because it is not possible to stop opioid administration in cancer patients with pain, a useful approach may be the use of parenteral analgesics in association with continuous subcutaneous infusion of metoclopramide using a syringe driver.[64,65] In patients treated with metoclopramide at a dose of 60 mg/day, significant improvements in nausea, vomiting, appetite, and abdominal distention were observed within 72 hours from the start of therapy; and with this therapy, some patients could return to the original oral therapy.[65]

Irritable bowel syndrome

Irritable bowel syndrome (IBS), or "irritable colon," presumably produces pain and discomfort through muscular spasm. In IBS, the whole gut is involved; the gut is both hypersensitive and hyperreactive to mechanical and chemical stimuli. Even contractile waves that are apparently "normal" in amplitude can evoke the discomfort.[66] In addition to pain, the characteristic symptoms of IBS are constipation, abdominal distention, flatulence, and tenesmus. IBS is frequently associated with psychosomatic complaints affecting other organ systems. Cisapride has proved effective in treating the symptoms of IBS in a small number of placebo-controlled clinical trials.[67–69]

Some studies indicate that 5-HT3 receptor activation may be involved in the etiology of IBS. In 12 patients, the intravenous administration of granisetron increased the threshold volumes at which the perceptions of gas, tenesmus, and discomfort were perceived, without affecting rectal compliance or motility during distention.[70]

Bowel obstruction

Although cancer patients may develop bowel obstruction at any time, patients with more advanced disease are predisposed to this, with an incidence of 5.5% to 25% in ovarian carcinoma[71–75] and 4.4% to 24% in colorectal cancer.[76,77] In terminal cancer patients, the incidence of bowel obstruction is 42% in ovarian cancer,[72] and 10% in colorectal cancer.[78] Several physiopathologic mechanisms may be involved in the onset of gastrointestinal obstruction (Table 4.5).

Table 4.5. Physiopathologic mechanism of GI obstruction

Extrinsic occlusion of the lumen

    Enlargement of the primary tumors or recurrence
    Mesenteric and omental masses
    Abdominal or pelvic adhesions
    Post-irradiation fibrosis

Intraluminal occlusion of the lumen

    Polypoid lesions due to primary cancer or metastases
    Annular tumoral dissemination

Intramural occlusion of the lumen

    Intestinal linitis plastica

Intestinal motility disorders (pseudo-obstruction)

    Infiltration of the mesentery or bowel muscle and nerves
    Malignant involvement of the coeliac plexus
    Paraneoplastic neuropathy in patients with lung cancer:[95,182]
        Chronic intestinal pseudo-obstruction[86,87]
        Paraneoplastic pseudo-obstruction[91]

Bowel obstruction can be partial or complete, and single or multiple, due to benign or malignant causes. Pancreatic cancer spreads directly to the duodenum or stomach; colon cancer spreads to the jejunum and ileum; and prostate and bladder cancers spread to the rectum.[79] Tumors at the splenic flexure cause an obstruction in 49% of cases, and tumors of the right and left colon obstruct in 25% of cases; only 6% of tumors of the rectum and rectosigmoid junction cause bowel obstruction.[76] In patients with ovarian carcinoma, the small bowel is more commonly involved than the large bowel (61% vs. 33%), and in 6% to 22% of cases, both are obstructed.[80,81] In ovarian cancer, the cause of the intestinal blockage is usually recurrent tumor and less often adhesions or radiation-associated strictures or fibrosis.

In the majority of patients with advanced cancer, there appears to be a slow progression from partial to complete bowel obstruction. Symptoms gradually worsen until they become continuous and their presence and intensity depend on the site of the gastrointestinal tract. Vomiting can be intermittent or continuous; it develops early and in large amounts in gastric, duodenal, and small bowel obstruction, and develops later in large bowel obstruction. The prevalence of vomiting ranges from 68% to 100%.[78,82] Pain is due to abdominal distention, tumor mass, hepatomegaly, or to abdominal colic in small and large bowel obstruction. The prevalence of colicky pain is 72% to 76%, whereas continuous abdominal pain is present in more than 90% of the patients.[78,82] In cases of complete obstruction there is no evacuation of feces and no flatus. Sometimes overflow diarrhea results from bacterial liquefaction of the fecal material blocked in the sigmoid or rectum. Other symptoms associated with bowel obstruction include abdominal distention, visible peristalsis, intermittent borborygmi, and anorexia.

To diagnose a mechanical obstruction, one must first rule out the presence of constipation and paralytic ileus. Constipation is often the sole cause of obstructive symptoms when patients complain of hard feces and infrequent bowel movements; these symptoms may follow the use of constipating drugs (opioids, belladonna, alkaloids, antispasmodics, antidepressants) without the use of laxatives. This situation may be worsened by inactivity, a low-fiber diet, and weakness or inability to reach the toilet when feeling the urge to evacuate. Physical examination shows feces in the rectum and palpable fecal masses in the abdomen. When the rectum is empty and impaction is high, abdominal radiographs are needed for diagnosis.

Abdominal radiographs taken with the patient in a supine or a standing position are the first investigations to be performed in patients with suspected small bowel obstruction. This is done to document the dilated loops of intestine, air–fluid interfaces, or both. Studying the small bowel with a contrast medium can distinguish obstruction from metastases, radiation injury, or adhesions. The diagnosis of a motility disorder is revealed by the slow passage of barium through undilated bowel, with no demonstrable point of obstruction. Abdominal radiographs in different positions are necessary when large bowel obstruction is suspected. This examination can be carried out with a barium enema and colosigmoidoscopy.[83,84] When duodenal obstruction is suspected, tests using oral barium or endoscopy may be needed to evaluate the cause.

Chronic intestinal pseudo-obstruction

Chronic intestinal pseudo-obstruction (CIP) is a heterogeneous group of nerve and muscle disorders that share a common clinical presentation of bowel obstruction with no demonstrable anatomical lesion.[85–89] CIP is characterized by nausea, vomiting, abdominal distention, and diffuse abdominal pain. Severe constipation or diarrhea, or both, may also be present. CIP is mainly due to diabetes mellitus, previous gastric surgery, and varied neurologic disorders. These factors may affect extrinsic neural control to viscera. Vagal dysfunction is confirmed in a majority of patients with CIP associated with diabetes or neurologic disorders.

Acute pseudo-obstruction of the colon was first described by Ogilvie.[90] It is characterized by massive colonic dilatation with a clinical and radiological picture of colonic obstruction in the absence of any mechanical obstruction. Colonic dilatation is most marked in the cecum and may be rapidly progressive, leading to cecal necrosis and perforation.

Autonomic neuropathy

Autonomic neuropathy (AN) is a rare syndrome that occurs alone or with other neurologic disorders. It is usually associated with small cell lung cancer (SCLC) and may occur with other cancers (pancreas, breast, pulmonary carcinoid, and adenocarcinoma of undetermined origin). Autonomic neuropathy may occur before or after the diagnosis of cancer. Patients present a subacute onset of intestinal dysmotility characterized by chronic nausea and anorexia secondary to gastroparesis with delayed gastric emptying, marked small and large intestinal dilatation and poor propulsive activity, and sometimes symptoms and signs consistent with intestinal pseudo-obstruction (IPO). Other manifestations associated with neuropathic and autonomic disorders are cardiovascular alterations (postural hypotension, syncopal episodes, painless myocardial infarction, and fixed heart rate), pupillary abnormalities, sensory disturbances, and neurogenic bladder.[91–94]

The association between neuropathy and GI disorders was originally described by Denny Brown in 1948.[95] However, the autonomic instability and paralysis of the digestive tract was initially found in cancer patients many years later.[96] The initial description depicted a patient with small cell lung cancer who had tumor infiltration of autonomic nerves, mainly in the myenteric plexus. Subsequently, other authors have described cases of cancer associated with GI neuropathies.[97–99] Chinn and Schuffler[100] reported seven patients with dysautonomia, myenteric plexopathy, pseudo-obstruction, and neurologic disorders (two patients manifested encephalopathy, ataxia, neurogenic bladder, and polyneuropathy). The histological changes in the esophagus, stomach, small bowel, and colon showed neuronal and axonal degeneration, lymphoplasmocytic infiltration, and glial cell proliferation within the myenteric plexus.

Lennon and coworkers[101] reported on patients with SCLC, myenteric plexopathy, and AN whose serum contained the specific antibody Anti-Hu (antinuclear neuronal antibody I). These antibodies also reacted with antigens found in SCLC and were identical to the Anti-Hu antibody associated with paraneoplastic encephalomyelitis and sensory neuropathy reported by Dalmau and coworkers.[102] Anti-Hu antibody is a polyclonal, complement-fixing IgG that reacts strongly with the nuclei of virtually all neurons in the peripheral nervous system and in the CNS.[92]

Treatment of AN, using steroids, plasmapheresis, or immunosuppressants, does not appear to improve the paraneoplastic symptoms. In the majority of patients, death is caused by neurologic failure.[101-103]

The clinical presentation of paraneoplastic AN and IPO usually begins with GI symptoms, including progressive anorexia and nausea, early satiety, vomiting, and constipation. Patients usually report GI discomfort and often reveal a history of an abdominal surgical procedure and substantial weight loss. After several weeks or months, neurologic dysfunction, such as paresthesias of the distal extremities, may appear. This may progress to a severe peripheral asymmetric sensory neuropathy with postural instability (ataxia), neuropathic pain, distal weakness, and urological symptoms.[91,104]

Autonomic neuropathy and IPO are increasingly recognized in clinical practice, particularly with the introduction of antroduodenojejunal manometry, scintigraphic transit, electrophysiological studies, and autonomic function tests. Bruera and coworkers[93,94,105] have demonstrated that cardiovascular autonomic insufficiency is a frequent finding in patients with advanced cancer and should be suspected mainly in patients with a combination of heart rate > 100/min, Karnofsky index score of < 60 (deconditioning syndrome), and malnutrition. In patients with advanced cancer, AN is probably a multifactorial syndrome in which malnutrition, decreased activity, drugs (vinca alkaloids, opioids, and tricyclic antidepressants), or paraneoplastic syndromes are all possible causes. Hence, the differential diagnosis of IPO is like any intestinal motility disorder: mechanical obstruction, pseudo-obstruction or dysmotility due to visceral myopathy, familial pseudo-obstruction, connective tissue diseases, endocrine disorders, treatment with anticholinergics, or other neurologic diseases that affect the autonomic nervous systems.[106]

The prognosis for IPO patients is poor. Most patients die within a year after diagnosis without regaining either GI or neurologic function. Several reports include patients who survived and had some return of GI activity, but not neurologic function. Treatment with prokinetic agents in patients with such extensive destruction of the myenteric plexus is very difficult; drugs and surgical interventions are probably of little use. Early detection of paraneoplastic syndromes could help the identification of the primary cancer, thus allowing earlier treatment.

Pharmacological Approach to Motility Disorders

Prokinetic drugs promote transit throughout the gastrointestinal tract by means of various mechanisms (Table 4.6). Transit may be enhanced by increasing peristalsis or by inhibiting segmental contractions, by promoting and coordinating gastroduodenal contractile activity, or by increasing slow-wave function. Serotoninergic neurons appear to play an important role in maintaining the balance between contractile and relaxant activity that permits normal peristalsis to occur. Prokinetic agents are believed to enhance luminal transit by producing or altering this balance.[30]

Prokinetic drugs are used in the treatment of gastro-esophageal reflux, diabetic gastroparesis, irritable bowel syndrome, bile reflux gastritis, postoperative ileus, nonmechanical pseudo-obstruction of the colon, chronic lower gastrointestinal motility disorders associated with systemic disease, and constipation.[107–110] Although the mechanism of action of prokinetic drugs is not fully understood, it is thought that these drugs enhance intestinal function by either promoting the effect of a motility agonist or antagonizing the effect of an inhibitory transmitter.[30]

Prokinetic drugs increase the motility of the GI tract and modify the absorption and bioavailability of other concomitantly orally administered drugs. For narrow therapeutic range drugs or other drugs that require careful titra-

Table 4.6. Prokinetic agents

Drugs	*Mechanism of action*
Bethanechol	Cholinergic agonism
Pyridostigmine	Anticholinesterases
Metoclopramide	Dopamine antagonism Cholinergic agonism
Cisapride	Serotonin antagonism Cholinergic agonism
Domperidone	Dopamine antagonism
Erythromycin	Motilin agonism
Naloxone	μ-Receptor antagonism
Octreotide	Inhibition of gut hormone release

tion, plasma concentrations should be monitored closely during concomitant therapy with prokinetic drugs.[111]

Cholinergic agonists and anticholinesterases

The prototypes of these classes are bethanechol and pyridostigmine. The peristaltic activity of the bowel and tone and amplitude of the contractions are mediated by the action of ACh upon muscarinic cholinergic receptors (M1, M2). Bethanechol is a cholinergic agonist that binds to the M2 receptor on smooth muscle gastrointestinal cells.[112,113] Pyridostigmine prevents the breakdown of endogenously released ACh. Bethanechol increases both the pressure of the LOS and the magnitude of the esophageal contractions.[114] In patients with gastro-esophageal reflux, bethanechol provoked a symptomatic and endoscopic improvement in esophagitis[115] without accelerating small bowel transit or facilitating gastric emptying.[116] The recommended doses are 10 to 25 mg four times daily for bethanechol and 60 mg three times daily for oral pyridostigmine.

Generalized parasympathetic side effects are seen in 10% to 15% of patients treated with bethanechol. These effects include abdominal cramps, diarrhea, salivation, flushing, bradycardia, blurred vision, fatigue, and bronchospasm. These unwanted effects are particularly marked in those patients with cholinergic denervation due to autonomic neuropathy.

Substituted benzamides: cisapride and metoclopramide

Substituted benzamides represent the first class of true prokinetic agents.

Cisapride is a substituted piperidinyl benzamide, chemically related to metoclopramide. Unlike metoclopramide, cisapride does not have dopamine-blocking activity, and therefore has no antidopaminergic effects on the CNS. For the same reason, the drug has no antiemetic effects. Cisapride stimulates GI motor activity through an indirect mechanism involving the release of ACh mediated by postganglionic nerve endings in the myenteric (Auerbach's) plexus of the gut.[117] The drug has no direct cholinergic properties, nor does it sensitize muscarinic receptors or interact with acetylcholinesterase. It is an agonist of serotonin at the 5-HT4 receptor (located on cholinergic neurons of the myenteric plexus), as well as an antagonist at the 5-HT3 receptor.[117] Cisapride also increases levels of endorphins, motilin, and pancreatic polypeptide, and decreases the concentration of substance P and cholecystokinin.[118]

Most of the clinical studies have shown an effect of cisapride on gastro-esophageal reflux disease (GERD), functional (non-ulcer) dyspepsia, gastroparesis, or constipation. Administered orally or intravenously at the dose of 5 to 20 mg, cisapride is able to increase the pressure of the LOS by 20% to 50% in patients with GERD.[117–122] The effects are most pronounced when basal LOS pressure is low, during the night or when lying down. In controlled studies, endoscopically confirmed response rates of 57% to 73% have been reported with 10 mg 4 times daily for 6 to 16 weeks and compared to a response rate of 12% to 53% in the placebo group.[117] Cisapride is also able to control symptoms such as pyrosis.[123]

In a double-blind placebo-controlled crossover study, cisapride 20 mg twice a day administered in association with ranitidine 150 mg twice a day produced a further reduction of acid reflux from 6.4% obtained with only ranitidine to 3.7% in 24 hours[124] in patients with GERD. In other studies comparing cisapride (40 mg daily) and ranitidine (300 mg daily) a similar efficacy in improving esophagitis was observed.[125] Cisapride also showed a similar or superior efficacy in reducing esophageal exposure time to acid in comparison to metoclopramide.[123] In one study, cisapride was as efficacious as H2-receptor antagonists in the treatment of GERD.[126] Various studies have evaluated the effects of cisapride on gastric emptying in healthy subjects and in patients with gastroparesis (idiopathic or diabetic origin).[117,123] In all these studies, cisapride proved to be effective in accelerating gastric emptying. In contrast, cisapride did not work in nine patients with anorexia nervosa and delayed gastric emptying.[127]

The effect of cisapride on gastric emptying seems to be related to the dose. For example, 10 mg administered twice daily showed no effect in 17 patients with idiopathic gastroparesis, but increasing the drug to 30 or 40 mg daily resulted in a significant increase in gastric emptying.[128] In comparison to metoclopramide, cisapride showed similar or superior efficacy in reducing the time of gastric emptying in healthy volunteers as well as in patients with idiopathic or diabetic gastroparesis.[129–131]

In patients with functional dyspepsia the superiority of cisapride in comparison to standard doses of metoclopramide or domperidone is still controversial. Cisapride was more effective than metoclopramide in reversing delayed gastric emptying due to intramuscular administration of morphine.[132]

In a double-blind, placebo-controlled study, the efficacy of 20 mg of cisapride orally on the absorption of controlled-release morphine, 20 mg, was evaluated.[133] Cisapride significantly increased plasma morphine concentrations after 1 hour when both drugs were taken simultaneously. There was no significant change in time of peak concentration. It is not possible to conclude that the increase in plasma morphine concentration was due to increased gastric emptying. Another study showed the effect of 10 mg of oral metoclopramide[134] on plasma concentrations of morphine in patients treated with MST 20 mg. While metoclopramide did not modify the maximum plasma morphine concentration, there was a significant reduction in the time to maximum concentration. This shows that metoclopramide increases morphine absorption, probably by accelerating gastric emptying.

Unlike drugs such as metoclopramide and domperidone, cisapride also stimulates motility of the lower gastrointestinal tract.[135,136] Compared with placebo, cisapride significantly reduced the transit time through the small and large bowel in both healthy subjects and patients.[123,137,138] In a double-blind crossover study[137] carried out on patients suffering from constipation, the time of emptying of the cecum and ascending colon was significantly reduced after cisapride administration. Furthermore, cisapride (20 mg twice daily) was found to significantly increase spontaneous stool frequency and consistency and to reduce the laxative intake in 126 patients with idiopathic constipation.[139] In the latter study, both cisapride and placebo improved constipation, as assessed by means of a patient-rated visual analogue scale, but cisapride did so to a larger extent than placebo. This is the first study showing an effect on bowel movements of a drug that is not classified as a laxative. The mechanism underlying these laxative effects has not yet been well defined.

Metoclopramide is a dopamine antagonist at both central and peripheral levels, a cholinergic agonist at 5-HT4 receptors,[117] and a weak antagonist at the 5-HT3 receptors. At high doses, metoclopramide produces 5-HT3 receptor blockade, which may contribute to its antiemetic activity.[140] Metoclopramide inhibits the inibitory effect of dopamine at the dopaminergic receptors in the GI tract, promoting the release of ACh. Metoclopramide increases the pressure of the LOS as well as the amplitude of esophageal contractions.[141]

In controlled clinical studies, metoclopramide has been shown to be efficacious in the treatment of GERD.[142,143] Because of its dopamine antagonism and cholinergic agonism, the effects of metoclopramide on gastrointestinal motility are antagonized by anticholinergic drugs (e.g., scopolamine hydrobromide and butylbromide) and opioid analgesic drugs. Metoclopramide increases the tone and strength of gastroduodenal contractions. Its prokinetic action is less in the jejunum, ileum, and colon. It does not stimulate gastric, enteric, pancreatic, or biliary secretions. It is a powerful antiemetic because of its combined actions on the chemoreceptor trigger zone (CTZ) and intestinal motility.

The efficacy of orally administered metoclopramide in treating delayed gastric emptying has been established in a number of controlled clinical trials.[144–147] Metoclopramide is also effective in reversing tumor-related gastroparesis,[31,148,149] nausea, and anorexia in advanced cancer patients.[36,65] There is no evidence that metoclopramide is efficacious in myopathic or neuropathic intestinal pseudo-obstruction.[86]

In a double-blind crossover study, controlled-release metoclopramide was able to reduce the intensity of nausea significantly more than immediate-release metoclopramide in advanced cancer patients.[150] Metoclopramide is not usually indicated for long-term use. The oral preparations are recommended for 4 to 12 weeks of therapy. Use of parenteral metoclopramide should be limited to 1 or 2 days because of the occurrence of CNS effects such as drowsiness, lassitude, anxiety, and extrapyramidal side effects.[151] Metoclopramide should be avoided in patients receiving monoamine oxidase inhibitors and used cautiously in patients receiving tricyclic antidepressants, sympathomimetics, or phenothiazines, and in patients with epilepsy or extrapyramidal syndromes.[135] Recommended doses of cisapride and metoclopramide are 10 to 20 mg, to be taken 30 minutes before each meal, and at bedtime.

Antidopaminergics: domperidone

Domperidone is a peripherally acting dopamine-2 receptor antagonist that acts like metoclopramide but does not cross through the blood–brain barrier, does not have extrapyramidal side effects, and has excellent tolerability. It blocks the inhibitory effects of dopamine on cholinergic neurons promoting ACh release. The efficacy of domperidone is predominantly limited to the stomach. Oral and intravenous domperidone increases peristaltic activity of the antrum and duodenum, and increases the gastric emptying of liquids and semisolids such as a barium meal. The drug has also been shown to be an effective symptomatic treatment in patients with chronic postprandial dyspepsia. The effect of oral domperidone on LOS pressure is also unclear because the results coming from controlled clinical studies are controversial.[152]

Domperidone 10 or 20 mg 3 to 4 times daily has been shown to be more effective than, or comparable to, an equal dose of metoclopramide in patients with symptoms of dyspepsia caused mainly by gastritis.[153] In this study, domperidone was better tolerated than metoclopramide. Domperidone 10 to 20 mg has also been shown to be more efficacious than placebo in controlling vomiting caused by gastritis, pancreatitis, uremia, and hepatitis.[154]

Domperidone is a well-tolerated drug in most patients. Occasionally reported side effects include dry mouth, transient skin rash or itching, and diarrhea.

Macrolide antibiotics: erythromycin

The macrolides are a new class of gastrokinetic compounds.[155,156] In clinical practice, their role in the treatment of motility disorders is not yet fully understood. Erythromycin and oleandomycin mimic the effects of motilin (a GI peptide hormone) by binding to motilin receptors located on smooth muscle cells distributed along the GI tract.[157] Intravenous infusion of erythromycin at doses of 200 mg in 10 patients with diabetic gastroparesis allowed normal gastric emptying of both liquid and solids;[158,159] the drug induced premature antral phase III activity and increased the frequency of antral contractions.[160] Oral and intravenous administration of erythromycin also improved gastrointestinal motility in colonic pseudo-obstruction.[161,162] Preliminary studies have suggested that, in the short term, erythromycin stimulates other regions of the digestive tract, including the esophagus, gallbladder, and colon.

A reduced production and/or release of motilin could have some effect on the pathogenesis of idiopathic constipation; such patients have lower plasma levels of motilin[163] than people with normal bowel function. It is reasonable to suppose that patients with chronic constipation can benefit from a trial with erythromycin.

Erythromycin appears to have limited clinical utility for long-term treatment. Tachyphylaxis often occurs and side effects may require discontinuation of the treatment. It may have a role in association with other prokinetic drugs, particularly because of its acute effects.

The most frequent side effects of erythromycin are abdominal cramps, gastric discomfort, nausea, vomiting, and diarrhea. Prolonged therapy can provoke overgrowth of bacteria or fungi. Intravenous administration can also cause cardiac side effects.[164] Tolerance to erythromycin appears to be related to motilin receptor down-regulation.

Opioid antagonists

Opioid administration results in numerous disorders of GI motility.[51,52] Mu (μ), δ, and κ opioid receptors are involved in the neuroregulation of smooth muscle of human colon, and opioid agonists modulate both excitatory and inhibitory neurotransmission through an action on cholinergic and non-adrenergic, noncholinergic neurons.[52] The subcutaneous administration of naloxone (a potent mu-receptor antagonist) at doses of 0.8 mg every 6 hours accelerates the transit in the transverse colon and rectosigmoid without increasing the frequency of bowel movements.[165] Naloxone slightly increases transit in the colon in healthy subjects.[165] Naloxone selectively normalizes gastrointestinal motor abnormalities and gastric stasis induced by exogenous opioids but not similar abnormalities otherwise produced.[166,167]

Oral naloxone has a bioavailability of less than 3%.[168] In a placebo-controlled, dose-ranging study the anticonstipation effect of oral naloxone was evaluated in constipated hospice patients receiving morphine or diamorphine by mouth.[168] Small-bowel transit time was assessed with the lactulose–hydrogen breath test.[169] Oral naloxone, given at a dose of at least 10% that of concurrent opioid analgesia, can reverse constipation without reversing analgesia.[168] Because very little oral naloxone appears in the systemic circulation, its mechanism is probably related to antagonism of opioid receptors in the gut. The small amount absorbed systemically may be sufficient to produce withdrawal in some physically dependent patients. For this reason, it should be used cautiously with appropriate dose titration.

Octreotide

Somatostatin is a polypeptide present in many tissues of the nervous system and gastrointestinal tract, including the pancreas. Somatostatin and its analogues have been shown to inhibit the release and activity of GI hormones. They also modulate GI function by reducing gastric acid secretion, decreasing bile flow, increasing mucus production, and reducing splanchnic blood flow.[170]

Octreotide is a synthetic analogue of somatostatin that has greater potency and a longer half-life. It has been shown to increase both enteric action potentials and the frequency of migrating myoelectric complexes.[171] Octreotide increases LOS tone amplitude and enhances the speed of esophageal contractions.[172] Octreotide stimulates motility in the rectosigmoid, speeding the transit in the colon.[173]

Conclusion

GI motility disorders cause symptoms that often necessitate medical consultation. The cancer patient presents GI symptoms, such as dysphagia, nausea, vomiting, early satiety, bloating, and constipation, that may be linked to an underlying incurable disease or a drug therapy that is essential for the control of pain and other symptoms. The GI motility disorders reduce food intake and may contribute to the anorexia–cachexia syndrome. Future studies are needed to assess the frequency, causes, and the intensity of symptoms related to GI motility disorders in cancer patients. The efficacy and tolerability of prokinetic drugs, particularly the laxative effect of cisapride, should be evaluated by means of controlled clinical studies to improve the treatment of GI symptoms in this population.

Acknowledgments

This work was supported in part by Italian National Research Council grants ACRO 92,02367 PF 39 and by Italian Association for Cancer Research grant AIRC 798572.

References

1. Cohen S. Gastrointestinal motility disorders. In: Fisher R, Krevsky B, eds. *Motor Disorders of the Gastrointestinal Tract.* New York: Academy Professional Information Services; 1993:1–5.
2. Bassotti G, Germani U, Morelli A. Human colonic motility: physiological aspects. *Int J Colorectal Dis* 1995; 10:173–180.
3. Sarna S. Gastrointestinal system: In vivo myoelectric activity: methods, analysis, and interpretation. In: Schultz S, Wood J, Rauner B, eds. *Handbook of Physiology.* Baltimore: Waverly Press; 1989:817–864.
4. Scratcherd T, Grundy D. The physiology of intestinal motility and secretion. *Br J Anaesth* 1984; 56:3–18.
5. Ryan JP. The biochemistry and mechanics of smooth muscle contraction. In: Fisher R, Krevsky B, eds. *Motor Disorders of the Gastrointestinal Tract.* New York: Academy Professional Information Services; 1993:7–11.

6. Makhlouf G. Regulation of muscle by neuropeptides. In: Fisher R, Krevsky B, eds. *Motor Disorders of the Gastrointestinal Tract*. New York: Academy Professional Information Services; 1993:13–16.

7. Daniel E, Collins S, Fox J, Huizinga J. Pharmacology of drugs acting on gastrointestinal motility. In: Schultz S, Wood J, and Rauner B, eds. *Handbook of Physiology*. Baltimore: Waverly Press; 1989:715–757.

8. Rao SSC, Schulze-Delrieu K. The stomach, pylorus and duodenum. In: Kumar D, Wingate D, eds. *Guide to Gastrointestinal Motility*. Edinburgh: Churchill Livingstone; 1993:373–391.

9. Kolbel C, Mayer E, Holtmann G, et al. Effects of neurokinins on human colonic motility. *Neurogastroenterol Motil* 1994; 6:119–127.

10. Sanford P. Digestive system physiology. In: Arnold E, ed. London: Hodder & Stoughton Press; 1992:41–45.

11. Sykes NP, Baines M, Carter RL. Clinical and pathological study of disphagia conservatively managed in patients with advanced malignant disease. *Lancet* 1988; 2:726–728.

12. Kahrilas PJ. Motility of the oropharynx and proximal esophagus. In: Fisher R, Krevsky B, eds. *Motor Disorders of the Gastrointestinal Tract*. New York: Academy Professional Information Services; 1993:29–35.

13. Carter RL, Pittam MR, Tanner NSB. Pain and dysphagia in patients with squamous carcinomas of the head and neck: the role of perineural spread. *J R Soc Med* 1982; 75:598–606.

14. Twycross R. Dysphagia, dyspepsia, and hiccup. In: Doyle D, Hanks G, MacDonald N, eds. *Oxford Textbook of Palliative Medicine*. Oxford: Oxford University Press; 1993:291–299.

15. Richter JE. Motor disorders of the smooth muscle esophagus. In: Fisher R, Krevsky B, eds. *Motor Disorders of the Gastrointestinal Tract*. New York: Academy Professional Information Services; 1993:37–44.

16. Vantrappen G, Janssens J, Ghillebert G. The irritable oesophagus—a frequent cause of angina-like pain. *Lancet* 1987; 1:1232–1234.

17. Clouse RE, Lustman PL, Eckert TC, et al. Low dose trazodone for symptomatic patients with esophageal contraction abnormalities: a double-blind placebo-controlled trial. *Gastroenterology* 1987; 92:1027–1032.

18. Castell D. Gastroesophageal reflux disease and its complications In: Fisher R, Krevsky B, eds. *Motor Disorders of the Gastrointestinal Tract*. New York: Academy Professional Information Services; 1993:45–49.

19. Silber W. Augmented histamine test in the treatment of symptomatic hiatus hernia. *Gut* 1969; 10:614–616.

20. Stanciu C. Gastric secretion, gastroesophageal reflux and esophagitis. *Am J Gastroenterol* 1975; 64:104–107.

21. Hirschowitz BI. A critical analysis, with appropriate control, of gastric acid and pepsin syndrome in clinical esophagitis. *Gastroenterology* 1991; 101:1149–1158.

22. Richter JE, Pandol SJ, Castel DO, McCarthy DM. Gastroesophageal reflux disease in the Zollinger-Ellison syndrome. *Gastroenterology* 1990; 98:341–346.

23. Miller L, Vinayek R, Frucht H, Gardner J, Jensen R, Maton P. Reflux esophagitis in patients with Zollinger-Ellison syndrome. *Ann Intern Med* 1981; 95:37–43.

24. Verlinden M. Review article: a role for gastrointestinal prokinetic agents in the treatment of reflux oesophagitis? *Aliment Pharmacol Ther* 1989; 3:113–131.

25. Lieberman DA. Medical therapy for chronic reflux esophagitis. *Arch Intern Med* 1987; 147:1717–1720.

26. McTavish D, Buckley MMT, Heel RC. Omeprazole: an updated review of its pharmacology and therapeutic use in acid-related disorders. *Drugs* 1991; 42:138–170.

27. Malagelada JR. Gastric emptying disorders: clinical significance and treatment. *Drugs* 1982; 24:353–359.

28. Lang I, Sarna S. Gastrointestinal system: Motor and mioelectric activity associated with vomiting, regurgitation, and nausea. In: Schultz S, Wood J, and Rauner B, eds. *Handbook of Physiology.* Baltimore: Waverly Press; 1989:1179–1197.

29. Drenth JPH, Engels LGLB. Diabetic gastroparesis: a critical reappraisal of new treatment strategies. *Drugs* 1992; 44(4):537–553.

30. Reynolds J. Agents that accelerate gastrointestinal transit. In: Fisher R, Krevsky B, eds. *Motor Disorders of the Gastrointestinal Tract.* New York: Academy Professional Information Services; 1993:17–23.

31. Kris MG, Yeh SDJ, Gralla RJ, et al. Symptomatic gastroparesis in cancer patients—a possible cause of cancer-associated anorexia that can be improved with oral metoclopramide. *Proc Am Soc Clin Oncol* 1985; 4:1038A. Abstract.

32. MacDonald N, Alexander R, Bruera E. Cachexia–anorexia–asthenia. *J Pain Symptom Manage* 1995; 10:151–155.

33. Nelson K, Walsh D, Sheehan FA. The cancer anorexia-cachexia syndrome. *J Clin Oncol* 1994; 12:213–225.

34. Ripamonti C, Sbanotto A, De Conno F. Oral complications of advanced cancer. In: Bruera E, Higginson I, eds. *Cachexia-Anorexia in Cancer.* Oxford: Oxford University Press; 1996:38–56.

35. Nelson K, Walsh D, Sheehan F. Assessment of upper gastrointestinal motility in the cancer associated dyspepsia syndrome. *J Palliat Care* 1993; 9:1:27–31.

36. Nelson K, Walsh D. Metoclopramide in anorexia caused by cancer-associated dyspepsia syndrome. *J Palliat Care* 1993; 9(2):14–18.

37. Holtmann G, Talley N. Functional dyspepsia: current treatment recommendations. *Drugs* 1993; 45(6):918–930.

38. Jones R, Lydeard S. Prevalence of symptoms of dyspepsia in the community. *Br Med J* 1989; 298:30–32.

39. Talley N. Drug treatment of functional dyspepsia. *Scand J Gastroenterol* 1991; 26 (suppl 182):47–60.

40. Talley N, Zinsmeister AR, Schleck CD, Melton III LJ. Dyspepsia and dyspepsia subgroups: a population-based study. *Gastroenterology* 1992; 102:1259–1268.

41. Malagelada JR. Gastrointestinal motor disturbances in functional dyspepsia. *Scand J Gastroenterol* 1991; 26 (suppl 182):29–32.

42. Johannssenn T, Peterson H, Kristensen P, Fosstvedt D, Kleveland PM, et al. Cimetidine on-demand in dyspepsia. Experience with randomized controlled single-subject trials. *Scand J Gastroenterol* 1992; 27:189–195.

43. Farup PG, Larsen S, Ulshagen K, Osnes M. Ranitidine for non-ulcer dyspepsia: a clinical study of the symptomatic effect of ranitidine and a classification and characterization of the responders to treatment. *Scand J Gastroenterol* 1991; 26:1209–1216.

44. Kairaluoma MI, Hentilae R, Alavaikko M, et al. Sucralfate versus placebo in treatment of non-ulcer dyspepsia. *Am J Med* 1987; 83 (suppl 3B):51–55.

45. Skuobo-Kritensen E, Funch-Jensen P, Kruse A, Hanberg-Sorensen F, Amdrup E. Controlled clinical trial with sucralfate in the treatment of macroscopic gastritis. *Scand J Gastroenterol* 1989; 24:716–720.

46. Holtmann G, Talley NJ. Functional dyspepsia: current treatment recommendations. *Drugs* 1993; 45(6):918–930.

47. Berstein JE, Kasih AM. A double-blind trial of simethicone in functional disease of the upper gastrointestinal tract. *J Clin Pharmacol* 1974; 14:617–623.

48. Kellow JE, Borody TJ, Phillips SF, Tucker RL, Haddad C. Human interdigestive motility: variations in patterns from esophagus to colon. *Gastroenterology* 1986; 91:386–395.

49. Ouyang A. Motor disorders of the gastrointestinal tract. In: Fisher R, Krevsky B, eds. *Small Bowel Motility Disorders*. New York: Academy Professional Information Services; 1993:97–107.

50. Konturek SJ. Action of enkephalins on the digestive system. In: Bloom SR, Polack JM, eds. *Gut Hormones*. 2nd ed. Edinburgh: Churchill Livingstone; 1981:432–440.

51. Jaffe J, Martin W. Opioid analgesics and antagonists. In: Gilman A, Goodman L, Rall T, Murad F, eds. *The Pharmacological Basis of Therapeutics*. New York: Macmillan; 1985:491–531.

52. Angel F, Chamouard P, Klein A, Martin E. Opioid agonist modulates excitatory and inhibitory neurotransmission in human colon. *Gastrointest Motil* 1993; 5:289–297.

53. Bueno L, Fioramonti J. Action of opiates on gastrointestinal function. *Baillieres Clin Gastroenterol* 1988; 2:123–139.

54. Porrecca F, Galligan JJ, Burks TF. Central opiod receptor involvement in gastrointestinal motility. *Trends Pharmacol Sci* 1986; 7:104–107.

55. Chavkin C. Electrophysiology of opiate and opioid peptides. In: Pastenark G, ed. *The Opiate Receptors*. Clifton, N.J.: Humana Press; 1988:273–306.

56. Simon EJ, Hiller JM. Opioid peptides and opioid receptors. In: Spiegel GJ, ed. *Basic Neurochemistry: Molecular, Cellular and Medical Aspects*. 4th ed. New York: Raven Press; 1989:271–285.

57. James S, Hoyle CHV, Burnstock J, Jass J, Jeffrey JM, Lennard-Jones JF. Autoradiographic localization of opioid bindings sites in human sigmoid colon. *Eur J Pharmacol* 1987; 142:185–186.

58. Sundler F, Bjartell A, Bottcher G, Ekblad E, Hakanson R. Localization of enkephalins and other endogenous opioids in the digestive tract. *Gastroenterol Clin Biol* 1987; 11:14B–26B.

59. Ruoff HJ, Flaudung B, Demol P, Weihrauch TR. Gastrointestinal receptors and drugs in motility disorders. *Digestion* 1991; 48:1–17.

60. Grider JR, Makhlouf GM. Suppression of inhibitory neural input to colonic circular muscle by opioid peptides. *J Pharmacol Exp Ther* 1987; 243:205–210.

61. Bauer AJ, Saar MJ, Szurszewski JH. Opioids inhibit neuromuscular transmission in circular muscle of human and baboon jejunum. *Gastroenterology* 1991; 101:903–906.

62. Sun EA, Snape J, Cohen S, and Renny A. The role of opiate receptors and cholinergic neurons in the gastrocolic response. *Gastroenterology* 1982; 82:689–693.

63. Sandgren J, McPhee M, Grenberger N. Narcotic bowel syndrome treated with clonidine. *Ann Intern Med* 1984; 101:331–334.

64. Bruera E, Brenneis C, Michand M, MacDonald N. Continuous subcutaneous infusion of metoclopramide for treatment of narcotic bowel syndrome. *Cancer Treat Rep* 1987; 71:1121–1122.

65. Bruera E, Brenneis C, MacDonald RN, et al. Continuous subcutaneous infusion of metoclopramide using a disposable portable pump. *Ann Intern Med* 1986; 104: 896–897.

66. Read NW. Irritable bowel syndrome (IBS) definition and pathophysiology. *Scand J Gastroenterol* 1987; 22:7–13.

67. Evans PR, Kellow JE, Bak YT, Jones MP. Effects of cisapride on small bowel motility in irritable bowel syndrome (IBS). *Gastroenterology* 1993; 104:A504. Abstract.

68. Hurlimann S, Shorvon P, Misiewicz JJ. Effects of cisapride on symptoms and ileo-caecal transit in patients with bloated irritable bowel syndrome. *Gastroenterology* 1992; 102 (Suppl):A460. Abstract.

69. Van Outryve M, Milo R, Toussaint J, Van Eeghem P. "Prokinetic" treatment of constipation-predominant irritable bowel syndrome: a placebo-controlled study of cisapride. *J Clin Gastroenterol* 1991; 13:49–57.

70. Prior A, Read NW. Reduction of rectal sensitivity and postprandial motility by granisetron, a 5HT3 receptor agonist, in patients with irritable bowel syndrome. *Gut* 1990; 31:A1174.

71. Tunca JC, Buchler DA, Mack EA, et al. The management of ovarian-cancer caused bowel obstruction. *Gynecol Oncol* 1981; 12:186–192.

72. Beattie GJ, Leonard R, Smyth JF. Bowel obstruction in ovarian carcinoma: a retrospective study and review of the literature. *Palliat Med* 1989; 3:275–280.

73. Lund B, Hansen M, Lundvall F, et al. Intestinal obstruction in patients with advanced carcinoma of the ovaries treated with combination chemotherapy. *Surg Gynecol Obstet* 1989; 169:213–218.

74. Castaldo TW, Petrilli ES, Ballon SC, et al. Intestinal operations in patients with ovarian carcinoma. *Am J Obstet Gynecol* 1981; 139:80–84.

75. Solomon HJ, et al. Bowel complications in the management of ovarian cancer. *Aust N Z J Obstet Gynaecol* 1983; 23:65–68.

76. Phillips RKS, Hittinger R, Fry JS, et al. Malignant large bowel obstruction. *Br J Surg* 1985; 72:296–302.

77. Kyllonen LEJ. Obstruction and perforation complicating colorectal carcinoma. *Acta Chir Scand* 1987; 153:607–614.

78. Baines M, Oliver DJ, Carter RL. Medical management of intestinal obstruction in patients with advanced malignant disease: a clinical and pathological study. *Lancet* 1985; 2:990–993.

79. Baines M. The pathophysiology and management of malignant intestinal obstruction. In: Doyle D, Hanks GWC, MacDonald N, eds. *Oxford Textbook of Palliative Medicine*. 2nd ed. Oxford: Oxford University Press; 1993:311–316.

80. Rubin SC, Hoskins WJ, Benjamin I, et al. Palliative surgery for intestinal obstruction in advanced ovarian cancer. *Gynecol Oncol* 1989; 34:16–19.

81. Clarke-Pearson DL, Chin NO, DeLong ER, et al. Surgical management of intestinal obstruction in ovarian cancer. Clinical features, postoperative complications, and survival. *Gynecol Oncol* 1987; 26:11–18.

82. Ventafridda V, Ripamonti C, Caraceni A, Spoldi E, Messina L, De Conno F. The management of inoperable gastrointestinal obstruction in terminal cancer patients. *Tumori* 1990; 76:389–393.

83. Ziter FMH. Radiologic diagnosis: small bowel. In: Welch JP, ed. *Bowel Obstruction.* Philadelphia: WB Saunders; 1990:96–108.

84. Markowictz SK. Radiologic diagnosis: colon. In: Welch JP, ed. *Bowel Obstruction.* Philadelphia: W.B. Saunders; 1990:108–121.

85. Hyman P. Chronic intestinal pseudo-obstruction: outcome of treatment with cisapride in adults and children. In: Heading RC, Wood JC, eds. *Gastrointestinal Dysmotility: Focus on Cisapride.* New York: Raven Press; 1992:281–287.

86. Schuffler MD, Rohrmann CA, Chaffee RG, et al. Chronic intestinal pseudo-obstruction. *Medicine* 1981; 60:173–196.

87. Faulk DL, Anuras S, Christensen J. Chronic intestinal pseudo-obstruction. *Gastroenterology* 1985; 88:1223–1231.

88. Hyman P, McDiarmid V, Napolitano J, Abrams C, Tomomasa T. Antroduodenal motility in children with chronic intestinal pseudo-obstruction. *J Pediatr* 1988; 112:899–905.

89. Hayman P, Di Lorenzo C, McAdams L, Flores A, Tomomasa T, Garvey III T. Predicting the clinical response to cisapride in children with chronic intestinal pseudo-obstruction. *Am J Gastroenterol* 1993; 8:832–836.

90. Olgivie H. Large intestine colic due to sympathetic deprivation. A new clinical syndrome. *Br Med J* 1948; 2:671–673.

91. Liang B, Albers J, Sima A, et al. Paraneoplastic pseudo-obstruction, mononeuropathy multiplex, and sensory neuropathy. *Muscle Nerve* 1994; 17:91–96.

92. Posner J. Paraneoplastic syndromes. In: Reinhardt R, Wissler B, Massey R, Forgione L, eds. *Neurologic Complications of Cancer.* New York: F.A. Davis Company Press; 1995:353–384.

93. Bruera E, Chadwick R, Hanson J, MacDonald N. Study of cardiovascular autonomic insufficiency in advanced cancer patients. *Cancer Treat Rep* 1986; 70:1383–1387.

94. Bruera E, Catz Z, Hooper R, Lentle B, MacDonald N. Chronic nausea and anorexia in advanced cancer patients: a possible role for autonomic dysfunction. *J Pain Symptom Manage* 1987; 2:19–21.

95. Denny-Brown D. Primary sensory neuronopathy with muscular changes associated with carcinoma. *J Neurol Neurosurg Psychiatry* 1948; 11:73–87.

96. Ahmed MN, Carpenter S. Autonomic neuropathy and carcinoma of the lung. *Can Med Assoc J* 1975; 113:410–412.

97. Lhermitte F, Gray F, Lyon-Caen O, Pertuiset BF, Bernard P. Paralysis of digestive tract with lesions of myenteric plexus: a new paraneoplastic syndrome. *Rev Neurol (Paris)* 1980; 136:825–836.

98. Schuffler M, Baird H, Fleming C, et al. Intestinal pseudo-obstruction as the presenting manifestation of small cell carcinoma of the lung. *Ann Intern Med* 1983; 98:129–134.

99. Sodhi N, Camillieri M, Camoriano JK, Low PA, Fealey RD, Perry MC. Autonomic function and motility in intestinal pseudo-obstruction caused by paraneoplastic syndrome. *Dig Dis Sci* 1989; 34:1937–1942.

100. Chinn J, Schuffler M. Paraneoplastic visceral neuropathy as a cause of severe gastrointestinal motor dysfunction. *Gastroenterology* 1988; 95:1279–1286.

101. Lennon V, Sas D, Busk M, et al. Enteric neuronal autoantibodies in pseudoobstruction with small-cell lung carcinoma. *Gastroenterology* 1991; 100:137–142.

102. Dalmau J, Graus F, Rosenblum M, Posner J. Anti-Hu-associated paraneoplastic encephalomyelitis/sensory neuropathy. *Medicine* 1992; 71:59–72.

103. Dalmau J, Furneaux H, Gralla R, Kris M, Posner J. Detection of the anti-Hu antibody in the serum of patients with small cell lung cancer—a quantitative western blot analysis. *Ann Neurol* 1990; 27:544–552.

104. Graus F, Boventura I, Uchuya M, et al. Indolent anti-Hu-associated paraneoplastic sensory neuropathy. *Neurology* 1994; 44:2258–2261.

105. Bruera E. Autonomic failure in patients with advanced cancer. *J Pain Symptom Manage* 1989; 3:163–165.

106. Phillips S. Disorders of gastrointestinal motility. In: Wyngaardes JB, Smith LH eds. *Cecil Textbook of Medicine.* Philadelphia: Saunders; 1985:702–712.

107. Bright-Asare P, El Bassoussi M. Cimetidine, metoclopramide or placebo in the treatment of symptomatic gastroesophageal reflux. *J Clin Gastroenterol* 1980; 25:750–755.

108. Muller-Lisner SA, Fraels C, Hartl A. Cisapride offsets dopamine-induced showing of fasting gastric emptying. *Dig Dis Sci* 1986; 31:807–810.

109. Bailey LD, Stewart WR, McCallum RW. New directions in the irritable bowel syndrome. *Gastroenterol Clin North Am* 1991; 20:335–349.

110. McCallum RW. Review of the current status of prokinetic agents in gastroenterology. *Am J Gastroenterol* 1985; 80:1008–1016.

111. Greiff J, Rowbotham D. Pharmacokinetic drug interactions with gastrointestinal motility modifying agents. *Clin Pharmacokinet* 1994; 27(6):447–461.

112. Burks TF. Actions of the drugs on gastrointestinal motility. In: Johnson LR, ed. *Physiology of the Gastrointestinal Tract.* Vol 1. New York: Raven Press; 1987:723–743.

113. Hammer R, Giachetti A. Muscarinic receptor subtypes: M1 and M2. Biochemical and functional characterization. *Life Sci* 1982; 31:2991–2998.

114. Cohen S, Green F. Force velocity characteristics of esophageal muscle: effect of acetylcholine and norepinephrine. *Am J Physiol* 1974; 226:1250–1255.

115. Thanik DI, Chey WY, Shah AN, et al. Reflux esophagitis: effect of oral bethanechol on symptoms and endoscopic findings. *Ann Intern Med* 1980; 93:805–808.

116. McCallum RW, Fink SM, Lerner M, et al. Effects of metoclopramide and bethanechol on delayed gastric emptying present in gastroesophageal reflux patients. *Gastroenterology* 1983; 84:1573.

117. Wiseman L, Faulds D. Cisapride: an updated review of its pharmacology and therapeutic efficacy as a prokinetic agent in gastrointestinal motility disorders. *Drugs* 1994; 47(1):116–152.

118. Koop H, Monnikes H, Koop I, et al. Effect of the prokinetic drug cisapride on gastrointestinal hormone release. *Scand J Gastroenterol* 1983; 21:907–913.

119. Corazziari E, Scopinato F, Bontempo G, et al. Effects of R–51619 on distal esophageal motor activity and gastric emptying. *Ital J Gastroenterol* 1983; 15:185–186.

120. Ceccatelli P, Janssens J, Van Trappen G, et al. Cisapride restores the decreased lower esophageal sphincter pressure in reflux patients. *Gut* 1988; 29:631–635.

121. Janssens J, Ceccatelli P, Van Trappen G. Cisapride restores the decreased lower esophageal sphincter pressure in reflux patients. *Digestion* 1984; 34:139.

122. Smout AJ, Bogaa WJ, Grade AC, Thije OJ, Akkermans LM, Wittebol P. Effects of cisapride, a new gastrointestinal prokinetic substance, on interdigestive and postprandial motor activity of the distal esophagus in man. *Gut* 1985; 26:246–251.

123. McCallum RW, Prakash C, Campoli-Richards DM, Goa K. Cisapride. A preliminary review of its pharmacodynamic and pharmacokinetic properties, and therapeutic use as a prokinetic agent in gastrointestinal motility disorders. *Drugs* 1988; 36:652–681.

124. Inauen W, Emda C, Weber B, Armstrong D, et al. Effects of ranitidine and cisapride on acid reflux and oesophageal motility in patients with reflux oesophagitis: a 24-hour ambulatory combined pH and manometry study. *Gut* 1993; 34:1025–1031.

125. Otten MH, Geldof H, Hazelhoff B, Reyntjens A. Double-blind comparison of the effect of two dosage schedules of cisapride with that of ranitidine on endoscopic healing rates in reflux oesophagitis. *Neth J Med* 1991; 39:A2. Abstract.

126. Galmiche JP, Fraitag B, Filoché B, et al. Double blind comparison of cisapride and cimetidine in treatment of reflux esophagitis. *Dig Dis Sci* 1990; 35:649–655.

127. Young GP, Miller G, Szmulder G. Gastric symptoms and gastric emptying in anorexia nervosa: effect of cisapride. *Gastroenterology* 1992; 102 (suppl 4):537.

128. Corinaldesi R, Stanghellini V, Tosetti C, Rea E, et al. The effect of different dosage schedules of cisapride on gastric emptying in idiopathic gastroparesis. *Eur J Clin Pharmacol* 1993; 44:429–432.

129. Corinaldesi R, Raiti C, Stanghellini V, et al. Comparative effects of oral cisapride and metoclopramide on gastric emptying of solids and symptoms in patients with functional dyspepsia and gastroparesis. *Curr Ther Res* 1987; 42:428–435.

130. McHugh S, Lico S, Diamant N. Cisapride vs. metoclopramide: an acute study in diabetic gastroparesis. *Dig Dis Sci* 1992; 37:997–1001.

131. De Caestecker JS, Ewing DJ, Tothill P, Clarke BF, Heading RC. Evaluation of oral cisapride and metoclopramide in diabetic autonic neuropathy: an eight-week double-blind crossover study. *Aliment Pharmacol Ther* 1989; 3:69–81.

132. Rowbotham DJ, Bamber PA, Nimmo WS. Comparison of the effect of cisapride and metoclopramide on morphine-induced delay in gastric emptying. *Br J Clin Pharmacol* 1988; 26:741–746.

133. Rowbotham DJ, Milligan K, McHugh P. Effect of cisapride on morphine absorption after oral administration of sustained-release morphine. *Br J Clin Anaesth* 1991; 67:421–425.

134. Manara AR, Shelly MP, Quin K, Park GR. The effect of metoclopramide on the absorption of oral controlled release morphine. *Br J Clin Pharmacol* 1988; 25:518–521.

135. Longo W, Vernava III A. Prokinetic agents for lower gastrointestinal motility disorders. *Dis Colon Rectum* 1993; 36:696–708.

136. Reboa G, Arnulfo G, Frascio M, et al. Colon motility and colo-anal reflexes in chronic idiopathic constipation. Effects of a novel enterokinetic agent cisapride. *Eur J Pharmacol* 1984; 26:745–748.

137. Krevsky B, Maurer AH, Malmud LS, Fisher RS. Cisapride accelerates colonic

transit in constipated patients with colonic inertia. *Am J Gastroenterol* 1989; 84:882–887.

138. Rajendran SK, Reiser JR, Bauman W, Zhang RL, Gordon SK, et al. Gastrointestinal transit after spinal cord injury: effect of cisapride. *Am J Gastroenterol* 1992; 87:1614–1617.

139. Muller-Lissner SA and The Bavarian Constipation Study Group. Treatment of chronic constipation with cisapride and placebo. *Gut* 1987; 28:1033–1038.

140. Harrington RA, Hamilton CW, Brogwden RN, Linkewich JA, Romankiewics JA, Heel RC. Metoclopramide: an updated review of its pharmacologic properties and clinical use. *Drugs* 1983; 25:451–494.

141. Wallin L, Boesby S, Madsen T. Effects of metoclopramide on oesophageal peristalsis and gastroesophageal sphincter pressure. *Scand J Gastroenterol* 1979; 14:923–927.

142. Fuch B. Prevention of meal-induced heartburn and regurgitation with metoclopramide in patients with gastroesophageal reflux. *Clin Ther* 1982; 5:179–185.

143. McCallum RW, Fink SM, Winnan GR, et al. Metoclopramide in gastroesophageal reflux disease: a double blind trial. *Am J Gastroenterol* 1984; 79:165–172.

144. Perkel MS, Moore C, Hersh T, Davidson ED. Metoclopramide therapy in patients with delayed gastric emptying: a randomized, double-blind study. *Dig Dis Sci* 1979; 24:662–666.

145. Snape WJ, Battle WM, Schwartz SS, et al. Metoclopramide to treat gastroparesis due to diabetes mellitus. *Ann Intern Med* 1982; 96:444–446.

146. McCallum RW, Ricci DA, Rakatansky H, et al. A multicentre placebo controlled clinical trial of oral metoclopramide in diabetic gastroparesis. *Diabetes Care* 1983; 6:463–467.

147. Schade RR, Dugas MC, Lhotsky DM, Gavaler JS, Aan Thiel DH. Effect of metoclopramide on gastric liquid emptying in patients with diabetic gastroparesis. *Dig Dis Sci* 1985; 30:10–15.

148. Shivshanker K, Bennett RW, Haynne TP. Tumor-associated gastroparesis: correction with metoclopramide. *Am J Surg* 1983; 145:221–225.

149. Thomas J, Shields R. Associated autonomic dysfunction and carcinoma of the pancreas. *Br Med J* 1970; 4:32.

150. Bruera E, MacEachern T, Spachynski K, et al. Comparison of the efficacy, safety and pharmacokinetics of controlled release and immediate release metoclopramide for the management of chronic nausea in patients with advanced cancer. *Cancer* 1994; 74:3204–3211.

151. Ganzini L, Casey E, Hoffman WF, McCall L. The prevalence of metoclopramide-induced tardive diskinesia and acute extrapyramidal movement disorders. *Arch Intern Med* 1993; 153:1469–1475.

152. Brogden RN, Carmine AA, Heel RC, Speight TM, Averly GS. Domperidone: a review of its pharmacological activity, pharmacokinetics and therapeutic efficacy in the symptomatic treatment of chronic dyspepsia and as an antiemetic. *Drugs* 1982; 24:360–400.

153. O'Shea M. A double-blind comparison of Domperidone and Metoclopramide in the treatment of postprandial dyspepsia. *Curr Ther Res* 1980; 26:367.

154. Agarostos I, Zissis NP, Kaprinis I, Goulis G. Double-blind evaluation of Domperidone in acute vomiting and dyspeptic disorders. *J Int Med Res* 1981; 9:143.

155. Annese V, Janssens J, Vantrappen G, et al. Erythromycin accelerates gastric emptying by inducing antral contractions and improved gastroduodenal coordination. *Gastroenterology* 1992; 102:823–828.

156. Fraser R, Shearer T, Fuller J, et al. Intravenous erythromycin overcomes small intestinal feedback on antral, pyloric and duodenal motility. *Gastroenterology* 1992; 103:114–119.

157. Peeters TL, Matthijs G, Depoortere I, et al. Erythromycin is a motilin receptor agonist. *Am J Physiol* 1989; 257:G469–474.

158. Janssens J, Peeters TL, Vantrappen G, et al. Improvement of gastric emptying in diabetic gastroparesis by erythromycin: preliminary studies. *N Engl J Med* 1990; 322:1028–1031.

159. Urbain JLC, Vantrappen G, Janssens J, et al. Intravenous erythromycin dramatically accelerates gastric emptying in gastroparesis diabeticorum and normals, and abolishes the emptying discrimination between solids and liquids. *J Nucl Med* 1990; 31:1690–1693.

160. Tack J, Janssens J, Vantrappen G, et al. Effects of the erythromycin on gastric motility in controls and in diabetic gastroparesis. *Gastroenterology* 1992; 103:72–79.

161. Armstrong DN, Ballantyne GH, Modlin IM. Erythromycin for reflux ileus in Ogilvie's syndrome. *Lancet* 1991; 337:1991.

162. Miller SM, O'Dorsio TM, Thomas FB, Mekhjian HS. Erythromycin exerts a prokinetic effect in patients with chronic idiopathic intestinal pseudoobstruction. *Gastroenterology* 1990; 98:A375.

163. Sjolund K, Ekman R, Akre F, Linden P. Motilin in chronic idiopathic constipation. *Scand J Gastroenterol* 1986; 21:914–918.

164. Catnach SM, Fairlough PD. Erythromycin and the gut. *Gut* 1992; 33:397–401.

165. Kaufman PN, Krevsky B, Malmud LS, et al. Role of opiate receptors in the regulation of colonic transit. *Gastroenterology* 1988; 94:1351–1356.

166. Konturek SJ. Opiates and the gastrointestinal tract. *Am J Gastroenterol* 1980; 74:285–291.

167. Lefebvre RA, Willems JL, Bogaert MG. Gastric relaxation and vomiting by apomorphine, morphine and fentanyl in the conscious dog. *Eur J Pharmacol* 1981; 69:139–145.

168. Sykes NP. Oral naloxone in opioid-associated constipation. *Lancet* 1991; 337:1475.

169. Basilisco G, Gamboni G, Bozzani A, Paravicini M, Bianchi PA. Oral naloxone antagonises loperamide-induced delay of orocaecal transit. *Dig Dis Sci* 1987; 32:829–832.

170. Katz MD, Erstad BL. Ocreotide, a new somatostatin analogue. *Clin Pharm* 1989; 8:255–273.

171. Peeters TL, Janssens J, Van Trappen FT. Somatostatin and the interdigestive migrating motor complex in man. *Regul Pept* 1983; 5:209–217.

172. Harstock M, Little AG. Somatostatin stimulation of the normal oesophagus. *Am J Surg* 1992; 163:159–162.

173. Soudah HC, Hasler WL, Owyang C. Somatostatin analog stimulates rectosigmoid motility and promotes colonic transit in humans via a cholinergic pathway. *Gastroenterology* 1991; 180:A497.

174. Grond S, Zech D, Diefenbach C, Bischoff A. Prevalence and pattern of symptoms

in patients with cancer pain: a prospective evaluation of 1635 patients referred to a pain clinic. *J Pain Symptom Manage* 1994; 9:372–382.

175. Twycross RG, Lack SA. Control of alimentary symptoms in far advanced cancer. Edinburgh: Churchill Livingstone: 1986.

176. Reuben DB, Mor V, Hiris J. Clinical symptoms and length of survival in patients with terminal cancer. *Arch Intern Med* 1988; 148:1586–1591.

177. Brescia FJ, Adler D, Gray G, Ryan MA, Cimino J, Mamtani R. Hospitalized advanced cancer patients: a profile. *J Pain Symptom Manage* 1990; 5:221–227.

178. Seale C. Death from cancer and death from other causes: the relevance of the hospice approach. *Palliat Med* 1991; 5:12–19.

179. Ventafridda V, De Conno F, Ripamonti C, Gamba A, Tamburini M. Quality-of-life assessment during palliative care programme. *Ann Oncol* 1990; 1:415–420.

180. Curtis EB, Krech R, Walsh TD. Common symptoms in patients with advanced cancer. *J Palliat Care* 1991; 7:25–29.

181. Coyle N, Adelhardt J, Portenoy RK, Foley KM. Character of terminal illness in the advanced cancer patient: pain and other symptoms during the last four weeks of life. *J Pain Symptom Manage* 1990; 5:83–93.

182. Addison NV. Pseudo-obstruction of the large bowel. *J R Soc Med* 1983; 76:252–255.

5

Assessment and Management of Opioid-Induced Constipation

SUSAN DERBY AND RUSSELL K. PORTENOY

In 1995, approximately 547,000 people in the U.S. died of cancer and several million lived with their disease.[1] Of those with metastatic solid tumors, more than two thirds had pain severe enough to necessitate opioid therapy. Opioid analgesics are highly effective, but produce side effects that may limit therapy or contribute to impaired quality of life. Constipation, a particularly common side effect with multiple contributing etiologies, may be difficult to treat.

Constipation should be defined as a symptom (that is, a subjective phenomenon) characterized by diminished frequency of defecation associated with difficulty or discomfort.[2-4] It is usually distressing when present, and occasionally poses serious risks.[5] Associated symptoms include abdominal pain, bloating and distention, and sometimes anorexia and nausea. Untreated constipation may progress to obstipation, which may potentially lead to life-threatening complications associated with bowel obstruction. Constipation is also a risk factor for intestinal perforation in patients receiving corticosteroids for the management of intracranial lesions.[6]

In recent years, cancer therapy has shifted to the ambulatory setting. As a result, more responsibility for symptom management has devolved from the healthcare professional to patients and their families. Families have varying resources and abilities. Many patients are older than age 65, and the responsibility for symptom assessment, intervention, and monitoring must be assumed by elderly spouses. As part of the assessment of patients and their families, healthcare professionals must clarify reasonable expectations for care, determine supportive services that may be needed, and ascertain the extent of caregiver burden that may result. The potential for serious comorbidity in the family must be recognized. For example, studies that compare the psychological responses of cancer patients and their families indicate that families experience similar, if not greater, negative emotional responses than the patient with chronic illness.[7] The burden of caregiving frequently leads to conflict and guilt.

Although home-based symptom management is preferable to hospitalization, necessary resources to assess and aid caregivers are scarce. Various models of continuing care that could potentially provide expert symptom control have been described, but these services are not available to the majority of cancer patients. In one study, two thirds of patients with advanced cancer who were receiving chemotherapy had never used a community service, and nearly one half were unaware that such services existed.[8] These observations raise some troubling questions about the quality of assessment and treatment, and the adequacy of education for these patients and families.

The need for palliative care, with competent symptom management in the ambulatory setting, highlights several unresolved issues. Who should provide ongoing assessment and intervention for symptoms such as constipation? What role should nursing play? Advanced Practice Nurses (Nurse Practitioners, Clinical Nurse Specialists) trained in symptom management could provide this care, but in many ambulatory settings, there are few, if any, nurses. Who will bear the financial burden associated with symptomatic therapies? Research is needed to clarify the implications of these issues for the treatment of constipation and other symptoms.

Pathophysiology and Etiology of Constipation

Normal bowel function requires the coordination of motility, mucosal transport, and defecation reflexes.[9] Motility, in turn, depends on central nervous system mechanisms, activity in the peripheral autonomic nervous system (both parasympathetic and sympathetic), and the function of a variety of gastrointestinal hormones.[9-12] Three types of motility have been distinguished: segmental, nonpropulsive; short-segment propulsive; and long-segment propulsive (mass movements). Segmental movements of the colon churn and mix the contents, and propulsive movements, or peristalsis, drive the contents forward. Increases in segmental, nonpropulsive motility of the bowel are associated with the development of constipation.[13]

Mucosal transport of electrolytes and fluids is complex and poorly understood. Increased absorption could potentially cause constipation, although it is more likely that desiccation of bowel contents is due to prolonged transit time, rather than mucosal processes. Interference in defecation reflexes can also cause constipation and may have particular impact in patients with structural lesions of the pelvis.

Opioids augment the tone and nonpropulsive motility of both the ileum and colon,[14,15] thereby increasing transit time. Specific opioid receptors in the central nervous system and gastrointestinal tract presumably mediate these actions. Changes in gut motility observed during experimental administration of opioid drugs into the cerebral ventricles indicate the importance of central opioid effects.[16] A local effect is clear in the response of the bowel to oral administration of nonabsorbable opioids,[17] the efficacy of poorly absorbed oral opioid antagonists in the treatment of opioid-related constipation,[18] and in the persistence of the gastrointestinal effects of systemic opioids even after extirpation of the neural supply to the bowel.[15] Several classes of endogenous opioids and their receptors have been identified in the intestine and also suggest a local effect of opioid drugs.[19,20] The existence of these receptors supports a role for the endorphins in normal gut physiology.

Exogenous opioid administration slows transit time and desiccates intraluminal contents. Desiccation occurs either by increased absorption of fluid and electrolytes or by increased absorption time due to slowing of bowel transit.

Constipation caused by opioids is dose-related and characterized by large interindividual variablity. Tolerance appears to develop slowly and most patients require laxative therapy for as long as they take opioids. This opioid effect adds to other factors that may be contributory. In the cancer population, constipation may develop from physiological disturbances that may or may not be disease-related, the use of constipating drugs other than the opioid, structural pathology that is either intraluminal or extraluminal, and neurological disorders (Table 5.1). A recent survey suggests the importance of these factors. In a hospice population, 50% of patients receiving no opioids required regular doses of laxatives.[21]

Table 5.1. Common causes of constipation in cancer patients

Physiologic abnormalities				
Nonspecific	*Metabolic disturbances*	*Structural deformities*	*Drugs*	*Neurologic disorders*
Advanced age	Hypercalcemia	Intraluminal or	Opioids	Damage from any
Inactivity	Hypokalemia	extraluminal	Drugs with anti-	cause to sacral
Dehydration	Hypothyroidism	masses	cholinergic	plexus, cauda
Depression		Adhesions	actions	equina, or spi-
Change in diet		Fibrosis	Antacids	nal cord
Physical or social			Diuretics	Autonomic neu-
impediments to			Anticonvulsants	ropathy caused
defecation			Iron	by cancer or
Rectal or abdomi-			Antihypertensives	concurrent dis-
nal pain				ease (e.g., dia-
				betes) or drug
				(e.g., vin-
				cristine)

Assessment of Constipation

The need to pursue a clinical evaluation of the constipated cancer patient depends on the course and medical setting. Many patients develop this symptom in close relation to a discrete event, such as the initiation of opioid therapy. In such cases, further evaluation is needed only if there is reason to suspect a previously unidentified contributing cause that may be amenable to treatment. In contrast, the patient who develops progressive constipation in the absence of a clear precipitating cause should be considered for an evaluation that may extend to sophisticated imaging procedures. Clinical judgments about the extent of evaluation must always consider the overall goals of care and desires of the patient.

Patients who become constipated immediately after receiving an opioid usually require no assessment other than a careful history. The relevant information includes the date of the last bowel movement, usual frequency of bowel movements, usual time of day for bowel movement, the difficulty of defecation, and associated symptoms, including presence of fullness, distention, pain in abdomen or rectum, or sensation of incomplete evacuation. Other queries may assess diet, including the amount of fiber and fluid intake, mobility, and activity level. In the inpatient setting, the assessment should be documented in the progress notes. In the ambulatory setting, patients receiving chronic opioid therapy who develop problems with constipation should be encouraged to keep a log documenting their bowel function.

A thorough physical examination of the abdomen should be performed on all patients who develop progressive or severe constipation, complain of unrelieved constipation despite therapy, or experience constipation associated with rectal pain, liquid diarrhea, or seepage of stool. In most cases, this examination should include a careful evaluation of the perianal region and a digital rectal examination.

Routine assessment of constipation is unusual, and clinicians must be encouraged to maintain a high level of vigilance. In one retrospective review of 122 patients admitted to a palliative care unit, 59% of patients did not undergo a rectal examination at admission and there was minimal documentation in the chart by either physician or nurse related to symptoms of constipation even in patients who were symptomatic.[22] In another study of 74 patients admitted to an oncology unit, discharge orders for laxatives were not written routinely for patients receiving opioids; rather, the laxative order was triggered by a history of constipation.[23]

Prevention of Opioid-Induced Constipation

Many specialists in palliative medicine believe that the prevalence of opioid-induced constipation warrants prophylaxis with a laxative when initiating opioid therapy.[24] Clinical observation in ambulatory cancer populations suggests, however, that some patients can manage a change in bowel function by simple dietary approaches and that some seemingly develop tolerance to the constipating effects of these drugs. The use of laxatives can be burdensome, and the need for prophylactic therapy must be carefully considered in every case. A reasonable approach limits prophylactic therapy to those patients with other predisposing factors. In patients at low risk, including younger ambulatory patients with relatively early disease, constipation can be managed expectantly.

Some nonpharmacologic interventions are appropriate in most cases. An increase in dietary fiber should be encouraged in ambulatory patients. Fiber may improve gut motility by increasing intraluminal volume. In the cancer patient, empiric therapy involves an increase in fiber intake to at least 10 g per day. Table 5.2 lists selected food with fiber contents.

In some patients, fiber is problematic. Patients who increase fiber consumption must also increase fluid intake, and those who are unable to increase fluids may experience a paradoxical worsening of constipation from high fiber intake. Patients with partial obstruction should not be given fiber because of the risk of increased obstructive symptoms, and those who are anorectic

Table 5.2. Fiber content of selected foods

Food	Amount	Fiber (grams)
Avocado	1/2 cup	3.0
Beans, kidney	1/2 cup	4.0
Beans, lima	1/2 cup	5.0
Broccoli, cooked	1/2 cup	2.0
Brussels sprouts, cooked	1/2 cup	3.0
Spinach	1/2 cup	2.0
Flour, whole wheat	3 tbsp	3.0
Flour, white	3 tbsp	1.0
Barley, cooked	1/2 cup	4.0
Bran, all varieties, uncooked	3/4 oz	11.0
Bread, whole wheat	1 slice	3.0
Carrots, cooked	1/2 cup	3.0
Guava	one medium	7.0
Blackberries	3/4 cup	7.0
Figs, fresh	one large	4.0
Peas, green, cooked	1/2 cup	4.0
Pistachio nuts	40 nuts (1 oz)	3.0
Potato	8 oz	6.0
Raspberries	3/4 cup	4.0
Squash	1 cup	6.0
Strawberries	1 cup	3.0
Tabouli	1/2 cup	8.0

Source: Adapted from Weight Watchers, 1994.

should be given fiber cautiously lest the satiety produced by a high-fiber diet worsen malnutrition.

Patients with opioid-induced constipation should also be encouraged to increase fluid intake irrespective of fiber consumption. Anecdotally, an intake of 2 to 3 liters per day is recommended. Water is preferred over coffee or tea because the latter beverages may act as diuretics.

Compliance with fiber intake or oral hydration can be very difficult, if not impossible, for many patients who are multisymptomatic and experience abdominal fullness or anorexia. Fluid intake may also be problematic for patients with peripheral edema.

Inactivity can be associated with decreasing colonic motility,[25] and regular exercise may also play an important role in prevention of constipation. If possible, patients who receive opioids should be encouraged to become active. An ongoing program of turning, positioning, sitting, standing, balancing, and walking short distances can be used for those with limited performance status.

Treatment of Opioid-Induced Constipation

The nonpharmacologic interventions used for prevention should also be encouraged as part of a treatment strategy for the patient with constipation. A second component of this strategy includes treatment of other contributing causes. This may involve the elimination of nonessential constipating drugs (e.g., antacids), treatment of metabolic disturbances (e.g., hypercalcemia), or other interventions.

Pharmacologic management of constipation varies with the medical status, expectations, and responses of the patient. In routine cases, clinicians should discuss the various options with the patient, initiate treatments that are consistent with patient preference, and provide an opportunity to change from one approach to another if the overall response is not favorable.

Most patients with opioid-induced constipation respond to current therapies. For the rare refractory patient, a trial of a nonoral route of opioid administration should be considered. In these cases, severe constipation could alter gastrointestinal absorption of the opioid and, theoretically, the nonoral administration could produce less constipation than the oral route. Very rarely, constipation necessitates the use of an invasive means of pain control, such as nerve block, in an effort to eliminate the need for opioids. In these cases, it is important to determine the impact of severe constipation on the patient's quality of life, identify the goals of care, and ascertain the cost of ineffective pharmacological management.

Routine laxative therapy should not be initiated in patients with severe constipation until fecal impaction has been excluded. Low impaction can be assessed by examination of the rectum; suspicion of a high impaction or another cause of bowel obstruction requires abdominal imaging for evaluation.

The urgent management of impaction may require physical disimpaction, repeated enemas, and a combination of rectal and oral laxatives, including a lubricant, softening agent, osmotic laxative, or a contact laxative. Routine laxative therapy can begin after impaction is cleared.

Therapeutic interventions for the routine management of constipation may be administered rectally or orally.[2–4] For most cancer patients, the use of enemas and rectal suppositories is limited to the acute short-term management of more severe episodes. Occasional patients who cannot tolerate oral laxatives may be able to use long-term rectal laxatives or enemas effectively; these are usually administered two to three times per week. Surveys of hospice populations suggest that more than 40% of this population use rectally administered laxative therapy on a regular basis.[26] Thus, access to rectally administered treatments for constipation should be retained for all who do not otherwise have contraindications to their use (e.g., thrombocytopenia). Rectal suppositories may be inert or active. Inert suppositories are usually fashioned from glycerin alone. They draw fluid into the rectum and act as a stimulus to defecation. Active suppositories contain a contact cathartic (e.g., bisacodyl). Enemas may consist of small volume or large volume. Small-volume enemas may contain sodium phosphate or oil. Larger-volume enemas can use tap water, soap suds, or saline (Table 5.3).

Table 5.3. Types of enemas

Enema	Mechanism	Indications/Comments
Small Volume		
Phospha Soda® (Fleets)	Stimulates lower bowel	May be used 1–3 times per week
Oil retention (Fleets)	Softens hard, impacted stool	Best, if can be retained; administer before large-volume enema
Milk and molasses	Stimulates lower bowel; sugar in the molasses is an irritant to the bowel lining; sugar and milk produce gas that distends bowel, causes pressure, peristalsis, and evacuation	Softens hard, impacted stool
Large Volume		Warming solution is helpful; mineral oil may be added to any large-volume enema to soften stool; difficult to self-administer
Tap water	Induces peristalsis	
Soap suds	Stimulates lower bowel; promotes evacuation	Can be irritating
Saline	Stimulates lower bowel; promotes evacuation	
Harris flush (up and down flush)	Lower bowel irrigation, promotes expulsion of flatus	Useful postoperatively

Oral laxatives comprise (1) bulk agents, (2) lubricants, (3) osmotic (saline) agents, (4) agents for colonic lavage, (5) contact cathartics, (6) prokinetic drugs, and (7) oral naloxone (Table 5.4). There have been no adequate comparative studies of long-term management of opioid-induced constipation, and, as noted previously, empirical therapy must be based on a comprehensive assessment of the patient's medical needs, capabilities, and expectations. Combination therapy is often used.

Bulk-forming laxatives

Preparations: The most commonly used preparations incorporate cellulose or psyllium seeds or bran.

Mechanism: Like dietary fiber, these agents increase stool bulk and soften its consistency by increasing the mass and water content of the stool. Transit time through the colon is decreased. Intraluminal fluid may be increased by an accumulation of osmotically active particles after catabolism by gut microflora.

Problems: These agents are generally safe, but anecdotal experience suggests that they may worsen symptoms, such as flatulence, distention, bloating, or abdominal pain, in some patients with intra-abdominal disease. They are best avoided in patients who are severely debilitated and those with partial bowel obstruction from any cause. Significant allergy to these substances has been reported.

Use: Bulk-forming laxatives should probably be added to most laxative regimens, except in the setting of suspected obstruction or extreme debilitation of the patient. They may also be useful in changing the character of the effluent from a functioning stoma.

Lubricants

Preparations: Mineral oil is the preferred preparation.

Mechanism: This agent lubricates the stool, allowing easier elimination.

Problems: Chronic use impairs the absorption of fat-soluble vitamins. Irritation of the perianal area may occur, and there is the serious potential for lipoid pneumonia should aspiration occur. Mineral oil should not be used in demented or obtunded patients.

Use: This substance has little role in the management of chronic constipation. It may be useful in management of transient acute constipation or fecal impaction.

Osmotic (saline) cathartics

Preparations: Magnesium salts (e.g., magnesium hydroxide, magnesium citrate), sodium salts (e.g., sodium phosphate), lactulose, and sorbitol.

Mechanism: Osmotically active particles draw fluid into the bowel lumen. The transit time of the resultant semiliquid stool is decreased.

Problems: Magnesium and phosphate salts are contraindicated in patients with renal insufficiency, because systemic electrolyte accumulation can occur. Similarly, the use of sodium salts, which may result in some salt and water retention, must be used cautiously in patients at risk from volume overload, such as those with congestive heart failure. Phosphate-containing salts have also been reported to cause a symptomatic increase in serum phosphate and a decrease in serum calcium caused by phosphate absorption. All of these agents can cause cramping and bloating, and dehydration can occur as a result of severe diarrhea.

Use: These agents are often used for bowel cleansing before or after radiological procedures, sigmoidoscopy, or colonoscopy. Some patients find these agents useful chronically (a dose every 1–3 days), but others find their rapid onset (3–6 hours) inconvenient or cannot tolerate their side effects. Lactulose and sorbitol, poorly absorbed sugars that also act as osmotic laxatives, have a slower onset and usually greater flexibility. A randomized comparison of lactulose 15 mL twice daily and a magnesium salt at the same dose in the postoperative management of hemorrhoidectomy patients demonstrated significantly better results in the former group.[27] Lactulose is used most often, but a recent controlled trial demonstrated that the less expensive alternative, sorbitol, was equally effective.[28] Most patients consume a dose once or twice daily (occasionally more often), following a period of dose adjustment. Patients who find the approach disagreeable usually complain of the taste or report an increase in flatulence. At a dose of 30 mL every hour, lactulose can also be useful for the urgent management of severely constipated patients.

Agents for colonic lavage

Consumption of small quantities of polyethylene glycol (Go Lytely®) (25–500 mL) can be used to reverse chronic constipation in patients who are refractory to other laxatives.[29] Some patients find the use of 8 oz to 1 quart every few days to be tolerable and effective.

Contact Cathartics

Contact cathartics include four drug classes that share, at least in part, a common mechanism of action. These drugs are probably the most commonly administered laxatives for opioid-induced constipation. They include the docusates, anthraquinone and diphenylmethane derivatives, and castor oil. All these compounds cause an increase in mucosal secretion and an increase in

Table 5.4. Classification of laxatives

Class of agent	Mechanism of action	Site of action*	Starting Dose	Effects/Comments
Saline (Osmotic) Cathartics	Increases water in the bowel, transit time decreased	SLI		
Magnesium citrate		SLI	1/2–1 bottle	3–6 hours
Magnesium sulfate (Epsom salts)		SLI	5–15 g	
Magnesium hydroxide (Milk of Magnesia®)		SLI	30–60 mL	30 minutes–6 hours
Sodium phosphate (Fleets Phospha Soda®)		SLI	45 mL	30 minutes–6 hours Useful as a prep for colonoscopy
Lactulose/Sorbitol	Attracts water into colon, acidifies contents	Colon	30 mL	24–48 hours
Polyethylene glycol (Go Lytely®)		SLI	240–1000 mL	1–4 hours
Bulk-Forming	Increases mass and water content of stool, transit time decreased	Colon		
Psyllium (Metamucil®)		Colon	1 tbsp. tid	2–4 days Must be taken with at least 8 oz of water
Methyl cellulose (Citrucel®)		Colon		Must be taken with fluids
Contact Cathartics	Increases propulsive activity through stimulation of myenteric plexus and reduction of net water absorption and electrolytes from intraluminal contents	Colon		
Diphenylmethane (phenolphthalein—[Ex-Lax®])	Increases secretions	Colon	1–2 tabs	6–12 hours

Drug	Mechanism	Site	Dose	Onset	Comments
Bisacodyl (Dulcolax®)	Affect mucosal electrolyte transport and motility	Colon	1–2 tabs	6–12 hours	
Anthraquinones		Colon		6–12 hours	
Cascara, senna (Senokot®, Danthron®)		Colon	2 tabs	6–12 hours	
Castor oil	Increases secretions	Small intestine	1–2 tbsp.	3–6 hours	May cause cramping; not recommended for chronic constipation
Docusates (Colace®)	Anionic surfactant with emulsifying properties; facilitate mixture of fat and lubricants	Colon	300 mg	1–3 days	
Emollients					
Mineral oil	Softens stool	Colon	1–2 tbsp.	1–3 days	
Prokinetic Agents	Improves colonic transit	SLI			
Metoclopramide (Reglan®)	Dopamine antagonist/cholinergic agonist, decreases transit time	Colon	10 mg qid		
Cisapride (Propulsid®)	Cholinergic agonist/dopamine antagonist increases bowel activity, stimulates colonic contractions and accelerates transit of stool from ileum to anus	SLI	10 mg qid		
Domperidone	Dopamine antagonist	SLI			
Oral Naloxone	Opioid antagonist	SLI	0.8 mg bid		Titrate dose; monitor for withdrawal symptoms

Abbreviations: SLI = small and large intestine; bid = twice daily; tid = thrice daily; qid = four times daily.

peristalsis.[30,31] There have been no comparative studies and data are largely limited to patients with advanced cancer treated in a hospice setting.[21]

Although there are survey data to the contrary,[21] clinical experience and observations in a small survey[32] suggest a relationship between the opioid and contact cathartic doses necessary to reverse constipation. However, this relationship, if it exists, is certain to be complex. Large interindividual variability exists in response to laxatives at baseline. The effects of a given dose may change over time because of the development of tolerance or changes in any of the numerous factors that can contribute to constipation. The most reasonable clinical approach begins with a relatively low dose, which can be increased every 2 to 3 days until constipation is relieved, the patient reports side effects, or the therapy becomes too burdensome or costly to continue. Once the correct dose is found, most patients continue with daily therapy. Some patients prefer to use a contact cathartic on an intermittent basis, such as every 3 to 4 days if needed. There are no established benefits or disadvantages to this approach.

The risks associated with short-term use of the contact cathartics are minimal. Long-term ingestion, however, may result in so-called "laxative bowel," a condition characterized by dependence on laxatives for bowel function. This syndrome, putatively the result of drug-induced damage to the myenteric plexus, should be considered in patients with long life expectancies, but is not a contraindication to therapy in the setting of advanced cancer.

Docusates (dioctyl sodium)

Preparations: Dioctyl sodium succinate is available in a wide variety of over-the-counter products.

Mechanism: Although docusate may be categorized as a contact cathartic based on mechanisms observed in vitro,[33] the relatively low doses used clinically only produce a surfactant effect that allows water and fats to mix with feces. As typically used, therefore, the docusates are detergents or surfactant laxatives. These agents are often combined with other contact cathartics as a first-line therapy for opioid-induced constipation. The potential advantage of this approach relates to the possibility that a combination of laxatives that act differently may increase efficacy.

Problems: The risks appear to be minimal, although there has been a case report that demonstrated liver toxicity from an interaction between docusate and danthron, a contact cathartic not currently available in the United States.[34]

Use: This drug is often added to other contact cathartics as a stool softener.

Castor oil

Mechanism: Castor oil is the only contact cathartic with a mechanism of action mediated in the small bowel. Castor oil is hydrolyzed by gut microflora to ricinoleic acid. This compound, in turn, acts on the small intestine, producing abundant mucosal secretions.

Problems: Cramping and diarrhea are common with this agent and it is not generally used in the cancer population. With chronic use, malabsorption of nutrients may occur.

Anthraquinone derivatives

Preparations: Cascara, senna, and danthron. The latter drug is not available in the United States.

Mechanisms: These drugs affect mucosal electrolyte transport and motility. They act primarily on the colon.

Problems: In addition to laxative bowel, overuse can produce melanosis coli, a benign and usually reversible dark pigmentation of the colonic mucosa. Dehydration can result from diarrhea.

Use: Chronic therapy is a common approach for opioid-induced constipation. Anecdotal reports specifically cite the utility of senna.[32,35] Intermittent use is preferred by some patients.

Diphenylmethane derivatives

Preparations: Phenolphthalein, bisacodyl, and oxyphenisatin. The latter drug is no longer available in the United States.

Mechanism: These drugs act primarily on the colon and produce effects similar to the anthraquinone derivatives.

Problems: Allergies to these substances have been reported and overuse may produce dehydration.

Use: Without controlled studies demonstrating differences, these drugs can be grouped with the anthraquinone derivatives as useful, generally safe, and well-tolerated medications for the management of chronic constipation. They are usually effective within 12 to 24 hours.

Prokinetic Drugs

Prokinetic agents promote transit through the gastrointestinal tract. The mechanism of action is incompletely understood, but it is speculated that these agents enhance intestinal function by either promoting the effect of a local transmitter that mediates motility or antagonizing the effect of an inhibitory transmitter.[36,37] Cisapride,[38] metoclopramide, or domperidone can be considered for trials in patients with opioid-induced constipation that has not responded to conventional measures.

Oral Naloxone

There is now evidence that oral administration of naloxone can ameliorate opioid-induced constipation without causing systemic opioid withdrawal in most patients.[39,40] The approach is not without risk, however, because some patients will absorb sufficient naloxone to develop uncomfortable signs of abstinence.[39] This potential adverse effect, presumably more likely to occur in patients who are receiving high systemic doses of an opioid, strongly suggests that oral naloxone should not be used until conventional therapies have failed. Treatment should always incorporate dose escalation that identifies a dose that can produce "bowel withdrawal" without concurrent systemic withdrawal. A reasonable approach begins with a dose of 0.8 mg twice daily and doubles the dose every 2 to 3 days until favorable effects occur or side effects are experienced.

Special Issues in the Management of Opioid-Induced Constipation

Constipation in the pediatric patient

Bowel continence is a complex process dependent on maturation of the external and internal anal sphincter, development of conscious awareness of rectal distention, rectal compliance, gastrointestinal transit time, and rectal expulsion.[41] By $2^{1}/_{2}$ years of age, maturation occurs and the child can be taught to consciously control defecation.[41]

There are no studies that focus on the management of opioid-induced constipation in the continent pediatric oncology patient. Anecdotally, practice has mirrored the adult models of assessment and intervention. A baseline elimination history should be obtained from the parents of young children and directly from older children and adolescents. Laxative approaches used in pediatric patients have included increasing fluids and fiber in the diet and promoting mobility if possible. In the inpatient setting, privacy is an essential part of any therapeutic effort to manage constipation.

Many children cannot swallow pills and creative interventions may be needed. These may include high-fiber cookies or snacks, and stool softeners or cathartics in liquid preparations that are chilled, frozen, or flavored. Rectal interventions, including suppositories or enemas, should not be used unless the need is overwhelming. Oral naloxone can be used in children, with guidelines identical to those for the adult population.

Constipation in the debilitated elderly patient

Elderly patients are prone to constipation, which can be life-threatening if unrecognized and untreated. The initial presentation of opioid-induced constipation may be confusing. Abdominal pain, distention, and nausea may be less notable than reduced appetite, depressed mood, or diminished activity. In addition, it may be difficult to obtain an elimination history from an elderly, debilitated patient.

Assessment of the elderly patient should include a careful evaluation of over-the-counter medication use, including iron preparations, antacids, laxatives, and drugs with anticholinergic properties. Management should include measures to ensure compliance and follow-up.

Cost

It is difficult to determine the cost of treatment for opioid-induced constipation. The relative efficacy of these agents has not been clearly documented. An economic analysis should include the cost per treatment or episode, cost of emergency room visits or hospitalization related to opioid-induced constipation, and indirect cost to patients and families (e.g., cost of medications or loss of income related to hospitalization).[42] Without this information, the cost-benefit ratio cannot be evaluated.

Prices for oral and rectal medications per unit dose vary among pharmacies and institutions. Third-party insurers reimburse at varying rates. In addition, many patients are prescribed sequential or combination therapies for opioid-induced constipation. These factors must also be considered in future economic analyses.

Compliance issues

Inherent in any opioid regimen is the provision for patient and family education about potential side effects, including constipation. Compliance with opioid regimens may be a significant problem if constipation has been poorly assessed and managed in the past and the patient finds the constipation intolerable. Patient and family education should be initiated at the start of opioid therapy with a careful history of elimination, diet, and activity.

Compliance with therapy for opioid-induced constipation depends on several factors, including complexity of the regimen, cost of medications, cognitive function of the patient, and level of support in the home. There has been no systematic evaluation of these factors, and this remains a goal of future research.

Table 5.5. Approaches in the management of opioid-induced constipation

Encourage:

Increased fluid intake as tolerated
Increased fiber in diet as tolerated
Mobility and ambulation
Comfort and privacy
Attempts at bowel movement at same time daily
Rule out or treat impaction if present

Consider various interventions:

1. Docusate sodium 300 mg PO daily with or without senna 2 tabs PO at bedtime or magnesium sulfate 30 mL PO at bedtime. If ineffective, increase the dose of senna (doses as high as 12 tabs per day have been used anecdotally).
2. Add lactulose 30 mL PO once or twice daily. If ineffective, gradually increase the dose until effects or side effects are noted.
3. For refractory cases, consider prokinetic drug, oral naloxone, or colonic lavage.
4. For severe constipation, first assess and treat impaction if present. Consider mineral oil and lactulose 30 mL PO every hour until bowel movement. If stool is soft, consider sodium phosphate enema. If stool is hard, consider glycerine and/or bisacodyl suppositories, or administer oil-retention or large-volume enema.

Conclusion

Constipation is extremely common in the palliative care setting. Opioid use is a prominent contributing factor in a majority of patients. The management of opioid-induced constipation begins with a careful assessment that may identify other, potentially treatable contributing factors. Preventive measures are indicated in most patients, and these are usually combined with ongoing therapy. Routine management is effective in most patients. For those with refractory constipation, new approaches, such as oral naloxone or intermittent lavage, may be useful (Table 5.5).

References

1. American Cancer Society. *Cancer Statistics 1995.*
2. Levy MH. Constipation and diarrhea in cancer patients. *Cancer Bull* 1991; 43:412–422.
3. Sykes NP. Constipation and diarrhoea. In: Doyle D, Hanks GW, MacDonald N, eds. *Oxford Textbook of Palliative Medicine.* Oxford: Oxford University Press; 1993:299–310.
4. Portenoy RK. Constipation in the cancer patient: causes and management. *Med Clin North Am* 1987; 71:303–311.

5. Rogers M, Cerda JJ. The narcotic bowel syndrome. *J Clin Gastroenterol* 1989; 11:132–135.

6. Fadul CE, Lemann W, Thaler HJ, Posner JB. Perforation of the gastrointestinal tract in patients receiving steroids for neurologic disease. *Neurology* 1988; 38:348–352.

7. Cassileth BR, Lusk EJ, Strouse TB, Miller DS, Brown LL, Cross PA. A psychological analysis of cancer patients and their next of kin. *Cancer* 1985; 55:72–76.

8. Guadagnoli E, Rice C, Mor V. Cancer patients' knowledge of and willingness to use agency based services: toward application of a model of behavior change. *J Psychosoc Oncol* 1991; 9(3):1–21.

9. Cohen S, Long WB, Snape WJ. Gastrointestinal motility. In: Crane RK, ed. *International Review of Physiology.* Vol 19. Baltimore: University Park Press; 1979:128–149.

10. Rostad H. Colonic motility in the cat: II, Extrinsic nervous control. *Acta Physiol Scand* 1973; 89:91–103.

11. Rostad H. Colonic motility in the cat III. Influence of hypothalamic and mesencephalic stimulation. *Acta Physiol Scand* 1973; 89:104–115.

12. Snape WJ, Matarazzo SA, Cohen S. The effect of eating and gastrointestinal hormones on human colonic myoelectrical and motor activity. *Gastroenterology* 1978: 75:373–378.

13. Connell AM. The motility of the pelvic colon. *Gut* 1962; 3:342–348.

14. Adler HF, Atkinson Aj, Ivy AC, et al. Effect of morphine and Dilaudid on the ileum, and of morphine, Dilaudid and atropine on the colon of man. *Arch Intern Med* 1942; 69:974–985.

15. Daniel EE, Sutherland WH, Gogoch A. Effects of morphine and other drugs on motility of the terminal ileum. *Gastroenterology* 1959; 36:510–523.

16. Parolaro D, Sala M, Gori E. Effects of intracerebroventricular administration of morphine upon intestinal motility in the rat and its antagonism with naloxone. *Eur J Pharmacol* 1977; 49:329–338.

17. Russel J, Bass P, Goldberg LI, et al. Antagonism of gut, but not central effects of morphine with quaternary narcotic antagonists. *Eur J Pharmacol* 1982; 78:255–261.

18. Kreek MJ, Schaeter RA, Hahn EF, et al. Naloxone, a specific opioid antagonist, reverses chronic idiopathic constipation. *Lancet* 1983; 1:261–262.

19. Kosterlitz HW, Lord JAH, Paterson SJ, et al. Effects of changes in the structure of enkephalins and of narcotic analgesic drugs on their interaction with mu and delta receptors. *Br J Pharmacol* 1980; 68:333–342.

20. Polak JM, Bloom SR, Sullivan SN, et al. Enkephalin-like immunoreactivity in the human gastrointestinal tract. *Lancet* 1977; 1:972–974.

21. Twycross RG, Harcourt JMV. The use of laxative at a palliative care centre. *Palliat Med* 1991; 5:27–33.

22. Bruera E, Suarez-Almazor M, Velasco A, Bertolino M, MacDonald SM, Hanson J. The assessment of constipation in terminal cancer patients admitted to a palliative care unit: a retrospective review. *J Pain Symptom Manage* 1994; 9(8):515–519.

23. Held JL, Anderson AV, Cohen MH. Constipation management on a medical oncology ward. (meeting abstract) *Proc Annu Meet Am Soc Clin Oncol* 1992; 11:1367.

24. Walsh TD. Prevention of opioid side effects. *J Pain Symptom Manage* 1990; 5:363–367.

25. Rader MC, Vaughen MD. Management of the frail deconditioned patient. *South Med J* 1994; 87:S61–S65.

26. Twycross RG, Lack SA. *Control of Alimentary Symptoms in Far Advanced Cancer.* London: Churchill Livingstone; 1986:166–207.

27. Porter N. The use of lactulose in post-hemorrhoidectomy patients. *Br J Clin Pract* 1975; 29:235–236.

28. Lederle FA, Busch DL, Mattox KM, West MJ, Aske DM. Cost-effective treatment of constipation in the elderly: a randomized double-blind comparison of sorbitol and lactulose. *Am J Med* 1990; 89:597–601.

29. Androsky RI, Goldner F. Colonic lavage solution (polyethylene glycol electrolyte lavage solution) as a treatment for chronic constipation: a double-blind, placebo-controlled study. *Am J Gastroenterol* 1990; 85:261–265.

30. Gaginella TS, Bass P. Laxatives: an update on mechanism of action. *Life Sci* 1978; 23:1001–1010.

31. Hardcastle JD, Wilkins JL. The action of sennosides and related compounds on human colon and rectum. *Gut* 1970; 11:1038–1042.

32. Maguire LC, Yon JL, Miller E. Prevention of narcotic-induced constipation. *N Engl J Med* 1981; 305:1651.

33. Binder HJ. Pharmacology of laxatives. *Annu Rev Pharmacol Toxicol* 1977; 17:355–367.

34. Tolman KG, Hammar S, Sannilla JJ. Possible hepatotoxicity of doxidan. *Ann Intern Med* 1976; 84:290–292.

35. Izard MW, Ellison FS. Treatment of drug induced constipation with a purified senna derivative. *Conn Med* 1962; 26:589.

36. Reynolds JC. Prokinetic agents: a key in the future of gastroenterology. *Gastroenterol Clin North Am* 1989; 18:437–457.

37. Reynolds JC, Putnam PE. Prokinetic agents. *Gastroenterol Clin North Am* 1992; 21:567–596.

38. Krevsky B, Maurer AH, Malmud LS, Fisher RS. Cisapride accelerates colonic transit in constipated patients with colonic inertia. *Am J Gastroenterol* 1989; 84:882–887.

39. Culpepper-Morgan JA, Inturrisi CE, Portenoy RK, Foley KM, Houde RW, Marsh F, et al. Treatment of opioid-induced constipation with oral naloxone: a pilot study. *Clin Pharmacol Ther* 1992; 52:90–95.

40. Sykes NP. Oral naloxone in opioid associated constipation. *Lancet* 1991; 337:1475.

41. Hatch T. Encopresis and constipation in children. *Pediatr Clin North Am* 1988; 35:257–280.

42. Portenoy RK: Issues in the economic analysis of therapies for cancer pain. *Oncology* 1995; 11 (suppl):71–78.

6

Assessment and Management of Mechanical Bowel Obstruction

SEBASTIANO MERCADANTE

Mechanical bowel obstruction is a well-recognized complication in cancer patients. Depending on the setting and criteria for diagnosis, its prevalence ranges from 3% to 15%.[1–3] Colorectal, gastric, ovarian, and uterine carcinomas are the common associated tumors, but many other primary neoplasms may be responsible. Although bowel obstruction can develop at any time during the course of the disease, it occurs most frequently in the advanced stages.

In patients with active disease, bowel obstruction is usually caused by intra-abdominal tumor masses or diffuse carcinomatosis, which may be part of the primary tumor or result from tumor recurrence after surgery, chemotherapy, or radiotherapy. Mechanical obstruction may be caused by different mechanisms.[4] An extrinsic, intramural, or intraluminal occlusion is common, and a pseudo-obstruction from an intestinal motility disorder without a mechanical block is often recognized. Strangulation and bowel ischemia are rarely found in advanced cancer patients.[4]

Extrinsic occlusion of the lumen may result from enlargement of the primary tumor or recurrence, fibrosis, or adhesions. Polypoid lesions or anular narrowing due to dissemination may cause an intraluminal occlusion. Infiltration of the intestinal wall due to intestinal linitis may produce an intramural occlusion of the lumen or pseudo-obstruction. Pseudo-obstruction may also be produced by paraneoplastic syndromes, diabetic neuropathy, or any other cause of autonomic neuropathy. Other factors that may contribute to mechanical obstruction include constipation, which is often due to the illness or drugs, and surrounding inflammatory edema. The coexistence of multiple factors may lead to obstruction at several sites, an outcome that is especially common in ovarian cancer.[5]

Pathophysiology

An occlusion of the lumen prevents or delays the propulsion of the intestinal contents from passing distally. As luminal contents accumulate proximal to the obstruction, the bowel becomes distended, which stimulates intestinal fluid secretion. This further stretches the bowel wall. Swallowed air provides a source of gas, which can further distend the bowel. Carbon dioxide is the predominant gas in the duodenum, but in contrast to nitrogen, it is rapidly absorbed. Intestinal bacteria normally produce hydrogen and methane in the colon, but in bowel obstruction, the abnormally increased flora may also produce gases in the small intestine, further contributing to the distention.[5]

The increasing intraluminal pressure obstructs venous drainage from the obstructed segment, which may interfere with oxygen consumption and eventually lead to intestinal gangrene or perforation. The accumulation of secretions causes more abdominal distention and intermittent peristaltic activity, which attempts to surmount the obstacle and may be associated with colic.

Although there is little or no through-movement of intestinal contents, the bowel continues to contract with increased incoordinated peristaltic activity. A vicious circle represented by distention–secretion–motor activity leads to a worsening of the clinical picture. The hypertensive intraluminal state can damage the intestinal epithelium, which in turn can produce an inflammatory response that enhances the cyclo-oxygenase pathway and the release of prostaglandins. The prostaglandins are potent secretagogues that act either by a direct effect on enterocytes or via activation of enteric nervous reflexes.[6]

The pathophysiology of bowel obstruction may also include the release of vasoactive intestinal polypeptide (VIP) into the portal and peripheral circulation. The primary stimulus for VIP release may be hypoxia, which could be caused by the redistribution of blood flow in the obstructed segment and the distal site of the obstruction, or, alternatively, by intraluminal bacterial overgrowth. In the experimental animal bowel obstruction model, higher VIP content is present in the duodenal tissue than in colon. High portal levels of VIP are known to cause hypersecretion and splanchnic vasodilatation.[7] VIP may mediate local intestinal and systemic pathophysiologic alterations that accompany intestinal obstruction, such as hyperemia and edema of the intestinal wall and an accumulation of fluid in the lumen.

Multiorgan failure may accompany bowel obstruction. In some cases, this complication may be caused, or worsened, by systemic hypotension associated with splanchnic vasodilatation and other mechanisms. The splanchnic flow seems relatively less responsive to vasoactive drugs, and disturbances of the autoregulatory local and neurohumoral control mechanisms during bowel obstruction may cause hypotension by impairing blood pressure regulation.[8] Furthermore, fluids and electrolytes are sequestered in the gut wall and lumen in the presence of vasodilatation, which may also contribute to hypotension. These outcomes further lead to multiorgan system failure, which is the cause of death in patients with bowel obstruction.

The relationship between bowel obstruction and renal failure is illustrative. The hypovolemic state associated with bowel obstruction may induce renal failure due to a decrease in renal blood flow and, as a consequence, glomerular filtration. Oliguria, hyperazotemia, and hemoconcentration may accompany dehydration, and hyponatremia and a total protein below the normal range are common laboratory findings in obstructed patients.[3] Abdominal distention may reduce venous return, worsening hypotension, and concurrently impair pulmonary ventilation by elevating the diaphragm. Secondary circulatory changes such as tachycardia, low central venous pressure, and a reduced cardiac output may lead to severe hypotension.

Bowel obstruction may also lead to sepsis as a result of bacterial translocation through the bowel wall. Toxins produced by the intestinal contents may also pass through the intestinal wall into the lymphatic and systemic circulation. This phenomenon is facilitated by an increase in endoluminal pressure, stasis, and intestinal ischemia, characteristic conditions present in bowel obstruction.

Metabolic disorders in intestinal obstruction depend on the site and duration of the obstruction. These disorders may be related to dehydration, electrolyte losses, and disorders of acid–base balance.[9] Different types of acid–base disturbances may be observed, depending on the level of obstruction. Where the level is high, metabolic alkalosis, hypochloremia, and hypokalemia can occur as a result of lost gastric secretions and hypoventilation. If the level of obstruction is distal, the secondary deficit is global, including chloride, sodium, potassium, and bicarbonate. These changes can be attributed to stasis of biliary, pancreatic, gastric, and intestinal secretions. Acidosis may also occur from the effects of ischemic lesions or septic complications.[5]

Clinical Syndrome

Bowel obstruction may be a mode of presentation for an intra-abdominal malignancy or a feature of recurrent disease or other pathologies in patients with a history of malignancy. At operation, the etiology is benign (e.g., adhesions or radiation enteritis) in 10% to 48% of cases; if the cause is malignant, there may be single or multiple sites of disease, or diffuse disease.[5]

Varying patterns of symptoms occur with bowel obstruction. The clinical presentation is influenced by the level of obstruction, which is associated with specific tumor types, and the tempo of progression from partial to complete occlusion. These factors also influence the intensity of symptoms and outcome. For example, the level of obstruction may determine, in part, the accumulation of secretions; the extent of secretions contributes to the development of abdominal pain, vomiting, constipation, abdominal distention, and the failure to pass flatus. Regardless of the site of pathology, however, crampy pain of this type may subside after a long period, possibly because bowel distention may inhibit motility.

A proximal jejunal obstruction can cause profuse and early vomiting, not associated with abdominal distention. Moreover, abdominal distention may be minimal in the presence of fixed tumors extensively infiltrating the small bowel. Pancreatic cancer can directly involve the upper tract of the gastrointestinal system, cancer of the colon mainly spreads in the small intestine, and pelvic cancer (e.g., prostate and ovary) can compress the rectum. In a distal obstruction, such as that observed in pelvic cancer, abdominal distention is more likely, and vomiting may be late or less frequent and become feculent owing to a greatly increased bacterial population of the intestinal contents.

Continuous pain associated with bowel obstruction is usually related directly to a tumor mass. Usually, this type of pain can be ascribed to compression of the intestine or hepatomegaly.

Examination of the patient with bowel obstruction may reveal hyperactive high-pitched or musical bowel sounds on abdominal auscultation. In a prolonged obstruction, the sounds often disappear as bowel motility decreases.[1,4–6]

Some cases of bowel obstruction are characterized by the eventual appearance of paradoxical diarrhea. This generally occurs in a large bowel obstruction and results from a leak of fluid stool around a fecal impaction.

The diagnosis of an intestinal obstruction is established or suspected on clinical grounds and usually confirmed by plain abdominal radiography. An abdominal radiograph reveals abnormally large quantities of gas in the bowel (Figs. 6.1 and 6.2). A small bowel obstruction is associated with minimal colonic gas, while a colonic obstruction with a competent ileocecal valve shows colonic distention but little small bowel gas. If the ileocecal valve is incompetent, there will be radiographic evidence of small intestinal and colonic distention. Plain abdominal radiographs may be misleading in patients with the proximal jejunal obstruction or a proximal closed loop obstruction by failing to show dilated loops and air–fluid levels.

A contrast study, such as a careful barium enema, may help in distinguishing the level or the causes of the obstruction. A paralytic ileus is radiographically characterized by a uniform gaseous distention of the stomach, small bowel, colon, and rectum.[5] Bowel obstruction may be suggested by deformity and kinking, which may demonstrate an extramural obstruction from tumors spreading directly to the bowel, such as the extension of pancreas or stomach cancers to the duodenum or the extension of prostate or bladder cancers to the rectum.

It is often very difficult to differentiate between a complete and a partial bowel obstruction. The majority of patients appear to experience a slow progression from a partial to a complete obstruction; some experience intermittent obstructive symptoms with resolution. When intestinal symptoms, such

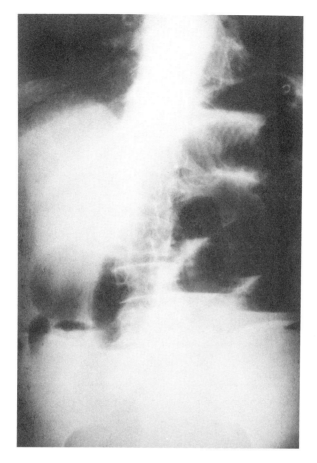

Figure 6.1. Abdominal x-ray film showing bowel obstruction (courtesy of Corrado Reina, MD, Service of Radiology, Buccheri La Ferla FBF Hospital, Palermo).

as colicky or continuous pain, abdominal distention, or nausea and vomiting, continuously worsen, an irreversible complete obstruction is likely.

Surgical Therapy

Treatment of a large bowel obstruction is primarily surgical, and surgery should be considered in all cases of bowel obstruction caused by known malignant disease. Most patients can be relieved of mechanical obstruction and, in some cases, surgery will reveal a benign etiology. A distinction should be made between patients with unproven intra-abdominal malignancy and those

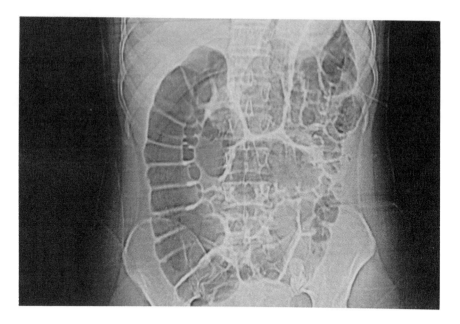

Figure 6.2. Abdominal x-ray film showing a pseudo-obstruction (courtesy of Corrado Reina, MD, Service of Radiology, Buccheri La Ferla FBF Hospital, Palermo).

with documented advanced intra-abdominal disease, some of whom may have a benign cause of obstruction.[9]

Urgent operation is rarely necessary in the management of patients with bowel obstruction. If the patient is a candidate for surgery, monitoring is still justified as long as serial radiographs and clinical evaluation indicate improvement of the intestinal distention.[10,11] A conservative approach for up to 5 days may result in spontaneous resolution of the obstruction in a relatively high percentage of patients, with no significant increase in mortality.[12]

In patients with advanced intra-abdominal malignancy, a more prolonged trial of conservative management should be offered before surgery. Conservative treatment has been reported successful in 30% to 50% of patients, although half of these patients may re-obstruct.[9,13,14] In one survey that described a "drip and suck" technique (drainage of gastric fluids and the replacement by intravenous fluids) in 13 patients, the median survival was 2 months (range 2 weeks to almost 2 years).[9]

Conservative management includes gastrointestinal intubation for removal of gases and secretions. This intervention is valuable even while the patient is being prepared for surgery. Gastrointestinal intubation has resolved bowel obstruction in 25% of cases, obviating the need for surgery temporarily or indefinitely, especially in the presence of postoperative adhesions of inflammatory strictures.[10] There may also be a therapeutic role for the nasogastric administration of oral gastrografin, a hyperosmolar water-soluble contrast agent, which has been reported to prompt the resolution of the obstructive episode while a treatment decision is under consideration.[15]

In preparation for surgery, the administration of the somatostatin analogue octreotide may be useful. Preoperative treatment with octreotide appears to limit the intraoperative pathological findings due to the accumulation of fluids in the lumen, such as edema, erythema, necrosis, and cyanosis of the bowel above the obstruction.[11] This may increase the chances of successful anastomosis.[11]

Decompression of a severely distended colon may be achieved by a temporary colostomy. The most common interventions, however, are lysis of adhesions, resection of the obstructed bowel segment and reanastomosis, bypass of the obstructed bowel, and enterostomy. Selection of the most appropriate approach depends on the level and causes of obstruction. More than two thirds of patients who are approached surgically have the obstruction relieved and can be discharged with a restored intestinal passage.[16] Radical surgery, such as pelvic exenteration, should be considered in a small minority of highly selected younger patients who have the prospect of prolonged survival or even the possibility of a cure despite extensive disease, such as in the case of Hodgkin's disease.

Reports of mean survival after palliative surgery for malignant obstruction have ranged from 2.5 to 11 months.[17–20] Benefit from surgery is mainly defined as at least 2 months of survival after operation.[21] However, symptoms that are frequently attributed to a partial obstruction can develop after surgery and persist until death, regardless of the duration of survival time.[4]

A surgical perspective to the problem of bowel obstruction should consider the aim of intervention. The aim may include relief of a mechanical obstruction, a gain in survival, symptomatic palliation, or the need for a diagnosis. If surgery can successfully achieve the most important objective or objectives, and there are no strong countervailing arguments, surgery must be strongly considered.

Although about one third of obstructed patients have a history of palliative surgery,[1,3] and surgery is generally considered in all, surgery should not be automatically undertaken in patients with far-advanced cancer. In some cases, surgical relief of the obstruction is not possible or surgery is not warranted in view of the limited prognosis. Surgical intervention does not always help and is associated with substantial perioperative mortality and morbidity rates. Indeed, in some populations, a postoperative mortality as high as 40% has been reported.[9] The survival rates of medically versus surgically treated patients may not be significantly different.[21]

Recent studies have tried to define which patients are suitable candidates for operation and which are not.[22] The poor results of surgery support the use of conservative management of intestinal obstruction due to widespread malignancy.

Criteria for surgery include a good general performance status (e.g., a score of ≥50 on the Karnofsky Performance Status Scale, or a score of 2 or better on the World Health Organization's [WHO] reference scale), no previous abdominal cancer surgery other than resection of the primary tumor, and recent onset of symptoms.[3,11] Absolute contraindications to surgery include a recent laparotomy demonstrating that corrective surgery was not possible, re-obstruction, intra-abdominal carcinomatosis as evidenced by diffuse intra-abdominal tumors or multiple palpable tumor masses, poor nutritional status, poor general performance status (Karnofsky Performance Status Scale score ≤40 or WHO scale of 3 or worse), and gross ascites that re-accumulates rapidly after paracentesis.[11] The development of a reobstruction signifies a uniformly grim outcome and surgery offers limited benefit.[9] Peritoneal carcinomatosis may cause motility problems because of intestinal paralysis secondary to extensive tumor involvement of the intestinal mesentery, which cannot be cured by bypass procedures.[23] A slow small bowel transit time without a mechanical obstruction, demonstrated radiologically with a contrast medium by a small bowel series and follow-through, may confirm the latter suspicion; this type of investigation, however, should not be regarded as routine.

Some conditions present relative contraindications to surgery, even when a tumor is present and not extensive enough to make a patient technically inoperable. Liver or distant extra-abdominal metastases, marked weight loss and hypoalbuminemia, a low lymphocyte count, and advanced age may worsen the prognosis. The decision to operate should be based upon the patient's fitness for the procedure and consent rather than the results of investigations that cannot predict palliative operability. Consent for surgery should be based on complete information, including specific discussion of a stoma, which may be the only surgical means of palliation in some cases.

Although nasogastric suction is the mainstay of the treatment of a temporary bowel obstruction, it is poorly suited to the management of patients with complete nonresolved bowel obstruction. Patients may be troubled by the nasal tube, and accidental or intentional dislodgement is a common occurrence, even in a supervised medical setting.

A percutaneous gastrostomy is the method of choice for patients with inoperable intestinal obstruction. It offers patients the opportunity to return home[22] and, with intermittent venting of the gastrostomy, allows the patient to continue oral intake and maintain an active lifestyle without the inconvenience of a nasal tube.[24] This technique usually requires only a brief period of hospitalization; it can also be performed on an outpatient basis (Fig. 6.3). The tube may also be placed at the time of surgical exploration if the intraoperative impression is that complete, permanent obstruction is imminent.

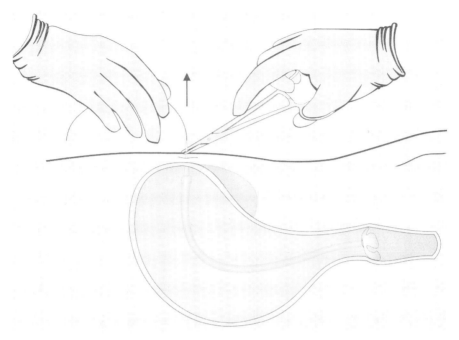

Figure 6.3. Gastrostomy by percutaneous endoscopy (drawn by Leonardo Salvaggio, MD).

Placement of the gastrostomy is performed using a fiber-optic endoscope. In a darkened room, maximal light transillumination through the anterior gastric wall is obtained and the maximal indentation in a relatively flat section of the anterior gastric wall is chosen for the skin incision. The stomach is distended with air and a sheathed needle is directed into the stomach under the entry site. After the needle is removed, a guidewire is introduced through the sheath. The endoscope is then removed, and the gastrostomy catheter is tightened to the guidewire and pulled through the mouth and into the stomach, until resistance is felt from the fixation plug in the stomach. Then the catheter is fixed to the skin.

Appropriate training in the use of gastrostomy tubes is necessary before the patient is discharged from the hospital. Following tube placement, average reported patient survival is 64 days (median 33 days), during which high volumes of electrolyte solution, opioids, antiemetics, and antispasmodics can be administered to the advanced cancer patient with a partial or complete bowel obstruction.[22,25] Recognized complications of gastrostomy include a gastric perforation, hemorrhage, gastrocolic fistula, infection of the stoma site, and aspiration pneumonia.[26,27]

The high success rate coupled with the low morbidity and mortality have made the percutaneous gastrostomy procedure attractive.[26,27] However, previous surgery or extensive carcinomatosis may technically impede the gastrostomy. Although there are no absolute contraindications, ascites, previous gastric surgery, or a coagulopathy may represent relative contraindications.[28] Anatomical or pathological difficulties may preclude the use of fluoroscopic guidance. The reasons for an unsuccessful percutaneous endoscopic gastrostomy include esophageal obstruction, previous gastric surgery, and the inability to insufflate the stomach.

Computed tomographic (CT) guided cannulation has been described in patients who had an esophageal or a pharyngeal obstruction.[29] CT assistance is useful in patients with a variety of abdominal problems, including masses compressing the stomach, a previous partial gastrectomy, and ascites. High costs, lack of availability, and lack of real-time monitoring are the disadvantages of CT guidance.

Medical Therapy

Patients who are unfit for surgery, who have inoperable disease, or who refuse consent are candidates for a palliative and supportive care regimen. The utility of a primary chemotherapy approach has not been recognized. Indeed, chemotherapy should be considered a contraindication in bowel obstruction because of the relatively poor performance status of these patients and the major problems that occur in the distribution of body fluids. The degree to which body fluids accumulate in the so-called "third space" may induce unpredictable toxicity from chemotherapy. Furthermore, many cytotoxic drugs, such as tamoxifen and aminogluthetimide (used in hormone-dependent cancer, such as in breast cancer) are available only in oral form and require some weeks to become effective. They are clearly not suitable in a patient with an intestinal obstruction. In patients with chemosensitive tumors, such as ovarian cancer, chemotherapy is seldom active after failure of second-line treatment in any case. Nonetheless, patients with tumors that can potentially respond favorably to chemotherapy or hormone therapy should have this approach reconsidered when bowel transit has been restored.[11]

Nasogastric tube

The "drip and suck" approach is still the first response in most clinical settings for an intestinal obstruction. However, there are no studies that describe the ability of patients to tolerate such treatment, the number who require hospitalization, and the proportion who can continue it until death. Nasogastric suction is invasive and may be more a burden than a benefit. For some patients, nasogastric tubes are poorly tolerated, difficult to place, or temporary because of blockage or displacement. Replacement of a nasogastric tube is uncomfortable in patients already distressed by the clinical situation.[1] Moreover, a long-term drainage by this technique is associated with nasal decubitus lesions.

Nonetheless, nasogastric drainage can be a holding measure for some days before proceeding to surgery. As mentioned previously, it can obviate the need for surgery temporarily or indefinitely for some patients, who experience resolution of the obstruction. Moreover, patients with a gastric outflow obstruction or high intestinal obstruction may benefit from a nasogastric tube if nausea and vomiting cannot be satisfactory controlled with medical therapy. The tube may be removed after days of gastric decompression to continue medical therapy, if gastric secretion is reduced.[2,30]

Hydration

Dehydration may increase the distress of the patient. It causes dryness of the mouth, changes in plasma osmolarity, and low cardiac output, all of which can contribute to a sensation of thirst. Notwithstanding, there has been no demonstrable association between the severity of thirst and fluid intake.[31]

Dehydration may also cause or worsen delirium and trigger pre-renal failure, which itself can result in the accumulation of morphine metabolites and other pharmacokinetic changes that further aggravate neurological disturbances.[32,33]

These complications associated with dehydration suggest that it should be treated. Treatment, however, is not always in the best interest of the patient. There is some anecdotal evidence that intravenous hydration results in more gastrointestinal secretions and, consequently, a worsening of the symptoms, but this has never been confirmed. More important, hydration should be avoided if it merely or mainly serves to prolong the process of dying. The care plan should be individualized and adjusted in collaboration with the patient, the patient's family, and the palliative care team.

Thus, the value of hydration for terminally ill patients is controversial. In some cases, the decision to proceed or not with this approach can be delayed by encouraging patients to eat and drink freely. Oral intake of water, other fluids, and small amounts of foods may be feasible when symptoms are under control. Additionally, moistening the mouth may reduce the thirst sensation for some time.

If hydration is pursued, an easier approach than intravenous fluids is hypodermoclysis, in which fluids are delivered subcutaneously. It is relatively simple to deliver a volume of 1 liter per day on average to a terminally ill patient. Gradual tapering of fluid intake can be accomplished in this way during the process of natural death, and this is probably less distressing than a sudden suspension of hydration.[33]

Most terminally ill patients do not benefit from parenteral nutrition, although there are some exceptions. Some patients, for example, who develop bowel obstruction relatively early in their disease, or who have the possibility of spontaneous resolution, may be appropriate candidates.[34,35] Life expectancy is an important parameter when considering parenteral nutrition, but, unfortunately, estimates of survival may be unreliable and biased due to several factors.

Often, personal belief and emotions influence the decision-making process concerning nutritional support. In many cases, parenteral nutrition is started in the hospital and the decision to stop it is difficult because of the adverse psychological impact of treatment withdrawal. The patient's desire regarding the choice of therapy must be considered despite the general attitude of the palliative care team in favor of a less aggressive treatment. For these patients, nutrition is often abandoned after the patient can no longer cooperate and the family is informed of the issues.

Special Issues in Populations with Very Short Life Expectancies

The inadequacy of prolonged conservative management of bowel obstruction with nasogastric suction and intravenous fluids alone has long been recognized.[36] A different approach has been advocated, which forgoes nasogastric tubes and intravenous fluids, and emphasizes aggressive treatment of the most distressing symptoms using analgesics, anticholinergics, and antiemetics. In this way, most advanced cancer patients who develop an inoperable bowel obstruction can be successfully managed with minimal use of a nasogastric tube and an intravenous line. This conservative management is well tolerated and, above all, can be performed at home. The vast majority of patients can continue this treatment until death. Dry mouth and drowsiness are the major problems encountered, but they can be treated with local measures or careful titration of the medications.

The delivery of drugs for symptom control cannot be via the oral route due to the unpredictability of drug absorption. Although the rectal and sublingual routes can be effective, not all the drugs are available in these formulations. The subcutaneous route (using either continuous or bolus delivery) or the intravenous route (if a central venous catheter was previously placed) are the preferred routes. Syringe drivers have become popular in the palliative care setting because they are easy for family to use at home, and are cheap and reliable.

Various surveys have reported survivals of 2 days to 7 months for patients treated with this type of medical approach.[2,3,36–39] This wide variation may reflect differences in assessment, methodology, and setting. For example, average survival would be expected to be relatively longer if patients with intermittent obstruction were included. In populations with complete obstruction, the average survival usually ranges from 10 to 20 days.

The therapeutic response to medical management can be assessed using a WHO scale, in which 0 is defined as no nausea and vomiting, grade 1 is nausea, grade 2 is transient vomiting, grade 3 is vomiting requiring therapy, and grade 4 is intractable vomiting. A good response can be considered a reduction in the WHO grade to below 2. In patients with a nasogastric tube in place, a favorable response can be considered a reduction in the volume of effluent during a 48-hour period to below one third of the level during the previous 48 hours.[39]

A comprehensive score for symptom distress, which includes pain, has also been used to assess the efficacy of therapy.[2] In this approach, nausea and vomiting were scored as follows: nausea or fewer than two episodes of vomiting = 3; 2 to 5 episodes of vomiting = 6; and > 5 episodes of vomiting = 9. This scale is similar to the WHO recommended scale. Multiplication by 3 is used to relate the score to the pain scale, which is a traditional visual analogue scale (VAS) score. The sum of these values gives a number expressing the distress due to symptoms of intestinal obstruction: intestinal score + pain VAS (from 0 to 19). A score under 7 means that the principal symptoms of bowel obstruction are well controlled. A significant decrease in the score of symptom distress has been shown after 1 week of medical treatment with different combinations of drugs.[2]

Antiemetics

Different combinations of drugs have been proposed to control gastrointestinal symptoms in terminally ill patients with a bowel obstruction (Table 6.1). Antiemetics are often needed to control nausea and vomiting. A reasonable goal may be the reduction and not the abolition of vomiting. Phenothiazines (e.g., cyclizine, chlorpromazine, methotrimeprazine) have been proved effective in controlling nausea and vomiting.[1,36,37,40] However, severe hypotension, som-

Table 6.1. Drugs used in inoperable bowel obstruction

Drug	Usual dose	Comment
Haloperidol	5–15 mg/day	Extrapyramidal side effects at higher doses
Cyclizine	150 mg/day	Crystallization may occur during continuous infusion
Methotrimeprazine	50–150 mg/day	Skin reactions necessitating frequent site changes during subcutaneous dosing
Chlorpromazine	50–100 mg/day	Marked sedative effects
Hyoscine butylbromide	80–120 mg/day	Tachycardia, hypotension, dry mouth
Metoclopramide	60–120 mg/day	Extrapyramidal side effects; should not be used in complete obstruction
Octreotide	0.3 mg/day	No important side effects; expensive
Morphine	Variable	Dose must be titrated against response

nolence, or parkinsonian side effects may occur, particularly with higher doses; opioid-induced myoclonus may also be worsened.[1,41] Moreover, long-term parenteral administration of cyclizine is compromised by the occurrence of crystallization, and subcutaneous methotrimeprazine can cause irritation.[1]

If somnolence is a problem, the use of haloperidol may be preferable. Haloperidol causes less sedation and anticholinergic effects than the phenothiazines. It can be given subcutaneously, either as a bolus or as a continuous infusion in combination with other drugs. In many cases, however, sedation may be required in agitated patients close to death, and the side effect of somnolence is not a problem, but furthers the goals of the therapy.

Effective emesis control sometimes requires trials of different drug combinations. Combinations can be administered that simultaneously block dopamine, muscarinic cholinergic, and histamine H_1 receptors.[42]

There is controversy regarding the use of some antinauseant drugs, such as metoclopramide, that have the capacity to increase gastric motility. These drugs could potentially increase colic pain and vomiting in the presence of a complete obstruction by driving stomach contents into a paralyzed intestine.[1] However, high doses of metoclopramide may reduce nausea and vomiting in patients with a low level of intestinal obstruction.[38] Candidates for metoclopramide should be patients with an incomplete bowel obstruction, the resolution of which may be possible.[3]

The role of corticosteroids in the management of an intestinal obstruction or its symptoms has still not been confirmed.[40,43] Peritumoral inflammatory edema may be reduced and, theoretically, this could improve intestinal passage. In reported series, higher doses of dexamethasone, ranging from 8 to 100 mg (median 40 mg), seem to be effective in managing nausea and vomiting, and, in some circumstances, restoring bowel function.[3,44] The degree of symptomatic improvement has been questioned when low doses of methylprednisolone (e.g., 150 mg per day) were used.[43] Oral candidiasis is the most common side effect reported.

Antisecretory drugs

Intestinal colic may be controlled using smooth muscle relaxants, such as atropine and scopolamine.[1] These drugs decrease the tone and peristalsis in the smooth muscle through their anticholinergic activity, which includes both a competitive inhibition of the muscarinic receptors at the smooth muscle level and an impairment of ganglionic neural transmission in the bowel wall. Hyoscine butylbromide penetrates the blood–brain barrier less than atropine or hyoscine hydrobromide (scopolamine), reducing the risk of central nervous system side effects.[30] Hyoscine butylbromide 80 mg to 120 mg per day has been successfully used in combination with haloperidol and morphine;[37] although this therapy reduced colicky pain, nausea, and vomiting, patients with an upper abdominal obstruction continued to require nasogastric suction to control vomiting. The quantities of gastrointestinal fluids drained through a nasogastric tube can also be significantly reduced by this treatment.[30] Hyoscine butylbromide is commonly combined in the same syringe with haloperidol and morphine.

Typical anticholinergic effects, such as tachycardia, dry mouth, blurred vision, drowsiness, and hypotension, can occur with the use of these drugs. Sucking ice cubes and drinking sips of water can reduce the discomfort of a dry mouth.

Octreotide, an analogue of somatostatin with a more favorable pharmacokinetic profile, seems to be useful in controlling gastrointestinal secretions and vomiting. It, too, is commonly combined in one syringe with haloperidol and morphine. The rationale for the use of octreotide in malignant bowel obstruction derives from the physiologic actions of the parent drug, which include inhibited release of the hormones gastrin, secretin, VIP, pancreatic polypeptide, insulin, and glucagon, and inhibited secretion of gastric acid, pepsin, pancreatic enzyme, bicarbonate, intestinal epithelial electrolytes, and water.[45] The inhibitory effect of octreotide on gastrointestinal secretions appears to break the vicious cycle of distention and secretion present in bowel obstruction, thereby reducing vomiting and pain. The effect can be likened to an artificial secretory bowel rest.[46] An indirect analgesic effect due to a reduction in distention and colicky pain might allow reduction of concurrent opioid therapy.[2,6]

Several reports have confirmed the effectiveness of octreotide 0.3 to 0.6 mg per day in controlling symptoms due to bowel obstruction.[39,46–48] The drug may also be effective in upper bowel obstruction, a situation that often warrants a nasogastric tube[37]; with this treatment, gastric drainage is reduced.[47] Patients with gastrointestinal obstruction due to chemosensitive or radiosensitive tumors may be treated with octreotide while undergoing chemotherapy or radiotherapy and then discontinue the drug once the response is obtained.

Octreotide has a prolonged action due to its relatively long half-life. It can be administered subcutaneously by bolus injection or infusion. Various drugs can be combined with octreotide in the same syringe-driver with no apparent reduction in efficacy.[49] No side effects have been reported, even at doses of 1.2 mg per day.[50]

Although octreotide is expensive and should not be considered first-line therapy, it can be cost-effective when several drug trials have already been unsuccessful. The distress to the patient and family must be weighed against the drug's cost.

Analgesics

As expected, a wide range of opioid doses has been reported to relieve the pain associated with malignant bowel obstruction. Subcutaneous morphine is the most common drug used,[2,3,37,38] although buprenorphine, available also as sublingual tablets, has equally been reported.[2] As an intestinal obstruction becomes evident, it is necessary to switch from the oral to the parenteral route, and opioid doses must be titrated to yield continued benefit.

Epidural morphine may alter intraluminal pressure, increasing retrograde pressure and delaying gastric emptying and orocecal transit time.[51] Epidural local anesthetics not only alleviate pain in situations of ischemic injury to the bowel, but may also hasten the recovery of gastrointestinal motility in states of incomplete obstruction.[52] However, spinal administration of local anesthetics is rarely considered in obstructed patients. If a spinal catheter has previously been placed, this treatment may have a rationale, although the hypovolemic state of obstructed patients represents a relative contraindication. Bedridden patients appear to tolerate epidural analgesia.[53]

References

1. Baines M. The pathophysiology and management of malignant bowel obstruction. In: Doyle D, Hanks GW, MacDonald N, eds. *Oxford Textbook of Palliative Medicine.* Oxford: Oxford Medical Publications; 1993:311–316.

2. Mercadante S. Bowel obstruction in home care cancer patients: four years of experience. *Suppl Care Cancer* 1995; 3:190–193.

3. Fainsinger R, Spachynski K, Hanson J, Bruera E. Symptom control in terminally ill patients with malignant bowel obstruction (MBO). *J Pain Symptom Manage* 1994; 9:12–18.

4. Ripamonti C. Management of bowel obstruction in advanced cancer. *J Pain Symptom Manage* 1994; 9:193–200.

5. Scott Jones R, Schirmer BD. Intestinal obstruction, pseudo-obstruction and ileus. In: Sleisinger MH, Fordtran JS, eds. *Gastrointestinal Disease.* Philadelphia: J.B. Lippincott Co; 1989:369–381.

6. Mercadante S. Pain in inoperable bowel obstruction. *Pain Digest* 1995; 5:9–13.

7. Basson MD, Fielding P, Bilchick A, et al. Does vasoactive intestinal polypeptide mediate the pathophysiology of bowel obstruction? *Am J Surg* 1989; 157:109–115.

8. Neville R, Fielding P, Cambria RP, Modlin I. Vascular responsiveness in obstructed gut. *Dis Colon Rectum* 1991; 34:229–235.

9. Chan A, Woodruff RK. Intestinal obstruction in patients with widespread intraabdominal malignancy. *J Pain Symptom Manage* 1992; 7:339–342.

10. Krebs HB, Goplerud DR. Mechanical intestinal obstruction in patients with gynecologic disease: a review of 368 patients. *Am J Obstet Gynecol* 1987; 157:577–583.

11. Consensus Conference on Bowel Obstruction in Advanced and Terminal Cancer Patients. October 28–29, 1994; Athens.

12. Seror D, Feigin E, Szold A, et al. How conservatively can postoperative small bowel obstruction be treated? *Am J Surg* 1993; 165:121–126.

13. Gallick HL, Weaver DW, Sachs RJ, Bouman DL. Intestinal obstruction in cancer patients. *Am Surg* 1986; 52:434–437.

14. Soo KC, Davidson T, Parker M, et al. Intestinal obstruction in patients with gynaecological malignancies. *Ann Acad Med Singapore* 1988; 17:72–73.
15. Assalia A, Schein M, Kopelman D, et al. Therapeutic effect of oral gastrografin in adhesive, partial small bowel obstruction: a prospective randomized trial. *Surgery* 1994; 115:433–437.
16. Rubin SC, Hoskins WJ, Benjamin I, Lewis JL. Palliative surgery for intestinal obstruction in advanced ovarian cancer. *Gynecol Oncol* 1989; 34:16–19.
17. Osten RT, Guyton S, Steele G, Wilson RE. Malignant intestinal obstruction. *Surgery* 1980; 87:611–615.
18. Piver MS, Barlow JJ, Lele SB, Frank A. Survival after ovarian cancer induced intestinal obstruction. *Gynecol Oncol* 1982; 12:44–49.
19. Ketcham AS, Hoye RC, Pilch YH, Morton DL. Delayed intestinal obstruction following treatment for cancer. *Cancer* 1970; 25:406–410.
20. Walsh HPJ, Schofield PF. Is laparotomy for small bowel obstruction justified in patients with previously treated malignancy? *Br J Surg* 1984; 71:933–935.
21. Larson JE, Podczaski ES, Manetta A, et al. Bowel obstruction in patients with ovarian carcinoma: analysis of prognostic factors. *Gynecol Oncol* 1989; 35:61–65.
22. Van Ooijen B, Van der Burg MEL, Planting AST, et al. Surgical treatment or gastric drainage only for intestinal obstruction in patients with carcinoma of the ovary or peritoneal carcinomatosis of other origin. *Surg Gynecol Obstet* 1993; 176:469–474.
23. Krebs HB, Helmkamp BF. Management of intestinal obstruction in ovarian cancer. *Oncology* 1989; 3:25–31.
24. Ashby MA, Game PA, Devitt P, et al. Percutaneous gastrostomy as a venting procedure in palliative care. *Palliat Med* 1991; 5:147–150.
25. Gemlo B, Rayner AA, Lewis B. Home support of patients with end-stage malignant bowel obstruction using hydration and venting gastrostomy. *Am J Surg* 1986; 152:100–104.
26. Waye JD. Percutaneous endoscopic gastrostomy. In: Waye JD, Geenen JE, Fleisher D, Venu RP, eds. *Techniques in Therapeutic Endoscopy*, vol. 4. Philadelphia: JB Lippincott; 1987:1–14.
27. vanSonnenberg E, Casola G, D'Agostino H. Radiologic percutaneous gastrostomy and gastroenterostomy. *Am J Gastroenterol* 1990; 85:1561–1562.
28. Willis JS, Oglesby JT. Percutaneous gastrostomy. *Radiology* 1988; 167:41–43.
29. Sanchez RB, vanSonnenberg E, D'Agostino HB, et al. CT guidance for percutaneous gastrostomy and gastroenterostomy. *Radiology* 1992; 184:201–205.
30. De Conno F, Caraceni A, Zecca E, et al. Continuous infusion of hyoscine butylbromide reduces secretions in patients with gastrointestinal obstruction. *J Pain Symptom Manage* 1991; 6:484–486.
31. Burge FI. Dehydration symptoms of palliative care cancer patients. *J Pain Symptom Manage* 1993; 8:454–464.
32. Fainsinger R, Bruera E, Miller MJ, et al. Symptom control during the last week of life on a palliative care unit. *J Palliat Care* 1991; 7:5–11.
33. Fainsinger R, MacEachern T, Miller M, et al. The use of hypodermoclysis (HDC) for rehydration in terminally ill cancer patients. *J Palliat Care* 1992; 8:70–72.
34. Fainsinger R, Chan K, Bruera E. Total parenteral nutrition for a terminally ill patient. *J Palliat Care* 1992; 8:30–32.

35. Mercadante S. Parenteral nutrition at home in advanced cancer patients. *J Pain Symptom Manage* 1995; 10:476–480.

36. Baines M, Oliver DJ, Carter RL. Medical management of intestinal obstruction in patients with advanced malignant disease. *Lancet* 1985; 2:990–993.

37. Ventafridda V, Ripamonti C, Caraceni A, Spoldi E, Messina L, De Conno F. The management of inoperable gastrointestinal obstruction in terminal cancer patients. *Tumori* 1990; 76:389–393.

38. Isbister WH, Elder P, Symons L. Non-operative management of malignant intestinal obstruction. *J R Coll Surg Edinb* 1990; 35:369–372.

39. Khoo D. Hall E, Motson R, et al. Palliation of malignant intestinal obstruction using octreotide. *Eur J Cancer* 1994; 30:28–30.

40. Twycross RG, Lack SA. Gastrointestinal obstruction. In: Twycross RG, Lack SA, eds. *Control of Alimentary Symptoms in Far Advanced Cancer*. New York: Churchill Livingstone; 1986:239–257.

41. Mercadante S. Opioids and akathisia. *J Pain Symptom Manage* 1995; 10:415.

42. Perutska SJ, Snyder SH. Antiemetics: neurotransmitter receptor binding predicts therapeutic actions. *Lancet* 1982:658–659.

43. Farr WC. The use of corticosteroids for symptom management in terminally ill patients. *Am J Hosp Care* 1990; 7:41–46.

44. Steiner N. Controle des symptomes en soins palliatifs: l'ileus terminal. *Med Hygiene* 1991; 49:1182–1192.

45. Mercadante S. The role of octreotide in palliative care. *J Pain Symptom Manage* 1994; 9:406–411.

46. Mercadante S, Maddaloni S. Octreotide in the management of inoperable gastrointestinal obstruction in terminal cancer patients. *J Pain Symptom Manage* 1992; 7:496–498.

47. Mercadante S, Spoldi E, Caraceni A, et al. Octreotide in relieving gastrointestinal symptoms due to bowel obstruction. *Palliat Med* 1993; 7:295–299.

48. Khoo D, Riley J, Waxman J. Control of emesis in bowel obstruction in terminally ill patients. *Lancet* 1992; 339:375–376.

49. Mercadante S. Tolerability of continuous subcutaneous octreotide used in combination with other drugs. *J Palliat Care* 1995; 11:14–16.

50. Riley J, Fallon MT. Octreotide in terminal malignant obstruction of the gastrointestinal tract. *Eur J Palliat Care* 1994; 1:23–25.

51. Thorn SE, Wattwil M, Lallander A. Effects of epidural morphine and epidural bupivacaine on gastroduodenal motility during fasted state and after food intake. *Acta Anesthesiol Scand* 1994; 38:57–62.

52. Udassin R, Eimerl D, Schiffman J, Haskel Y. Epidural anesthesia accelerates the recovery of postischemic bowel motility in the rat. *Anesthesiology* 1994; 80:832–836.

53. Mercadante S. Intrathecal morphine and bupivacaine in advanced cancer pain patients implanted at home. *J Pain Symptom Manage* 1994; 9:201–207.

III

ADVANCES IN THE PHARMACOTHERAPY OF PAIN

Introduction: What Might the Future Hold for Opioid Pharmacotherapy?

RUSSELL K. PORTENOY

"Translational" research, the stream of scientific endeavors that leads from basic discoveries in the laboratory to practical applications, has captured the attention of the scientific community. It is an appropriate label for research in opioid pharmacology during the past three decades. During this time, the ongoing elucidation of opioid-mediated antinociceptive processes and related opioidergic systems has provided the impetus for many advances in analgesic therapies. This part describes some of the most important advances and offers guidelines for opioid pharmacotherapy. An extensive clinical experience in the treatment of cancer pain suggests that these guidelines can provide sustained benefit to a large proportion of patients with chronic pain.

Although understanding of the endogenous opioid systems that mediate the effects of exogenously administered drugs has advanced at a remarkable rate, the complexity of these systems is truly staggering and many discoveries have opened new areas for research.[1] Studies in an expanding array of experimental models have confirmed that opioid receptors involved in analgesia have numerous subtypes, which can be found in both the periphery and multiple sites in the central nervous system. Supraspinal and spinal opioid systems can be activated independently or function in an additive or synergistic fashion. The outcomes produced by each of these opioid systems depend on the activation of complex second messenger systems, manipulation of which can influence analgesia and other opioid-mediated phenomena, such as physical dependence and tolerance. These second messenger systems interact with other receptor-mediated events that involve a very large number of nonopioid transmitters and modulators. The complexity of the interactions among opioid and nonopioid systems results in a remarkable degree of flexibility and feedback control in opioid mechanisms.

Many of these fascinating developments in basic pharmacology have been investigated in clinical models. Some have already yielded new techniques of clinical management. For example, the development of intraspinal techniques of opioid administration followed the elucidation of spinal opioid systems in animals. Similarly, studies of receptor-selective agonists have already yielded a group of drugs, the agonist-antagonist opioids, that complement the more widely used pure μ agonists.

Many other discoveries are likely to generate clinical advances in the future. These therapeutic advances will largely occur in the areas of new drug development, better use of current drugs, and novel techniques for opioid delivery. The overriding goal of this effort is the development of new therapies that improve the therapeutic index (the balance between analgesia and side effects) of current approaches.

New opioid drugs could potentially offer better side effect profiles than those currently available. Novel receptor-selective drugs or drugs with mixed mechanisms (like the currently available opioid tramadol) may offer advantages in some settings, and may be supplemented by the combined use of receptor-selective opioids and delivery approaches that optimize the exposure of the drug to the receptors with which they interact. For example, the δ receptor is involved with spinal analgesia and it is possible that spinal administration of a new δ agonist could become an important clinical advance.

The review of morphine metabolites included in this part underscores the importance of new findings related to pharmacokinetic–pharmacodynamic interactions. Intense investigation of morphine has yielded information that could result in new drug development and improved methods for the administration of morphine itself. Studies of other opioids might similarly yield information about clinically relevant metabolic products.

Differences in metabolites may be one factor that contributes to drug-selective differences in clinical effects. The existence of these drug-selective differences has never been systematically evaluated in repeated dose comparative trials. Clinical trials that are currently under way, or are planned, may allow more appropriate selection of an opioid based on the characteristics of the patient and the drug. For example, studies of interindividual variation in the activity of enzymes that metabolize specific opioids may yield information that aids in drug selection.[2] The review of interindividual variability in opioid response included in this part highlights the potential importance of these genetic factors. Future studies may be able to identify patient characteristics that increase or decrease the likelihood of a favorable response to specific opioids.

Clinical investigations of opioid drugs may also yield information about drug combinations that provide additive or synergistic effects, or improve side effect profiles. For example, such additive effects may occur during intraspinal administration of an opioid and a local anesthetic, a strategy that has become accepted for the management of highly selected patients with refractory pain. Future clinical trials are likely to identify other drug combinations that improve the outcome of opioid therapy.

The therapeutic index of an opioid drug can also be improved by diminishing the side effect burden, and studies of treatments for common side effects represent another avenue of clinically relevant research in opioid pharmacotherapy. For example, the co-administration of psychostimulants for opioid-induced somnolence or cognitive impairment is now widely accepted. Additional studies of this approach are needed to identify the best drug and appropriate dosing regimen. Future studies may similarly offer effective prophylactic approaches to other problems, such as the use of oral opioid antagonist therapy for constipation.

Much of the progress in opioid pharmacotherapy achieved during the past decade has occurred as a result of research in drug delivery technologies. The oral controlled-release formulations of morphine have achieved worldwide popularity and will be used to deliver other drugs in the future, including codeine, oxycodone, and hydromorphone. Other types of controlled release oral formulations are in development and are likely to yield drugs that can be given once daily, or even less frequently. In a similar way, the currently available controlled-release transdermal system for fentanyl is likely to be adapted for use with other drugs. As reviewed in this part, the use of fentanyl in the transdermal system has opened new treatment avenues for this drug and others in its class. Other delivery systems, including an oral transmucosal system, iontophoretic devices, and new techniques for subcutaneous and intraspinal administration, are also in development.

An important area of future clinical research will focus on comparative trials that evaluate new drugs and drug delivery systems in terms of both effectiveness and costs. Ultimately, the method of drug delivery will be based on empirical information that indicates the approach most likely to optimize the therapeutic index and minimize cost.[3]

References

1. Herz A, Akil H, Simon EJ, eds. *Handbook of Experimental Pharmacology.* New York: Springer-Verlag; 1993.
2. Sindrup SH, Brosen K, Bjerring P, et al. Codeine increases pain thresholds to copper vapor laser stimuli in extensive but not in poor metabolizers of sparteine. *Clin Pharmacol Ther* 1990; 48:686–693.
3. Portenoy RK. Issues in the economic analysis of therapies for cancer pain. *Oncology* 1995; 11 (suppl):71–78.

7

Pharmacology of Opioid Drugs: Basic Principles

ARTHUR G. LIPMAN AND MICHAEL E. GAUTHIER

The term *opium* is derived from the ancient Greek word for juice, because opium is obtained from the juicy exudate of the poppy plant. Opium has been used as an analgesic and euphoriant for over 5,000 years. *Opioid* is now the preferred term for both endogenous pain-modulating substances, such as beta endorphin and enkephalins, and exogenous drugs, such as morphine and codeine. In the past, these latter substances were called narcotics or opiates. *Narcotic*, derived from the Greek word for stupor, historically was used to indicate drugs that induce sleep. Narcotic now has been adopted as a legal term that includes many classes of substances that may be abused. Use of that word to describe opioid analgesics may cause confusion. *Opiate* was originally used to designate substances derived from opium. Later, the word was used for all exogenous opioids. It is now dated, because the distinction between endogenous and exogenous substances that act as opioid receptors is blurred.

Since the isolation of morphine from opium nearly 200 years ago by the German pharmacist Friedrich Serturner, ongoing research and development have provided dozens of natural, synthetic, and semisynthetic opioid analgesics. Over 20 such drugs are used clinically today (Table 7.1). Yet much of what we know about the pharmacology and appropriate therapeutic use of these very old and very effective analgesics has only been elucidated in the past three decades. Unfortunately, many clinicians still harbor untrue beliefs and biases about these drugs and many health professional schools continue to teach disproved concepts. This chapter briefly describes some of the basic pharmacological principles and newer findings about the clinical uses of these drugs. Application of these principles in clinical practice will lead to improved patient comfort, better treatment outcomes, and decreased adverse sequelae from pain.

Table 7.1. Opioids in Use

Drugs	Comments
Agonists	
Morphine	Prototypical μ agonist
Codeine	Acts like a partial agonist
Hydromorphone	
Oxymorphone	
Oxycodone	
Hydrocodone	Available only in combination with nonopioids in the United States
Levorphanol	
Meperidine	Use only for a few days due to accumulation of toxic metabolite
Methadone	Used also in opioid dependence maintenance and detoxification
Fentanyl	
Sufentanil	Used primarily perioperatively
Alfentanil	Used primarily perioperatively
Diphenoxylate	Used as antidiarrheal medication
Loperamide	Used as antidiarrheal medication
Propoxyphene	Less analgesic activity than other opioids
Diamorphine (heroin)	Used in other countries as an analgesic; not legal in the United States
Agonist–Antagonist Opioids	
Pentazocine	
Nalbuphine	
Butorphanol	
Dezocine	
Partial Agonist Opioid	
Buprenorphine	
Opioid Antagonists	
Naloxone	
Naltrexone	Used primarily in opioid detoxification

It is axiomatic that opioids are commonly underused in the management of acute pain and cancer pain, and that these drugs are often overused in the management of chronic nonmalignant pain syndromes. All pain is not opioid-responsive. Neuropathic pain due to deafferentation commonly does not respond to opioids to the same degree as acute and chronic malignant pain. But there is now general agreement that a subset of patients with chronic, nonmalignant pain have symptoms that are opioid-responsive. Chronic pain syndromes that include major psychological and deconditioning components are also opioid-resistant in many cases. Other types of pain that may respond to opioids are not appropriate indications for these drugs. For example, pain due to constipation may respond to opioids, but these drugs will exacerbate the underlying condition. However, other conditions that clinicians may consider contraindications to opioids should not necessarily be categorized as such. For example, respiratory impairment may be complicated more by severe pain than by appropriately dosed opioids that can control the pain.

A basic understanding of opioid pharmacology is helpful in using these drugs wisely. Pharmacology embraces the pharmacodynamics and pharmacokinetics of drugs on cellular and organ levels. Pharmacological information is derived largely from controlled animal experiments. Clinical use of opioids must be based on both pharmacological and therapeutic principles. Therapeutics deals with the effects of drugs and nonpharmacological modalities on an organism level. Patients' biases, beliefs, fears, and preferences influence medication compliance and outcomes. For subjective complaints such as pain, patients sometimes report poor results with drugs of choice and superior outcomes from drugs that are phamacologically inferior. This discussion attempts to address both pharmacological and therapeutic aspects of opioid analgesics.

Opioids are the most effective analgesics available. That they are not effective in the management of all types of pain can be explained in part by the pathophysiology of pain. Several pain mediators and multiple receptors are involved in this process, not all of which are affected by opioids.

Pain Impulse Transmission

Pain is a physiologic and emotional response to a noxious stimulus. Nociception is the perception of a painful stimulus. This process begins at specialized, peripheral nerve endings called nociceptors, which transmit impulses to the spinal cord via primary afferent nociceptive axons that include A δ (rapidly conducting) and C (slow conducting) fibers. The painful stimulus synapses in the dorsal horn of the spinal cord, a region rich in opioid receptors. Opioids directly inhibit synaptic transmission of noxious impulses in the spinal cord and brain, and indirectly produce analgesia by increasing descending inhibitory control of the stimuli. Recent studies have demonstrated that opioids also have peripheral activity, but the full implications of that activity on analgesia are not yet clear.

The second-order neurons then cross the midline of the spinal cord, where they form the ventral and lateral ascending spinothalamic tracts to the thalamus. The spinothalamic tracts are the principal, but not the only, pain-conducting pathways to the brain. The tracts eventually pass into the limbic system and cerebral cortex to synapse with third-order neurons. There is also an inhibitory descending pathway that passes through the periaqueductal gray (PAG) to the dorsal horn. Opioids can bind to receptors anywhere along this pathway and modulate the noxious stimulus (Fig. 7.1). Opioid receptors occur throughout the body, but the highest propensity for modulation of antinociception most probably occurs in the substantia gelatinosa of the dorsal horn and PAG.

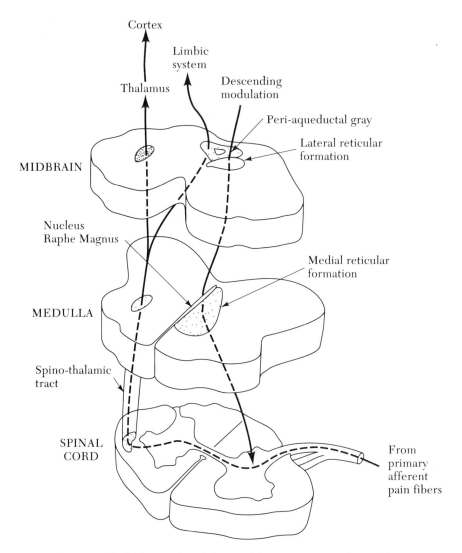

Figure 7.1. Simplified schema of modulation of the nociceptive pathway. The propensity of modulation occurs at the periaqueductal gray of the midbrain and the dorsal horn of the spinal cord. (Adapted with permission from Cousins MJ, Phillips GD, eds. *Acute Pain Management.* London: Churchill Livingstone, 1986.)

Opioid Mechanism of Action

It is not logical that morphine, an alkaloid isolated from the exudate of the opium poppy, would have a specific pharmacological receptor in the human central nervous system (CNS). Therefore, pharmacologists have long theorized the existence of endogenous, opioid-like substances. The isolation in 1975 of the endogenous opioid peptides met- and leu-enkephalin confirmed that theory. Endogenous opioid peptides act as the body's natural defense to noxious stimuli, including pain and stress. The pharmacological effects of endogenous and exogenous opioids are similar, but the latter can be administered in doses that provide more profound effects than those normally produced by the endogenous substances.

Three groups of endogenous opioids, β-endorphin, enkephalins, and dynorphin, have been identified. Each of these groups is derived from different, larger polypeptide precursors found in the adrenal medulla and pituitary. Each has different affinities for the distinct types of opioid receptors[1] (Table 7.2). Opioid receptors are glycoproteins located in cell membranes (Fig. 7.2) and are involved in potassium and calcium ion conduction. When an opioid agonist occupies and engages a receptor, an excitatory or inhibitory response may result from conformational changes in the receptor ion channel, or through a secondary messenger (e.g., cyclic AMP).

Table 7.2 Differentiated receptor affinity patterns for some opioid analgesics

Drug	μ	κ	σ
Morphine	AG + + + +	AG +	Minimal
Hydromorphone			
Meperidine			
Methadone			
Nalbuphine	ANT	pAG + + + +	Minimal
Pentazocine	ANT	AG + + + +	AG + +
Butorphanol	—	AG + + + +	AG +
Buprenorphine	pAG	Minimal	Minimal
Naloxone	ANT	ANT	ANT (incomplete)

AG = agonist, ANT = antagonist, pAG = partial agonist

+ + + + = major activity, + + = moderate activity, + = some activity, minimal = little or no activity demonstrated in laboratory studies but some activity may be seen clinically when the higher-affinity receptor types are relatively saturated.

In vitro studies of human CNS homogenates containing opioid receptors do not necessarily demonstrate all of the affinities listed in this table, e.g., morphine activity at the κ receptor. However, clinical evidence suggests that such low-level affinities do exist.

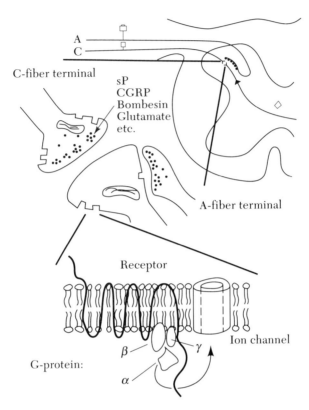

Figure 7.2. Illustration of synapse A δ and C fibers with second-order neurons in the dorsal horn of the spinal cord and proposed opioid receptor demonstrating the G protein subunits and close approximation to an ion channel. (Adapted with permission from Sabbe and Yaksh.[2])

The opioid receptor is coupled with a G protein. When that protein is coupled to an open potassium channel, neuronal inhibition occurs through hyperpolarization of the cell membrane.[2] That mechanism applies to μ and δ agonist receptor interactions. The κ agonist–receptor interaction results in inhibition when the G protein is coupled to a calcium channel. Activation of opioid receptors reduces transmission from peripheral primary afferent nerves to the higher CNS centers and also influences the processing of the pain stimulus.

The cardiovascular effects are usually inconsequential. However, opioids—morphine in particular—cause vasodilatation and histamine release that can be problematic in patients who have hypovolemia or limited cardiac reserve.

The pulmonary effects are usually not a clinical problem in patients receiving opioids chronically. Opioid-naive patients may experience respiratory depression when first exposed to large doses of the drugs. Opioids should be used with caution and titrated to effect in patients with serious pulmonary dysfunction because the drugs decrease the cough reflex, release histamine leading to bronchial constriction and possibly bronchospasm, and dry secretions.

The major gastrointestinal effect is decreased intestinal motility leading to constipation. Delayed gastric emptying appears to occur with both systemic and intrathecal opioid administration. Propulsive contractions are decreased in both the small and large intestines. Constipation should be anticipated and prevented. It should be treated aggressively with increased fluid intake and stimulating laxatives such as standardized senna concentrate or bisacodyl. Bulk laxatives, saline cathartics, and stool softeners are of limited usefulness in a narcotized gut. Opioids can cause spasm of the biliary tract.

Nausea and vomiting may occur with opioid treatment, primarily in the first few days of treatment. Many patients require concomitant antiemetic therapy only during the first few days after the opioid is initiated. Some patients actually report that they would rather suffer pain than nausea and vomiting. Effective treatment of this side effect improves patient compliance and pain control. The primary mechanism of opioid-induced nausea results from the drugs' action on the chemoreceptor trigger zone of the medulla. Therefore, most patients respond well to a centrally acting antiemetic (e.g., prochlorperazine). Motion potentiates opioid-induced nausea and vomiting in some patients through a vestibular mechanism. If that occurs, a motion sickness antiemetic (e.g., cyclizine, meclizine) should be added to the centrally acting antiemetic. When decreased gastrointestinal motility contributes to the nausea and vomiting, a gastrokinetic antiemetic (e.g., metoclopramide) can be administered orally or by the subcutaneous route.

Opioids can cause urinary retention by increasing sphincter tone. Bladder capacity is increased due to relaxation of the detrusor muscle, and μ and δ, but not κ, agonists inhibit the micturition reflex. This effect is seen more often with spinal opioids than with other routes of administration.

Pruritus usually involves the face and is more common with centrally administered opioids. It occurs in less than 10% of patients who receive epidural opioids, but nearly half of patients who receive intrathecal opioids.

Tolerance to CNS side effects including opioid-induced euphoria, dysphoria, sedation, drowsiness, confusion, and unsteadiness develops in a few days to weeks of initiating therapy for most patients.

Opioid receptors

Opioids activate (agonize) opioid receptors, which are found primarily in the central nervous system and intestinal tract, and perhaps in the periphery. Effects of opioid agonists include analgesia, sedation, decreased gastrointestinal motility, and autonomic and endocrine changes. Depressed mood, respiratory depression, nausea, and vomiting may occur. There are multiple types and subtypes of opioid receptors that have different affinities for endogenous and exogenous compounds that inhibit or excite some stimuli and not others.

Central sites

Opioids exert their analgesic (antinociceptive) effect by occupying and activating opioid receptors. Binding in the CNS occurs predominantly in the PAG and the dorsal horn. Opioid–receptor interactions in the PAG activate the descending inhibitory control system that blocks firing of the nociceptive neurons in the spinal cord. The other principal site in the CNS, the dorsal horn, continues to confound investigators. It remains uncertain whether the site of action is the presynaptic small-diameter primary afferent or the postsynaptic second-order neuron.[3,4] The evidence favors the presynaptic primary afferent neuron.[5]

Peripheral sites

Analgesia results from activation of a receptor-selective mechanism.[6] Autoradiography and receptor binding studies have demonstrated a dense localization of μ, κ, and δ opioid receptors in the dorsal horn of the spinal cord, with a significant proportion of those receptors located presynaptically on the primary afferent neurons.[7] Animal data support a dose-dependent, stereospecific, antagonist-reversible effect that is unlikely to result from local anesthetic-like action of the opioid. The peripheral antinociceptive effect of opioids is greater in inflammatory states than in normal controls in animal studies. Evidence of the efficacy of peripheral antinociception in humans is uncertain. While several human clinical trials support the peripheral mechanism, two studies of postoperative pain due to knee arthroscopy provide contradictory results. In one study, patients receiving 1 mg of intra-articular morphine had significantly less pain than patients receiving the same dose intravenously.[8] Another trial demonstrated no differences in postoperative visual analogue scale scores resulting from intra-articular injections of 3 mg of morphine in normal saline with 100 μg epinephrine and placebo injections consisting of 20 mL normal saline with 100 μg epinephrine.[9]

In 1964, the existence of three different types of opioid receptors was postulated.[10] These were then designated μ, κ, and σ based on different pharmacological profiles and differing affinities of the prototypical ligands morphine, ketocyclazocine, and the experimental agent SKF 10047 for the three receptor types, respectively. Subsequently, up to five opioid receptors and subtypes have been postulated. There is now evidence of three types of opioid receptors, two of which have known subtypes (Table 7.3). The existence of another receptor type designated the ϵ receptor has been postulated, but is still debated. The σ receptor is no longer considered an opioid receptor per se, because nonopioid substances also bind at the site, producing effects similar to

Table 7.3. Opioid receptor subtypes

Opioid receptors		
μ		Analgesia, supraspinal
		Dependence (withdrawal signs, drug-seeking behavior?)
		Sedation +
		Euphoria
		Respiratory depression
	μ_1	Analgesia
	μ_2	Undesirable effects
δ		Analgesia, spinal
		Euphoria, limbic
κ		Analgesia, spinal
		Sedation + + +
	κ_1	Kappa receptor subtypes have been demonstrated by differentiated
	κ_2	affinities for the receptors by experimental agonists. The clinical impli-
	κ_3	cations of the subtypes are not yet known.

Non–opioid-specific receptor

σ	Dysphoria
	Psychomotor stimulation (not clinically useful)
	Hallucinations

those of opioids. This receptor may be a part of the NMDA receptor and some of the actions previously attributed to the σ receptor may result from activation of one of the κ receptor subtypes.

The identification of different receptor populations is performed by correlating the pharmacological profile observed with physiologically defined effects.[3] Exogenous and endogenous μ receptor agonists are morphine, and β endorphin and met-enkephalin, respectively. Mu (μ) receptor agonists produce supraspinal analgesia, euphoria, respiratory depression, and physical dependence. The μ receptor modulates noxious thermal, pressure, and chemical stimuli. There is evidence for a high-affinity μ_1 receptor that mediates analgesia and a μ_2 receptor that mediates the adverse effects of dependence, respiratory depression, sedation, and euphoria commonly associated with morphine.[11] This work was done with experimental subtype-selective antagonists used in combination with morphine. Selective μ subtype receptor agonists have not been developed.

Kappa agonists modulate noxious stimuli, including pain and pressure, but are ineffective against thermal noxious stimuli at usual doses. The agonist–antagonist opioids are κ receptor agonists.

The δ receptor agonist leu-enkephalin mediates μ analgesia and seems to potentiate morphine analgesia. The δ receptor modulates thermal and chemical noxious stimuli, but to a lesser extent than the μ receptor. No commercially produced δ agonists are currently available.

Agonist, antagonist, partial agonist, and agonist–antagonists

The lock and key receptor occupation analogy is a good basic concept to illustrate the receptor–agonist interaction.[12] Agonists bind to receptors causing an action. Antagonists bind to receptors (competitive) or near receptors (noncompetitive) to prevent an action or displace the agonist, thereby terminating the action. Partial agonists bind to parts of the receptor, resulting in an action of lesser magnitude than a "pure" agonist. Such incomplete binding often produces a dose ceiling effect. As Figure 7.3 illustrates, agonist–antagonist and partial agonist opioids may precipitate withdrawal symptoms in a patient receiving a μ agonist. The figure also illustrates the dose ceiling effect that occurs with both agonist-antagonists and partial agonists. It is noteworthy that pure opioid agonists do not demonstrate a dose ceiling. Increasing doses provide increasing analgesia over a very broad dose range.

Common Opioid Controversies and Misconceptions

All of the pure μ agonist opioids are equianalgesic at appropriate dosing regimens (Table 7.4). However, some patients may experience better responses to one of these agents than to others.[13] Potency simply reflects the amount of drug needed for effect. Greater potency does not imply greater efficacy.

Many of the issues that clinicians find controversial about opioid therapy are due to outdated beliefs about the drugs. No caregiver wants his or her patients to suffer pain. But frequently, indicated opioids are not ordered, because of invalid fears of adverse events. Many persons extrapolate the experience of drug abusers to patients in pain. When abused as recreational substances, opioids have effects very different from those when they are used clinically. Opioids are abused to obtain a "high" or prevent withdrawal. The desired outcome of medical use of opioids is relief of symptoms while maintaining as normal a sensorium as possible. Applying drug abusers' experience to patients in pain produces invalid conclusions. Many pharmacological studies of opioids have used single doses that provide information that often does not apply to multiple dosing. Outcomes from studies utilizing "prn" dosing differ from outcomes obtained with scheduled dosing. Although animal models are valuable in characterizing the pharmacology of a drug, such models often provide data that do not apply to humans, in whom cognitive processes can profoundly influence outcomes. That is especially true when the drug is used for a complaint as subjective as pain. Artifacts from such studies are the basis for several common, false beliefs about opioids. For these reasons, among others, misconceptions about opioids often lead to less than optimal patient care. Some of these beliefs are described and refuted below.

Maximum doses

There is no maximum safe dose of morphine and other pure μ-agonist opioids. An interpatient variance of up to 50-fold has been reported for the dose of morphine required to provide pain relief.[14,15] Serum levels are not useful indicators of efficacy for opioids due to interpatient variability in response. Only titration to response will consistently and reliably determine the optimal dose for a specific patient. Median oral morphine doses that provide pain relief for advanced cancer patients have commonly been in the range of 10 to 20 mg every 4 hours,[16,17] but several hundred milligrams per dose may be required by some patients. Using median doses as a starting point, clinicians should increase the dose aggressively (i.e., 30%–50% at each dosing interval) until pain relief is obtained. It is important to increase opioid doses by the stated percentages of the previous dose, not by a fixed amount. Most clinicians would normally increase a 30 mg dose of morphine that is inadequate to 45 mg, a 50% increase. Likewise, a less-than-effective 150 mg dose should be increased to 200–225 mg, not by 15 to 30 mg. Inadequate dose increases often lead to the false conclusion that the pain is opioid-resistant or that tolerance has limited the usefulness of the drug.

Pure μ agonist opioid analgesic oral doses should be increased until either acceptable analgesia is achieved or unacceptable side effects occur. If sedation is problematic, addition of low doses of a central stimulant (e.g., methylphenidate 5 mg morning and noon) can be added.[18] Many patients experience nausea during the first few days of opioid administration, but become tolerant to that effect within 3 to 5 days. Addition of a centrally acting antiemetic (e.g., prochlorperazine) can be useful during the first few days of opioid therapy. If the patient experiences decreased GI motility, an antiemetic that acts both centrally and as a gastrokinetic agent (e.g., metoclopramide) may be more effective. One quarter to one third of patients experience vestibular disturbance when opioid therapy is initiated. If motion exacerbates the nausea, an antiemetic useful for motion sickness (e.g., cyclizine, meclizine) can be added to the centrally acting antiemetic.

These principles of dose titration do not apply to codeine, agonist–antagonist, or partial agonist opioids, however, because these drugs produce relative dose ceiling effects. There appears to be a diminishing return on increasing oral codeine doses above 65 or 100 mg per dose (clinical observation). Increasing the dose above 65 or 100 mg provides decreasing incremental analgesia, but full incremental side effects. The reason for this is not clear, but it suggests that codeine may be a partial μ-agonist. Therefore, once a 100-mg dose of oral codeine every 4 hours has been reached without adequate pain relief, a change to morphine or another potent pure μ-agonist opioid may be in order. The agonist–antagonist opioids (pentazocine, nalbuphine, butorphanol, dezocine) and partial agonist opioid (buprenorphine) have dose ceilings. Doses in excess of those ceilings produce little or no additional analgesia, but do

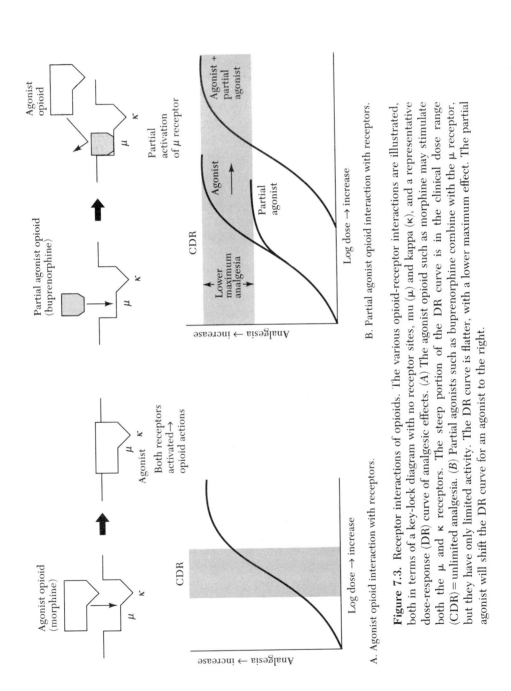

Figure 7.3. Receptor interactions of opioids. The various opioid-receptor interactions are illustrated, both in terms of a key-lock diagram with no receptor sites, mu (μ) and kappa (κ), and a representative dose-response (DR) curve of analgesic effects. (A) The agonist opioid such as morphine may stimulate both the μ and κ receptors. The steep portion of the DR curve is in the clinical dose range (CDR) = unlimited analgesia. (B) Partial agonists such as buprenorphine combine with the μ receptor, but they have only limited activity. The DR curve is flatter, with a lower maximum effect. The partial agonist will shift the DR curve for an agonist to the right.

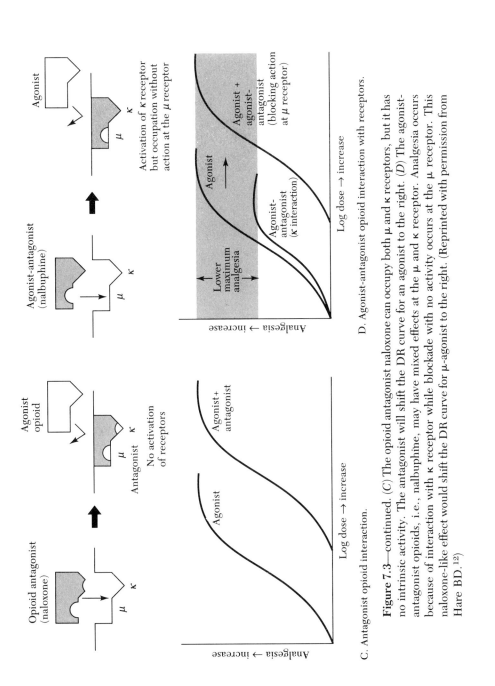

C. Antagonist opioid interaction.

D. Agonist-antagonist opioid interaction with receptors.

Figure 7.3—continued. (C) The opioid antagonist naloxone can occupy both μ and κ receptors, but it has no intrinsic activity. The antagonist will shift the DR curve for an agonist to the right. (D) The agonist-antagonist opioids, i.e., nalbuphine, may have mixed effects at the μ and κ receptor. Analgesia occurs because of interaction with κ receptor while blockade with no activity occurs at the μ receptor. This naloxone-like effect would shift the DR curve for μ-agonist to the right. (Reprinted with permission from Hare BD.[12])

Table 7.4. Comparative dosing data for selected opioid analgesics

Drug	Approximate equianalgesic oral dose (mg)	Approximate equianalgesic IM dose (mg)	Approximate Approximate onset PO IM (min)		Eauianalgesic dosing interval (hours)
Morphine	30 regular schedule	10	20	15	4–6
	60 prn dosing	10			
Methadone*	20	10	30	20	6–8
Levorphanol	4	2	30	20	6–8
Hydromorphone	4–6	1.5–2	20	15	4
Meperidine	150–250†	75–100	15	10	2.5–3.5
Codeine	130‡	75	20	15	4–6
Buprenorphine	Not available (sub-lingual available in Europe—in trials in U.S.)	0.3–0.4†	—	25	6–8
Butorphanol	Not available	2†	—	20	3–4
Nalbuphine	Not available	10†	—	20	3–6
Pentazocine	150†	60†	20	15	3–6
Oxycodone	10 mg is clinically equivalent to 10–20 mg of oral morphine. The maximum safe daily dose of oxycodone 5 mg/acetaminophen 325 mg is 12 tablets (~4 g of acetaminophen) due to potential for hepatotoxicity. Plain oxycodone can be titrated to higher doses much like morphine. OxyContin labeling recommends a dose ratio of oxycodone to morphine of 1:2. A ratio of 3:4 may be more accurate.					
Fentanyl, transdermal	a 50 μg/hr patch provides analgesia similar to 10 mg of oral morphine administered on a regular q 4 hour schedule, which is equal to 30 mg of sustained-acting morphine administered q 12 h. Patients with fever (e.g., tumor fever) may experience only about 48 hours of analgesia from a patch; fever or exogenous heat (e.g., heat lamps, electric blankets) may accelerate drug release. The patch requires a mean of 17 hours to reach peak blood levels and effects remain for 12–24 hours after removing a patch. Patches cannot be used effectively to titrate doses.					

*Due to its long and variable half-life, methadone must be administered cautiously; in practice, the potency is often assumed to be much greater than depicted in standard equianalgesic dose tables.

†Meperidine and agonist–antagonist analgesics are *not* recommended for cancer pain management because of potential adverse effects.

‡Codeine doses above 65 mg are usually not appropriate because of diminishing incremental analgesia with increasing doses but continually increasing constipation side effect.

Published tables vary in their suggested equianalgesic doses. Clinical response is the criterion that must be applied for each patient. Because there is not complete cross tolerance among these drugs, in patients whose pain is well controlled it is usually necessary to use a dose 10%–20% lower than equianalgesic doses when changing opioid drugs and then retitrate to response. If pain is not well controlled, use an equianalgesic or 10%–20% higher dose of the new opioid drug and then retitrate to response.

produce additional side effects. Therefore, the maximum doses listed in the labeling for these drugs should not be exceeded.

One pure μ-agonist opioid that should not be aggressively titrated is meperidine. This drug provides analgesia comparable to morphine at appropriate doses and dosing intervals, but it is metabolized to 6-desmethylmeperidine (normeperidine), a cerebral irritant[19] that has an elimination half-life more than four times longer than the parent compound. Therefore, this metabolite accumulates with continued dosing, especially in patients with impaired renal function, which can produce toxicities ranging from mood irritability to seizures. As a result, meperidine should not be used for more than 2 or 3 days and should be avoided in patients with severe renal impairment, especially the elderly.

Addiction and dependence

Many clinicians believe that opioids routinely cause addiction and therefore must be used with great restraint. This is patently false. Addiction is a compulsion or overpowering drive to take the drug in order to experience psychological effects.[20] Dependence is a pharmacological phenomenon that usually can be eliminated rapidly through tapering of the dose. Opioids cause dependence routinely when used for more than a few days, as do beta-blockers and other common drug classes. Dependence can be easily managed by titrating the patient off the drug over a period of about 5 days.[21] When opioids are used appropriately to treat patients in opioid-responsive pain, addiction is exquisitely rare. For chronic pain patients in whom opioids are indicated, addiction is rarely an issue. A study of 11,882 patients who received opioids for medical indications and were monitored for dependence revealed only four cases of addiction in patients who did not have a previous history of substance abuse.[22] Unnecessary fear of addiction is a major reason that opioids are underused.

Many caregivers assume that patients who demand increasing opioid doses are becoming tolerant or addicted. Patients in pain who demand more drug usually do so because of their pain. Mean dose and duration data are useful as starting points, but patients vary greatly in the amount of drug they require and the duration of relief that they receive from the opioids. The resulting phenomenon has been described as *pseudoaddiction*.[23] The most common reason for patients requesting seemingly inappropriate amounts of opioids is that insufficient amounts were ordered to manage their pain adequately. This occurs commonly with meperidine, which provides only 2.5 to 3.5 hours of relief for most patients. Morphine may provide only 3 hours of relief for some patients. Individualization of dosing times is important. An occasional patient will "scam" the system to obtain opioids. But that is not a reason for many other patients to suffer unnecessary pain.

Tolerance

Tolerance is a reduced effect from repeated doses of the same drug or repeated doses of drugs in the same class. Tolerance to opioids is widely believed to be a serious limitation on clinical use of the drugs. But consistent clinical experience does not support that belief. Tolerance has been documented by animal studies. In humans, the phenomenon does appear to occur with initial dosing, but it need not be a clinical problem. This effect is believed to result from second-messenger effects, not alterations in the opioid receptors per se. Most of the effects of tolerance appear to occur in the first week or two of therapy, and titration to response obviates clinical implications of tolerance. With continued opioid dosing as in cancer pain, patients' dose requirements usually remain stable over weeks to months unless the disease progresses.[24,25] Increased dose requirements may well indicate progressive disease, not tolerance. Dose requirements of many advanced cancer patients decrease with resolution of tumor size, decreased anxiety, destruction of nerve endings in painful organs or tissues secondary to disease or treatment, or other co-morbidity. Many patients, and some caregivers, believe that if morphine is used early in the course of a progressive, painful disease, there will be nothing left to treat the pain when it gets really bad. Morphine has a relatively straight-line dose response curve with a broad therapeutic range. Therefore, low-dose morphine may be appropriate when the pain is not very advanced and high-dose morphine may be used as the pain progresses. Since tolerance is not a clinical issue, morphine (or another potent opioid) should be started as soon as it is indicated. Additional research is needed to explain the inconsistent response to opioids that is commonly attributed to tolerance.

Respiratory depression

Fears of opioid-induced respiratory depression often prevent clinicians from using the analgesics, especially in patients with preexisting respiratory compromise. Opioids do depress respiration and must be used with caution in patients with impaired respiratory capability. However, pain impairs breathing in many patients, especially patients with chest disease or injury. Many patients breathe more deeply and efficiently only after their pain is controlled. Patients receiving opioids for severe pain may be wrongly thought to be in respiratory difficulty because their respiratory rate drops following initiation of the analgesic. The more probable explanation is that the patient can inspire more deeply and therefore no longer needs to take rapid, shallow breaths after pain management is achieved. Clinical appearance is often a better indicator than just the respiratory rate. A study of patients with lung cancer who received aggressive opioid analgesia to provide pain relief revealed that the drugs did not adversely affect the patients' arterial blood gases.[26]

Influence of route of administration

Many patients and caregivers falsely believe that parenteral opioids are more potent and more effective than oral analgesics. In acute postoperative or trauma pain when patients are unable to take medications orally, parenteral therapy is clearly indicated. Parenteral therapy offers more rapid onset of action than oral therapy for most drugs. However, injected opioids must be absorbed from intramuscular and subcutaneous injection sites and peak levels may not be reached for half an hour or more. Oral therapy requires a slightly longer time to reach analgesic and peak serum levels. When opioids are administered on a regular schedule (so that each subsequent dose takes effect before the previous dose loses all of its effect), there is no advantage of parenteral over oral administration. When patients are able to take medication orally, there are pharmacologic, economic, and psychological advantages to doing so. Oral doses often provide more consistent serum levels than subcutaneous or intramuscular doses, are equally effective if the appropriate dose is administered, and are less expensive than injections. When the oral route is not available, rectal suppositories and sublingual administration should be considered before resorting to the more invasive and expensive parenteral routes. Some patients may require intermittent parenteral therapy, but oral therapy should be restarted when the patient is able to take drugs by mouth again.

Intravenous administration provides more rapid peak serum levels than other parenteral routes. Intramuscular injection is painful. Subcutaneous administration offers increased patient comfort over IM administration and similar pharmacokinetics in most cases.

Morphine has been used by nebulization for analgesia and terminal dyspnea. This route provides effective serum levels, but may offer little advantage over sublingual or buccal administration of simple aqueous solutions of morphine or lactose-based (molded, not compressed) morphine tablets. These routes provide inconsistent bioavailability. Much of the drug administered buccally or sublingually may not be absorbed across oral muscosa; it may be absorbed from the GI tract after trickling down the throat in saliva. The bioavailability of opioids administered by these routes is not consistently high, but patients often experience good symptom control when the doses are titrated to response.

Fentanyl is commercially available in the United States as a transdermal patch and oral transmucosal dosage form. The former is useful when patients cannot or will not take drug orally or rectally and have a consistent opioid dose requirement. Although fentanyl is an inherently rapid-acting drug, the transdermal dosage form is very slow acting because the opioid is released at a controlled rate from the patch, depots in the subcutaneous fat, and must cross the stratum corneum to be absorbed. Due to the long time ($\sim$17 hours) to steady-state serum levels following application of a patch, this dosage form does not permit rapid dose titration. Oral, transmucosal fentanyl provides rapid serum levels and is useful both for sedation and analgesia prior to procedures and when patients who are taking consistent opioid doses experience breakthrough pain.[27]

Intranasal butorphanol is commercially available. This is a useful dosage form inasmuch as the drug cannot be administered orally. It is important that patients be instructed how to administer the intranasal drug correctly to prevent excessive and inappropriate use.

Opioids often are administered via patient-controlled analgesia (PCA) pumps that allow patients to self-administer predetermined doses no more often than predetermined "lockout" time intervals. PCA provides excellent analgesia for many patients postoperatively and is useful for determining opioid dose requirements.[28] PCA offers no clinical or pharmacokinetic advantage over regularly scheduled opioids[29] and there is a real risk of adverse outcomes if appropriate monitoring is not provided.[30] But PCA does provide a sense of control to many patients and, if the pump is properly programmed, assures that drug is available when needed. PCA is most commonly used intravenously, but epidural and subcutaneous PCA has also been used successfully.

Other false beliefs about opioid analgesics exist. Clinicians should ask patients and their families about their beliefs concerning opioids and should provide accurate information to refute those false beliefs.

Guidelines for Clinical Use of Opioids

Several important sets of clinical practice guidelines relating to the use of opioids have appeared. The World Health Organization published *Cancer Pain Relief*[31] in 1986, which was expanded to *Cancer Pain Relief and Palliative Care*[32] in 1990 and further expanded in 1996. The American Pain Society has now published three editions of *Principles of Analgesic Use in the Treatment of Acute Pain and Cancer Pain.*[33] The U.S. Department of Health and Human Services Agency for Health Care Policy and Research has published Clinical Practice Guidelines on Acute Pain Management[34] and Cancer Pain Management[35] in 1992 and 1994, respectively. In 1994, the International Association for the Study of Pain published *Management of Acute Pain:A Practical Guide.*[36] All of these documents support similar opioid use that can be summarized into five principles.

Use oral dosage forms whenever possible

The oral route of administration provides clinically effective opioid serum levels for most patients. The only advantage of parenteral administration is a slightly shorter time to onset of activity and peak serum levels. That advantage is obviated when oral drug is administered on a regular schedule. When oral administration is not feasible, rectal administration often provides comparable efficacy. When patients experience good analgesia but unacceptable sedation with oral opioids, epidural administration might be considered. This route provides excellent analgesia with fewer systemic side effects. However, the epidural space is vascular. Therefore, systemic uptake does occur. The intrathecal route bypasses that disadvantage, but carries greater risk of adverse events. The most serious of these are epidural abscesses and meningitis.

The oral-to-parenteral dose ratio for morphine often causes confusion. Single-dose studies indicate a 6:1 ratio—60 mg of oral morphine is equivalent to 10 mg of the drug administered parenterally. But the ratio for regularly scheduled dosing is closer to 3:1—30 mg of oral morphine is equivalent to 10 mg of parenteral drug. This was once thought to be due to a pharmacokinetic first-pass phenomenon. However, the metabolic pathways for morphine are not saturable. The different dose ratios are now attributed to accumulation of the active metabolite morphine-6-glucuronide (M-6-G), which has a longer half-life than the parent compound. The ratio of M-6-G to parent compound varies with the route of administration, being approximately two times greater with the oral route.[37] Other opioids do not have as large route-dependent dose ratio differences.

Dosing must be individualized

As noted above, titration to response is the only reliable way to determine the optimal opioid dose for a given patient.

Regularly scheduled dosing is indicated when there is an ongoing pain insult

Maintaining an effective opioid concentration at the receptors is essential to prevent recurrence of pain. It is important to note that pain sensitizes the primary afferent nerve fibers and causes biochemical changes in the dorsal horn of the spinal cord. These effects increase the patient's sensitivity to pain and can produce a chronic pain syndrome.[38] Most patients do not comply consistently with every-4-hour opioid dosing. The inherently long-acting opioids methadone and levorphanol allow dosing every 8 to 12 hours, but carry a risk of accumulation toxicity if the patients are not carefully monitored for insidious onset of CNS depressive symptoms. Pharmaceutically long-acting dosage forms (e.g., sustained-acting morphine and oxycodone) offer the advantage of every-12-hour dosing, providing consistent serum levels.

Chronic pain that is well controlled with regularly scheduled opioid dosing sometimes breaks through or is exacerbated by incidental events in the patient's life. Therefore, it is important to provide "prn" doses of opioid for breakthrough or incidental pain in addition to the regularly scheduled doses. A typical prn dose would be one half the amount of every-4-hour morphine every 2 hours prn in a rapid-acting dosage form (i.e., oral liquid or immediate-release tablets and capsules). If a patient is taking a 12-hour sustained-acting morphine tablet, one sixth of that dose should be available prn every 2 hours in a rapid-release form.

Opioid doses should be increased according to the analgesic ladder

The WHO defined an analgesic ladder consisting of three steps (Fig. 7.4); analgesia should be started on the appropriate step of the ladder for the patient. Often, that is not the first step. When a nonsteroidal anti-inflammatory drug (NSAID) or acetaminophen is insufficient to manage the pain, an opioid should be added to the nonopioid; the opioid should not replace the nonopioid.[39]

The ladder tends to oversimplify opioid use in many cases. It is important to treat the underlying cause of the pain, which may or may not be opioid responsive. Examples of such causes are listed in Table 7.5.

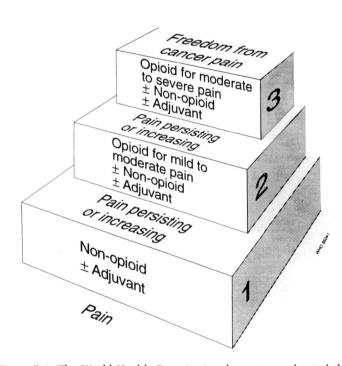

Figure 7.4. The World Health Organization three-step analgesic ladder.

Table 7.5. Examples of drugs that may be useful in pain of different etiologies

Etiology	Drug
Bone pain	NSAIDs with or without opioids
Deafferentation pain	Tricyclic antidepressants, anticonvulsants, topical capsaicin, oral systemic local anesthetics
Tissue damage due to infection	Antibiotics and analgesics
Gastrointestinal spasm	Anticholinergics
Constipation	Laxatives
Arterial ischemia	Peripheral vasodilators

Appropriate adjunctive drug therapy is essential for pain control

In addition to NSAIDs and opioids, many patients in pain require additional drugs as co-analgesics or to treat concomitant symptoms. Stimulating laxatives are essential adjuncts to regularly scheduled opioids because tolerance to opioid-induced constipation does not occur. Antidepressants, antianxiety agents, short courses of muscle relaxants, and other symptomatic agents may be needed to provide comfort to a patient in pain.

Barriers to Opioid Use

Opioids often are used less than optimally. This is not because clinicians want their patients to experience pain. It is due largely to misinformation, fears, and other barriers to the use of these drugs. Many of these barriers are more perceived than real. Prescribers, nurses, pharmacists, patients, their family members and friends, and society in general often present barriers to appropriate opioid use.

It is important that education programs on the evils of "drugs" for school-children differentiate between abused substances and legitimate medications. Billboards, placards on buses, and public service announcements in the broadcast media continually warn people to avoid drugs. Parents often induce fear of medications in their children through well-intentioned attempts to discourage the children's use of illicit drugs.

Clinicians' concerns about regulatory oversight often produce hesitancy to use indicated opioids. Today, many controlled-substance regulatory agencies and inspectors explicitly will not investigate cases of high-dose opioid use if the regulators know that the drugs are being used for appropriate indications.[40] When caregivers proactively inform regulators of intended opioid use for appropriate indications, all parties may benefit. Organizations such as the American Pain Society and State Cancer Pain Initiatives continue to work with legislatures and regulatory agencies to prevent inappropriate regulatory oversight.

Fear of addiction is a great barrier to many patients taking opioids. Often, patients are willing to take the medications after their caregivers explain the facts, but friends and family members discourage use of the medications because of their own inappropriate fear of addiction. Education and continual reminders to patients, families, and their support groups is needed. Refutation of inaccurate reports of iatrogenic addiction in the media also are important.

Fears of opioid-induced respiratory depression sometimes discourage the prescribing and administration of opioids. Commonly, opioid orders carry a notation to stop the drug and administer an opioid antagonist if the patient's respiratory rate drops below 10 or 12 per minute. More often than not, patients' respiratory rates drop and their gas exchange improves due to deeper breathing only after they get relief from their pain. Clinical observation and pulse oximetry are far better indicators of oxygenation than respiratory rate per se.

Fear of tolerance is usually misplaced. Many patients with progressive, painful diseases refuse to take opioids when they are needed because they fear

---

Numerical Rating Scale for Pain (NRS)

The patient is asked to rank present pain on a scale of zero to ten, with zero being no pain and ten being pain as bad as the patient can imagine.

Visual Analog Scale for Pain (VAS)

No   Pain as bad
pain   as it can be

Instructions: Make a mark on this line that indicates the level of your pain right now.

(The line is 10 cm long. To quantify the pain, measure the line with a mm rule and record the pain level as 1 to 100.)

Figure 7.5. Pain should be assessed and reassessed frequently, utilizing objective scales.

there will be nothing to take when the pain "really gets bad." It is important to educate patients that opioids will not lose their effect and that doses can be increased to comfort levels if the pain increases.

Many patients do not receive indicated opioids because they fail to communicate pain effectively to their caregivers. This may be due to fears that they will be labeled as "bad" patients if they complain. Clinicians should explain to patients why it is important to communicate pain and teach patients how to do so using objective indices such as visual analogue scales or numerical rating scales (Fig. 7.5). Clinicians should use these scales regularly and adjust analgesic doses when pain levels change.

Opioids sometimes are effective and should be used for indications in which they normally are not effective or appropriate. For example, patients with chronic myofascial and neurogenic pain who are unable to carry out activities of daily living without opioids, but who can do so with regularly scheduled, low-dose analgesics, may be good candidates for these drugs.[41] Use of pharmacological principles alone often will not result in optimal outcomes from opioid therapy. Nonpharmacological modalities should be used in combination with drug therapy. By applying sound pharmacology with good therapeutics, clinicians can manage pain far more effectively than often occurs today.

References

1. Franz DN. Pharmacology of analgesic receptors. *J Pharm Care Pain Symptom Control* 1994; 2(3):37–58.
2. Sabbe MB, Yaksh TL. Pharmacology of spinal opioids. *J Pain Symptom Manage* 1990; 5(3):191–203.
3. Yaksh TL. Spinal opiate analgesia: characteristics and principles of action. *Pain* 1981; 11:293–346.
4. Basbaum AI. Mechanisms of substance P-mediated nociception and opioid-mediated antinociception. In: Stanley TH, Ashburn MA, eds. *Anesthesiology and Pain Management*. Dordrecht, Netherlands: Kluwer Academic Publishers; 1994:1–17.
5. Dado RJ, Law PY, Elde R. Immunofluorescent identification of a delta opioid receptor on primary afferent nerve terminals. *Neuroreport* 1993; 5(3):341–344.
6. Hargreaves KM, Joris JL. The peripheral analgesic effects of opioids. *APS Journal* 1993; 2(1):51–59.
7. Taiwo YO, Levine JD. Opioid receptor subtype mediating peripheral antinociception. *APS Journal* 1993; 2(1):72–76.
8. Stein C, Comisel K, Haimerl E, et al. Analgesic effects of intraarticular morphine after arthroscopic knee surgery. *N Engl J Med* 1991; 325:1123–1126.
9. Raja SN, Dickstein RE, Johnson CA. Comparison of postoperative analgesic effects of intraarticular bupivacaine and morphine following arthroscopic knee surgery. *Anesthesiology* 1992; 77:1143–1147.
10. Goldstein A. Opioid peptides: function and significance. In: Collier HOJ, Hughs J,

Rance MJ, Tyers MB, eds. *Opioids: Past, Present and Future.* London: Taylor and Frances Ltd; 1984.

11. Pasternak GW, Wood PJ. Minireview: Multiple mu opiate receptors. *Life Sci* 1986; 38(21):1889–1898.

12. Hare BD. The opioid analgesics: rational selection of agents for acute and chronic pain. *Hospital Formulary* 1987; 22(1):64–86.

13. Galer BS, Coyle N, Pasternak GW, et al. Individual variability in the response to different opioids: report of five cases. *Pain* 1992; 49:87–91.

14. Walsh TD. Research in advanced cancer. In: Teller N, ed. *Hospice: The Living Idea.* London: Edward Arnold Ltd; 1981:101–122.

15. Twycross RG. Morphine and diamorphine in the terminally ill patient. *Acta Anaesth Scand* 1982; Suppl 74:128–134.

16. Aherne GW, Piall EM. Twycross RG. Serum morphine concentrations after oral administration of diamorphine hydrochloride and morphine sulfate. *Br J Clin Pharmacol* 1979; 8:577.

17. Walsh TD. Oral morphine in chronic cancer pain. *Pain* 1984; 18:1–11.

18. Bruera E, Brenneis C, Chadwick S, et al. Methylphenidate associated with narcotics for the treatment of cancer pain. *Cancer Treat Rep* 1987; 71:67–70.

19. Kaiko RF, Foley KM, Grabinsky PY, Heidrich G, Rogers, AG, Inturissi CE, Reidenberg MM. Central nervous system excitatory effects of meperidine in cancer patients. *Ann Neurol* 1983; 3:180–185.

20. Twycross RG. Opioids. In: Wall PD, Melzack R, eds. *Textbook of Pain.* 3rd ed. London: Churchill Livingstone; 1994:943–962.

21. Hare BD, Lipman AG. Uses and misuses of medication in the management of chronic, noncancer pain. *Problems in Anesthesia* 1990; 4:577–594.

22. Porter J, Jick H. Addiction rare in patients treated with narcotics (letter). *N Engl J Med* 1980; 302:123.

23. Weissman DE, Haddox JD. Opioid pseudoaddiction: an iatrogenic syndrome. *Pain* 1989; 36:363–366.

24. Twycross RG. Clinical experience with diamorphine in advanced malignant disease. *Int J Clin Pharmacol* 1974; 9:184–198.

25. Collins E, Poulain P, Gauvin-Piquard A, et al. Is disease progression the major factor in morphine "tolerance" in cancer pain treatment? *Pain* 1993; 55:319–326.

26. Walsh TD, Baxter R, Bowman KB, Leber B. High dose morphine and respiratory function in chronic cancer pain (abstract) *Pain* 1981; Suppl 1:S39.

27. Ashburn MA, Lipman AG. Management of pain in the cancer patient. *Anesth Anal* 1993; 76:402–416.

28. Bollish SJ, Collins CL, Kirking DM, Bartlett RH. Efficacy of patient-controlled versus conventional analgesia for postoperative pain. *Clin Pharm* 1985; 4:48–52.

29. Klieman RL, Lipman AG, Hare BD, MacDonald S. A comparison of morphine administered by patient-controlled analgesia and regularly scheduled intramuscular injections in severe, postoperative pain. *J Pain Symptom Manage* 1988; 3:15–22.

30. Ashburn MA, Love G, Pace N. Respiratory-related critical events with intravenous patient-controlled analgesia. *Clin J Pain* 1994; 10:52–56.

31. World Health Organization. *Cancer Pain Relief.* Technical Report Series. Geneva: World Health Organization; 1986.

32. WHO Expert Committee. *Cancer Pain Relief and Palliative Care*. Technical Report Series 804. Geneva: World Health Organization; 1990.

33. American Pain Society. *Principles of Analgesic Use in the Treatment of Acute Pain and Chronic Cancer Pain*. 3rd ed. Skokie, Ill.: American Pain Society; 1992.

34. Acute Pain Management Guideline Panel. *Acute Pain Management: Operative or Medical Procedures and Trauma; Clinical Practice Guideline*. AHCPR Publication Number 92–0032. Rockville, Md.: Agency for Health Care Policy and Research, U.S. Department of Health and Human Services, Public Health Service; 1992.

35. Jacox A, Carr DB, Payne R, et al. *Management of Cancer Pain. Clinical Practice Guideline*. AHCPR Publication Number 94–0592. Rockville Md.: Agency for Health Care Policy and Research, U.S. Department of Health and Human Services, Public Health Service; 1994.

36. Ready LB, Edwards WT, eds. *Management of Acute Pain: A Practical Guide*. International Association for the Study of Pain. Seattle: IASP Publications; 1992.

37. Tiseo PJ, Thaler HT, Lapin J, Inturissi CE, Portenoy RK, Foley KM. Morphine-6-glucuronide concentrations and opioid-related side effects: a survey in cancer patients. *Pain* 1995; 61:47–54.

38. Mendell LM. Physiological properties of unmyelinated fibre projections to the spinal cord. *Exp Neurol* 1966; 16:316–332.

39. Weingart WA, Sorkness CA, Earhart RW. Analgesia with oral narcotics and added ibuprofen in cancer patients. *Clin Pharm* 1985; 4:33.

40. Robinson DE. Prescribing controlled substances for cancer pain: position paper of the Utah Division of Occupational and Professional Licensing. *J Pharm Care in Pain Symptom Control* 1993; 1:109–112.

41. Portenoy RK. Chronic opioid therapy in non-malignant pain. *J Pain Symptom Manage* 1990; 5:S46–S62.

8

Clinical Implications
of Morphine Metabolites

PER SJØGREN

Morphine is the most widely used opioid analgesic and remains the "gold standard" when the effects of other analgesic drugs are to be compared. Morphine is a hydrophilic phenanthrene alkaloid, which is a natural constituent of opium. With its pKa of 7.9, 23% is unprotonized in plasma at physiological pH. About 30% of morphine is bound to plasma proteins. In humans, the mean volume of distribution ranges from 1.2 to 6.2 L/kg, the mean elimination half-life ranges from 1.7 to 4.5 hours, and the mean clearance ranges from 6.4 to 23 L/kg/min.[1,2] Absorption after parenteral administration averages 90% within 45 minutes, whereas oral bioavailability is low and variable (15%–65%).[3,4] In humans the predominant metabolic pathway for morphine is glucuronidation.[5] The high hepatic extraction rate of 0.7 indicates the important first-pass effect and explains the low oral bioavailability. To a much lesser extent, biotransformation takes place in the kidneys and lungs. The glucuronides, which are the main metabolites, are eliminated via bile and urine. Smaller amounts are excreted via sweat and breast milk. Ninety percent of the total elimination takes place within one day. The conjugation rate seems to increase gradually during chronic use of morphine.

The widely held view that only a single monoglucuronide, morphine-3-glucuronide (M-3-G), is formed from morphine was rejected by the observation over 20 years ago that morphine-6-glucuronide (M-6-G) is also produced in humans.[6,7] The first indication of the potential clinical relevance of M-6-G was the demonstration of its analgesic activity in mice, where subcutaneous injection of M-6-G proved to be four times as potent as morphine and intracerebral administration was approximately 45 to 200 times more potent than the parent drug.[8,9] However, evidence suggesting that M-6-G is produced from morphine in negligible quantities discouraged further investigation of its properties for years.[5]

The development of a sensitive and specific assay for morphine and its glucuronide metabolites by Svensson and coworkers[10] revealed for the first time that M-6-G was present in abundance after chronic oral morphine administration and that the area under the plasma concentration–time curve (AUC) exceeded that of morphine by many times. Single-dose studies of intravenous, oral, buccal, and sublingual morphine confirmed the quantitative significance of M-6-G relative to morphine. Although single doses of oral morphine yield relatively little M-6-G because of the poor bioavailability for unconjugated morphine and the delay in achieving adequate concentrations of M-6-G,[11] chronic oral morphine therapy produces an increasing concentration of this metabolite. Studies in cancer patients have also confirmed that the M-6-G:morphine ratio is higher with oral than parenteral administration;[12] this phenomenon is presumably a result of first-pass glucuronidation through the liver and, perhaps, the bowel wall. In patients with cancer pain, the molar M-6-G:morphine ratio during oral therapy has ranged from 4:1 to 9:1, and a linear relationship between morphine dose and both morphine and M-6-G concentration has been demonstrated.[12]

M-6-G has been demonstrated to be an extremely strong μ-opioid agonist, and its effects are easily reversed by naloxone.[13,14] However, the clinical effects of M-6-G, like other opioid agonists, would be predicted based on the ability of the compound to reach its site of action. Due to distribution, less than 0.1% of the dosage reaches sites of action in the central nervous system. This is probably one of many reasons for a poor correlation between pharmacokinetic data and pharmacodynamic effects. A study in cancer patients receiving chronic morphine therapy showed that M-6-G in plasma is distributed into cerebrospinal fluid (CSF), but to a far lesser extent than morphine itself; plasma contained approximately twice as much M-6-G as morphine, whereas CSF contained only one fifth to one third as much.[15] Another study showed that CSF concentrations of M-6-G were substantially higher in patients receiving chronic oral morphine, compared with those measured after single doses, and that M-6-G takes several hours to reach peak concentrations within the CSF after oral administration of morphine.[16]

Another study in cancer patients during chronic morphine therapy showed that morphine, M-6-G, and M-3-G were distributed into the CSF and that M-3-G has a similar CSF:serum distribution as M-6-G.[17] A recent study in cancer patients treated with chronic controlled-release oral morphine examined plasma and CSF minimum steady-state concentrations of morphine, M-6-G, and M-3-G;[18] both plasma and CSF morphine, M-3-G, and M-6-G concentrations were linearly correlated with dose of morphine, and the mean steady-state concentrations of M-3-G and M-6-G, in order of priority, substantially exceeded those of morphine in CSF as well as in plasma. These findings were in accordance with a study by Vandongen and coworkers,[19] who measured concentrations of morphine, M-6-G, and M-3-G in plasma and CSF in cancer patients receiving oral controlled-release morphine chronically; they found a close correlation between plasma and CSF morphine concentrations, both of which were correlated with morphine dose. Furthermore, M-3-G and M-6-G in plasma and CSF were correlated. Samuelsson and coworkers examined CSF and plasma concentrations of morphine and the glucuronides in cancer patients receiving chronic epidural morphine;[20] they found that the M-3-G and M-6-G metabolites in CSF were so low compared to unchanged morphine that they probably have little influence on analgesia. All these studies fail to confirm significant correlations between concentrations of morphine and the glucuronides in plasma and CSF and pharmacodynamic effect (e.g., analgesia).

M-3-G, the main glucuronide, shows no analgesic activity because the unoccupied 3-position seems to be necessary for opioid receptor binding.[13] However, M-3-G may combine with morphine and M-6-G to play a pathogenetic role in the phenomena of morphine-induced hyperalgesia, allodynia, and myoclonus described in cancer patients receiving high doses of morphine.[21] Furthermore, experimental work points out that M-3-G, in particular, has pronounced neuroexcitatory potency and that this metabolite may antagonize the analgesic effects of morphine and M-6-G. The latter effect has been hypothesized to contribute to the development of tolerance.[22]

Impaired liver function does not lead to prolonged or more potent morphine effects,[23,24] whereas accumulation of both glucuronides is pronounced in severe renal insufficiency.[25] Only 5% of the morphine dosage is demethylated in the liver to normorphine, a metabolite with no obvious practical importance.[26] Biotransformation of morphine to morphine-3,6-diglucuronide is also possible, but only of minor importance.[27] Methylation of morphine to codeine also occurs, but the amount is very small.

Pharmacodynamics of M-6-G

Analgesic efficacy

The first clinical evidence of analgesic properties of M-6-G in humans arose from studies by Osborne and coworkers, who investigated intravenous M-6-G injections in cancer patients.[28,29] They examined increasing doses (0.5–4 mg/70 kg) and followed plasma concentrations for up to 12 hours. The mean elimination half-life of M-6-G was 3.2 + 1.6 hours. The mean clearance of 96 + 38 mL/min correlated well with creatinine clearance and, interestingly, no transformation of M-6-G to morphine or M-3-G occurred. Seventeen of 19 patients reported pain relief after this single dose of M-6-G, which lasted from 2 to 24 hours. There was no evidence for correlation between blood concentrations of M-6-G and pharmacodynamic effects, including analgesia. Side effects were not encountered.[29] Other studies have yielded corresponding results. Thompson and coworkers reported that intravenously administered M-6-G in healthy volunteers was about 3 times more potent than morphine.[30] Side effects were fewer. Intrathecal administration of M-6-G in cancer patients was slightly more analgesic than morphine and remained in the CSF slightly longer.[31] There are some, albeit weak, indications that M-6-G is twice as potent as morphine when administered intrathecally.[31] M-6-G elimination half-life was less in healthy volunteers than in cancer patients; the subjective effects following intravenous injection of M-6-G 30 μg/kg resembled those of morphine 120 μg/kg but were shorter in duration.[32]

Portenoy and coworkers described chronic pain patients with normal renal function who received a loading infusion with morphine.[33] The analysis compared the molar concentration ratio of M-6-G:morphine from the start of the infusion until 240 minutes later. Time–effect plots showed that groups with increased M-6-G:morphine ratio had most pain relief, and that these parameters correlated significantly. The study suggested that M-6-G contributes to morphine analgesia in patients with normal renal function.[33]

Respiratory depression

Data concerning respiratory depression induced by M-6-G are conflicting. There is some evidence for less respiratory depression during M-6-G treatment. In a study performed by Gong and coworkers,[34] morphine, M-3-G, and M-6-G were given intracerebroventricularly to rats. M-6-G was found to be considerably more potent than morphine in antinociceptive assays (tail-flick and hot-plate). Furthermore, M-6-G was more potent in depressing central respiratory activity than morphine, while M-3-G stimulated ventilation. This action of M-3-G is in accordance with its known central excitatory activity. The ventilatory depression induced by morphine and M-6-G was readily reversed by naloxone, whereas the hyperventilation caused by M-3-G was slightly potentiated by the opioid antagonist.[34] In healthy volunteers, intravenous M-6-G 0.03–0.06 mg/kg caused less depression of the respiratory drive than did intravenous morphine 0.12 mg/kg.[34] This finding was in agreement with the above-mentioned study by Thompson and coworkers,[30] which reported less sedation and respiratory depression in healthy volunteers with M-6-G than morphine administered intravenously. Another double-blind study in six normal volunteers assessed the ventilatory effects of variable doses of morphine and M-6-G under resting conditions and CO_2 challenge. M-6-G had no effect on resting parameters or respiration (expired minute volume, end tidal CO_2, and respiratory rate) and produced significantly less respiratory depression than morphine during CO_2 challenge.[35]

Nausea and vomiting

The literature concerning nausea and vomiting after the administration of M-6-G is also conflicting. In case studies, high plasma levels of M-6-G caused by transient renal failure has been associated with chronic nausea.[36,37] But the clinical studies by Thompson and coworkers[30] and Osborne and coworkers[29] showed that nausea and vomiting were completely absent.

Tolerance

Few animal studies have evaluated the role of M-6-G in the development of tolerance.[38,39] Its clinical role in this respect is still unresolved

Myoclonus and cognitive function

A recent study in cancer patients did not demonstrate that myoclonus or cognitive impairment was correlated with M-6-G to morphine ratio.[40] Other studies have implicated M-3-G as the compound most responsible for the development of myoclonus, because of its pronounced neuroexcitatory potency. Another clinical study in 40 cancer pain patients receiving chronic oral morphine therapy showed that plasma morphine and metabolite concentrations were not correlated with nausea/vomiting or myoclonus.[41]

Pharmacodynamics of M-3-G

During the past 10 years, hyperalgesia, allodynia, and myoclonus have been reported at an increased frequency in humans treated with morphine. The side effects that have been reported to occur during treatment with any route of administration are most common in cancer patients treated with high doses. The mechanisms are largely unknown, but experimental work and both case series and clinical studies have focused on the causative role played by morphine, M-6-G, and, especially, M-3-G.

M-3-G does not have antinociceptive effects at the μ-opioid receptor due to its substituent on the phenolic hydroxyl site. It does, however, induce hyperalgesia when administered intrathecally.[42] In rats given low intrathecal doses (15 μg) of M-3-G, a low-threshold tactile stimulus elicited hyperesthesia and aggressive behavior, which was exaggerated by an opioid antagonist. Interestingly, this hyperalgesia/allodynia response, which has also been reported after high doses of intrathecal morphine,[42,43] occurs after a single dose of M-6-G 150 μg and is characterized by pain behavior involving biting or scratching the dermatomes corresponding to the spinal site of morphine application.[42]Another animal study has shown that central excitatory potency of morphine administered by cerebroventricular infusion is enhanced when using morphine derivatives substituted at the 3- and 6-position.[44] In particular, morphine derivatives substituted at the 3-position (phenolic group), such as M-3-G, showed such activity. In fact, M-3-G was several hundred times more potent than morphine in eliciting hyperactive motor behavior that could progress to lethal convulsions. The authors found a close negative correlation between excitatory potency and opioid receptor binding capacity, which could be interpreted as confirming the importance of a nonopioid receptor system. Furthermore, pretreatment with naloxone failed to diminish the central excitatory potency of morphine and its metabolites. A more recent study in rats confirmed the excitatory potency of intracerebroventricular M-3-G,[34] and other studies have shown that intrathecally administered M-3-G produces hyperesthesia and hyperalgesia in rats.[45]

Smith and coworkers found that intracerebroventricularly administered morphine in rats gave rise to allodynia, hyperalgesia, and "wet dog" shakes.[22] Although the mechanism for this action is not known, it is of interest that this response can be mimicked by intrathecal administration of the glycine antagonist strychnine.[46,47] Beyer and coworkers[47] showed that strychnine produced dose-dependent sensory and motor disturbances in rats. At all doses, strychnine-treated rats vocalized consistently in response to light cutaneous stimulation, whereas high doses of strychnine produced convulsive seizures, indicating that allodynia and myoclonus are induced by the same mechanisms. Glycine is known to mediate a postsynaptic inhibition on dorsal horn neurons and it is assumed that high doses of morphine or its metabolites may act via a spinal antiglycinergic effect to reduce postsynaptic inhibition, causing allodynia and myoclonus.

The activation of NMDA receptor complex by M-3-G, morphine, or even M-6-G, in this order of priority, is a tempting hypothesis that could explain the phenomena of hyperalgesia and allodynia. Interestingly, few animal studies have demonstrated in vitro binding of M-3-G and high-dose morphine to the NMDA receptor complex.[48,49] However, one study indicated that M-3-G and high-dose morphine probably do not elicit their effects through postsynaptic opioid, NMDA, AMPA, kainate, GABA, or glycine binding sites,[48] and another in vitro binding study showed that M-3-G has very low affinity for the known binding sites on the NMDA receptor complex.[49]

Clinically, hyperalgesia, allodynia, and myoclonus have been described primarily following high doses of morphine administered intrathecally and systemically in cancer patients.[21,50–52] The phenomenon is consistent with neuropathic pain, which can be an exacerbation of preexisting neuralgia. It can also present universal hyperalgesia and hyperesthesia associated with extreme tenderness of skin and muscles. The condition may be associated with myoclonus.[21] In case studies, segmental hyperalgesia and myoclonus have been described during intrathecal morphine in cancer patients.[50,52] There have also been case descriptions that associate high plasma and CSF concentrations of M-3-G with the side effects.[53,54] The terminology applied to morphine-induced pain, which is either unrelieved or worsened by further administration of the drug, is confusing. The terms "paradoxical pain" and "overwhelming pain syndrome" have been applied to it.[54] When morphine-induced allodynia, hyperalgesia, and myoclonus are encountered, it is rational, and in accordance with experimental data and the few case studies, to discontinue morphine and substitute another pure opioid agonist.[55] Animal studies have confirmed that high doses of methadone, fentanyl, alfentanil, and sufentanyl are devoid of these non-opioid receptor effects.[47,56] Furthermore, in vitro binding studies have indicated that drugs such as ketobemidone and methadone may have NMDA-receptor antagonistic properties.[57]

Another question concerning M-3-G is whether it antagonizes the analgesic effects of morphine and M-6-G, and thereby plays a role in the development of tolerance. Smith and coworkers showed that M-3-G was a potent antagonist of morphine analgesia when administered to rats by the intracerebroventricular route.[22] The antagonism was observed irrespective of whether M-3-G was administered prior to or after morphine administration. When M-3-G was administered intraperitoneally prior to morphine, antagonism was also demonstrated.[22] In accordance with these findings, Gong and coworkers showed in rats that M-3-G administered intracerebroventricularly may functionally antagonize both analgesia and ventilatory depression induced by M-6-G.[34] In other studies in rats, M-3-G did not significantly antagonize the antinociception induced by intrathecally administered morphine and M-6-G, although doses were comparable.[58,59] If M-3-G plays a role in antagonism of analgesia mediated by morphine and M-6-G, it also may be an essential factor in the development of morphine tolerance. A recent study in Sprague-Dawley rats, which were infused with intravenous morphine using three different dosing regimens, indicated that the M-3-G:morphine plasma concentration is a relatively reliable indicator of the degree of antinociceptive tolerance development.[60] Another study in Sprague-Dawley rats came to a quite different conclusion, however—namely, that M-3-G administered together with morphine prolonged and increased analgesia compared with the administration of morphine alone.[61] The hypothesis that M-3-G is involved in regulation of morphine analgesia and tolerance development is interesting, but at the moment, an unresolved matter. An important detail is the fact that the rats are unable to metabolize morphine to M-6-G.

In contrast to the increasing amount of information from animal studies concerning M-3-G, only a few clinical studies are available. A clinical study by Gourche and coworkers investigated steady-state concentrations of morphine, M-3-G, and M-6-G in serum and CSF in cancer patients who were receiving morphine but had morphine-resistant pain.[62] M-3-G:M-6-G ratios in the morphine-resistant patients were similar to published values in patients with well-controlled pain, suggesting that M-3-G does not play a major role in morphine resistance.[62] The hypothesis evaluated by this study is interesting, but there is virtually no clinical evidence that M-3-G plays a role in morphine antagonism, tolerance development, or analgesia regulation.

Morphine Metabolism, Renal Failure, and Aging

The elimination of unchanged morphine is not impaired during renal insufficiency, but both M-3-G and M-6-G have significantly prolonged elimination half-lives under this condition.[63–66] Säwe and Odar-Cederlöf studied the kinetics of morphine in seven patients with renal failure in comparison with patients with normal kidney function.[63] They found that metabolism of morphine was not significantly impaired in renal failure, but that the elimination half-life of M-3-G was 50 hours in uremics and 4 hours in patients with normal renal function. Peterson and coworkers demonstrated in a study of 21 cancer patients treated with oral or subcutaneous morphine that significant accumulation of both glucuronides occurred during renal insufficiency.[67] In patients with renal failure, M-6-G can be detected in plasma for more than 1 week.[25] Both M-3-G and M-6-G clearance were shown to be significantly correlated with creatinine clearance in intensive care patients.[68] Wolff and coworkers showed that patients with renal insufficiency had prolonged elimination of the glucuronides after an intravenous injection of morphine and that their clearance was significantly correlated with the Gr-EDTA clearance.[65] In a recent study by Tiseo and coworkers that examined 109 cancer patients receiving chronic oral or parenteral morphine, steady-state plasma concentrations of morphine and M-6-G were measured and confirmed the correlation between deteriorating renal function (blood urea nitrogen and creatinine) and increasing M-6-G:morphine ratio.[40] Osborne and coworkers showed that after intravenous morphine administration in patients with kidney failure, the increase in metabolites was severalfold greater than the increase of morphine, and that the metabolite accumulation was reversed by kidney transplantation.[69]

Morphine has a half-life of about 1 to 3 hours. The lower end of this range generally applies to young, healthy persons, whereas the upper end applies to older persons. In young, healthy patients (mean age, 30.2 years), morphine-6-glucuronide and morphine-3-glucuronide had half-lives of 2.6 and 3.9 hours, respectively, and in older patients (mean age, 49.4 years) the half-lives were 5.7 and 6.3 hours, respectively.[11,70] These data suggest that morphine should not be given to patients with renal failure because drug toxicity can occur and be prolonged by the inability to eliminate the glucuronides quickly. In elderly patients, renal function should be measured or estimated, and the morphine dosing interval should be extended accordingly. This would help to compensate for the normal decline in renal clearance associated with aging. Special caution should be applied during long-term morphine administration, because the slower the elimination of morphine-6-glucuronide, the higher its steady-state concentration, and the longer the time needed to achieve steady state. Thus, patients with poor renal function might respond favorably to morphine initially but could experience increasing respiratory depression and other side effects over the next several days as the metabolites accumulate.

Conclusion

Investigations of morphine and its metabolites, M-3-G and M-6-G, are currently revealing new pharmacological and clinical aspects. Although the clinical implications are far from clarified, some clues have been established. M-6-G undoubtedly has analgesic effects in humans, but more studies are needed to evaluate efficacy and side effects. The clinical relevance of the neuroexcitatory properties of M-3-G, M-6-G, and morphine demonstrated in animal models needs further investigation, as does the role of M-3-G in morphine antagonism, tolerance development, and analgesia regulation. Opioid drugs other than morphine may be more appropriate in patients with pronounced renal failure.

References

1. Glare PA, Walsh TD. Clinical pharmacokinetics of morphine. *Ther Drug Monit* 1991; 13:1–23.
2. Lehmann KA. Opioide und Antagonisten. *Klinische Pharmakologie für Anäs- thesisten, Intensivmediziner und Schmertztherapeuten.* Berlin: Springer-Verlag, 1990.
3. Vater M, Smith G, Aherne GW, Aitkenhead AR. Pharmacokinetics and analgesic effects of slow-release oral morphine sulfate in volunteers. *Br J Anaesth* 1984; 56:821–827.
4. Hoskin PJ, Hanks GW, Aherne GW, Chapman D, Littleton P, Filshie J. The bioavailability and pharmacokinetics of morphine after intravenous, oral and buccal administration in healthy volunteers. *Br J Clin Pharmacol* 1989; 27:499–505.
5. Boerner U, Abbott S, Roe RL. The metabolism of morphine and heroin in man. *Drug Metab Rev* 1975; 4:39–73.
6. Woods LA. Distribution and fate of morphine in non-tolerant and tolerant dogs and rats. *J Pharmacol Exp Ther* 1954; 112:158–175.
7. Oguri K, Ida S, Yoshimura H, Tsukamoto H. Metabolism of drugs. LXIX Studies on the urinary metabolites of morphine in several mammalian species. *Chem Pharm Bull (Tokyo)* 1970; 18:2414–2419.
8. Kamata O, Watanabe S, Ishii S, et al. Analgesic effect of morphine glucuronides. Proceedings 89th Meeting Pharmacology Society, Japan 1969:443.
9. Shimomura K, Kamata O, Ueki S, et al. Analgesic effect of morphine glucuronides. *Tohoku J Exp Med* 1971; 105:45–52.
10. Svensson JO, Rane A, Säwe J, Sjöqvist F. Determination of morphine, morphine-3-glucuronide and (tentatively) morphine-6-glucuronide in plasma and urine using ion-pair high-performance liquid chromatography. *J Chroma- togr A* 1982; 230:427–432.
11. Osborne R, Joel S, Trew D, Steven M. Morphine and metabolite behavior after different routes of administration: demonstration of the importance of the active metabolite morphine-6-glucuronide. *Clin Pharmacol Ther* 1990; 47:12–19.
12. Portenoy RK, Foley KM, Stulman J, et al. Plasma morphine and morphine-6-glucuronide during chronic morphine therapy for cancer pain: plasma profiles, steady-state concentrations and consequences of renal failure. *Pain* 1991; 47:13–19.

13. Pasternak GW, Bodnar RJ, Clark JA, Inturrisi CE. Morphine-6-glucuronide, a potent mu agonist. *Life Sci* 1987; 41:2845–2849.

14. Christensen CB, Jørgensen LN. Morphine-6-glucuronide has high affinity for the opioid receptor. *Pharmacol Toxicol* 1987; 60:75–76.

15. Portenoy RK, Khan E, Layman M, et al. Chronic morphine therapy for cancer pain: plasma and cerebrospinal fluid morphine and morphine-6-glucuronide concentrations. *Neurology* 1991; 41:1457–1461.

16. Hanks GW. Morphine pharmacokinetics and analgesia after oral administration. *Postgrad Med J* 1991; 67:60–63.

17. Gourche CR, Hackett P, Ilett K. Plasma and cerebrospinal fluid concentrations of morphine, morphine-6-glucuronide and morphine-3-glucuronide in cancer patients. 7th World Congress on Pain, Paris; 1993. Abstract 1410.

18. Wolff T, Samuelsson H, Hedner T. Morphine and morphine metabolite concentrations in cerebrospinal fluid and plasma in cancer pain patients after slow-release oral morphine administration. *Pain* 1995; 62:147–154.

19. Vandongen RTM, Crul BJP, Koopmanleimenai PM. Morphine and morphine glucuronide concentrations in plasma and CSF during long-term administration of oral morphine. *Br J Clin Pharmacol* 1994; 38:271–273.

20. Samuelsson H, Hedner T, Venn R, Michalkiewicz A. CSF and plasma concentrations of morphine and morphine glucuronides in cancer patients receiving epidural morphine. *Pain* 1993; 52:179–185.

21. Sjøgren P, Jonsson T, Jensen N-H, Drenck N-E, Jensen TS. Hyperalgesia and myoclonus in terminal cancer patients treated with continuous intravenous morphine. *Pain* 1993; 55:93–97.

22. Smith MT, Watt JA, Cromard T. Morphine-3-glucuronide—a potent antagonist of morphine analgesia. *Life Sci* 1990; 47:579–585.

23. Shelly MP, Cory EP, Park GR. Pharmacokinetics of morphine in two children before and after liver transplantation. *Br J Anaesth* 1986; 58:1218–1223.

24. Shelly MP, Quinn KG, Park GR. Pharmacokinetics of morphine in patients following orthotopic liver transplanation. *Br J Anaesth* 1989; 63:375–379.

25. Osborne RJ, Joel SP, Slevin ML. Morphine intoxication in renal failure: the role of morphine-6-glucuronide. *Br Med J* 1986; 292:1548–1549.

26. Sullivan AF, McQuay HJ, Bailey D, Dickenson AH. The spinal antinociceptive actions of morphine metabolites morphine-6-glucuronide and normorphine in the rat. *Brain Res* 1989; 482:219–224.

27. Yeh S, Gorodetzky CW, Krebs HA. Isolation and identification of morphine-3- and 6-glucuronides, morphine-3,6-diglucuronide, morphine-3-ethereal sulfate, normorphine, and normorphine-6-glucuronide as morphine metabolites in humans. *J Pharm Sci* 1977; 66:1288–1293.

28. Osborne R, Joel S, Trew D, Slevin M. Analgesic activity of morphine-6-glucuronide. *Lancet* 1988; 1:828.

29. Osborne R, Thomson P, Joel S, Trew D, Patel N, Slevin M. The analgesic activity of morphine-6-glucuronide. *Br J Clin Pharmacol* 1992; 34:130–138.

30. Thompson PI, John L, Wedzicha JA, Slevin ML. Comparison of the respiratory depression induced by morphine and its active metabolite morphine-6-glucuronide. *Br J Cancer* 1990; 62:484.

31. Hanna MH, Peat SJ, Woodham M, Knibb A, Fung C. Analgesic efficacy and CSF

pharmacokinetics of intrathecal morphine-6-glucuronide: comparison with morphine. *Br J Anaesth* 1990; 64:547–550.

32. Hanna MH, Peat SJ, Knibb AA, Fung C. Disposition of morphine-6-glucuronide and morphine in healthy volunteers. *Br J Anaesth* 1991; 66:103–107.

33. Portenoy RK, Thaler HT, Inturrisi CE, Friedlander-Klar H, Foley KM. The metabolite morphine-6-glucuronide contributes to the analgesia produced by morphine infusion in patients with pain and normal renal function. *Clin Pharmacol Ther* 1992; 51:422–431.

34. Gong Q-L, Hedner T, Hedner J, Björkman R, Nordberg G. Antinociceptive and ventilatory effects of the morphine metabolites: morphine-6-glucuronide and morphine-3-glucuronide. *Eur J Pharmacol* 1991; 193:47–56.

35. Peat SJ, Hanna MH, Woodham M, Knibb AA, Ponte J. Morphine-6-glucuronide: effects on ventilation in normal volunteers. *Pain* 1991; 45:101–104.

36. Hagen NA, Foley KM, Cerbone DJ, Portenoy RK, Inturrisi CE. Chronic nausea and morphine-6-glucuronide. *J Pain Symptom Manage* 1991; 6:125–128.

37. Zaw-Tun N, Bruera E. Active metabolites of morphine. *J Palliat Care* 1992; 8:48–50.

38. Olaso MJ, Fawa CC, Horga JF. Tolerance to morphine and M6G. 7th World Congress on Pain, Paris; 1993. Abstract 575.

39. Janichi PK, Erskine WAR, James FM. The route of morphine administration affects the development of tolerance in relation to gastric emptying in rats: is morphine-6-glucuronide involved? *Clin Exp Pharmacol Physiol* 1991; 18:193–194.

40. Tiseo PJ, Thaler HT, Lapin J, Inturrisi CE, Portenoy RK, Foley MK. Morphine-6-glucuronide concentrations and opioid-related side effects: a survey in cancer patients. *Pain* 1995; 61:47–54.

41. Ashby MA, Fleming BG, van Crugten J, Wood MM, Somogyi A. Plasma morphine, morphine-3-glucuronide and morphine-6-glucuronid concentrations in hospice patients receiving morphine for cancer pain: Absence of relationship to opioid side effects. 7th World Congress on Pain, Paris; 1993. Abstract 1002.

42. Yaksh TL, Harty GJ, Onofrio BM. High doses of spinal morphine produce a nonopiate receptor-mediated hyperesthesia: clinical and theoretic implications. *Anesthesiology* 1986; 64:590–597.

43. Woolf CJ. Intrathecal high dose morphine produces hyperalgesia in the rat. *Brain Res* 1981; 209:491–495.

44. Labella FS, Pinsky C, Havlicek V. Morphine derivatives with diminished opiate receptor potency show enhanced central excitatory activity. *Brain Res* 1979; 174:263–271.

45. Yaksh TL, Harty GJ. Pharmacology of the allodynia in rats evoked by high dose intrathecal morphine. *J Pharmacol Exp Ther* 1987; 244:501–507.

46. Werz MA, MacDonald RL. Opiate alkaloids antagonize postsynaptic glycine and GABA responses: correlation with convulsant action. *Brain Res* 1982; 236:107–119.

47. Beyer C, Roberts LA, Komisaruk BR. Hyperalgesia induced by altered glycinergic activity at the spinal cord. *Life Sci* 1985; 37:875–882.

48. Barlett SE, Dodd PR, Smith MT. Pharmacology of morphine and morphine-3-glucuronide at opioid, excitatory amino acid, GABA and glycine binding sites. *Pharmacol Toxicol* 1994; 75:73–81.

49. Barlett SE, Cramond T, Smith MT. The excitatory effects of morphine-3-glucuronide are attenuated by LY 274614, a competitive NMDA receptor antagonist, and by midazolam, an antagonist at the benzodiazepine site on the GABA$_A$ receptor complex. *Life Sci* 1994; 54:687–694.

50. Glavina JM, Robertshaw R. Myoclonic spasms following intrathecal morphine. *Anaesthesia* 1988; 43:389–390.

51. Potter JM, Reid DB, Shaw RJ, Hackett P, Hickmann PE. Myoclonus associated with treatment with high doses of morphine: the role of supplemental drugs. *Br Med J* 1989; 299:150–153.

52. Parkinson SK, Bailey SL, Little WL, Mueller JB. Myoclonic seizure activity with chronic high-dose spinal opioid administration. *Anaesthesiology* 1990; 72:743–745.

53. Sjøgren P, Dragsted L, Christensen CB. Myoclonic spasms during treatment with high doses of intravenous morphine in renal failure. *Acta Anaesth Scand* 1993; 37:780–782.

54. Morley JS, Miles JB, Wells CJ, Bowscher D. Paradoxical pain. *Lancet* 1992; 340: 1045.

55. Sjøgren P, Jensen NH, Jensen TS. Disappearance of morphine-induced hyperalgesia after discontinuing or substituting morphine with other opioid agonists. *Pain* 1994; 59:313–316.

56. Frenk H, Watkins LR, Mayer DJ. Differential behavioral effects induced by intrathecal microinjection of opiates: comparison of convulsive and cataleptic effects produced by morphine, methadone, and D-ala$_2$-methionine-enkephalinamide. *Brain Res* 1984; 299:31–42.

57. Ebert B, Andersen S, Krogsgaard-Larsen P. Ketobemidone, methadone and pethidine are non-competitive N-methyl-D-aspartate (NMDA) antagonists in the rat cortex and spinal cord. *Neurosci Lett* 1995; 187:165–168.

58. Suzuki N, Kalso E, Rosenberg PH. Intrathecal morphine-3-glucuronide does not antagonize spinal antinociception by morphine or morphine-6-glucuronide in rats. *Eur J Pharmacol* 1993; 249:247–250.

59. Hewett K, Dickenson AH, McQuay HJ. Lack of effect of morphine-3-glucuronide on the spinal antinociceptive actions of morphine in the rat: an electrophysiological study. *Pain* 1993; 55:59–63.

60. Smith GD, Smith MT. Morphine-3-glucuronide: evidence to support its putative role in the development of tolerance to the antinociceptive effects of morphine in the rat. *Pain* 1995; 62:51–60.

61. Lipkowski AW, Carr DB, Langlade A, Osgood PF, Szyfelbein SK. Morphine-3-glucuronide: silent regulator of morphine actions. *Life Sci* 1994; 55:149–154.

62. Gourche CR, Hackett LP, Ilett KL. Concentrations of morphine, morphine-6-glucuronide and morphine-3-glucuronide in serum and cerebrospinal fluid following morphine administration to patients with morphine resistant pain. *Pain* 1994; 56:145–149.

63. Säwe J, Odar-Cederlof I. Kinetics of morphine in patients with renal failure. *Eur J Clin Pharmacol* 1987; 32:377–382.

64. Aitkenhead AR, Vater M, Achola K, Cooper CMS, Smith G. Pharmacokinetics of single-dose intravenous morphine in normal volunteers and patients with end-stage renal failure. *Br J Anaesth* 1984; 56:813–818.

65. Wolff J, Bigler D, Christensen CB, Rasmussen SN, Andersen HB, Tønne-

sen HK. Influence of renal function on the elimination of morphine and morphine glucuronides. *Eur J Clin Pharmacol* 1988; 34:353–357.

66. Woolner DF, Winter D, Frendin DJ, Begg EJ, Lynn KL, Wright GJ. Renal failure does not impair the metabolism of morphine. *Br J Clin Pharmacol* 1986; 22:55–59.

67. Peterson GM, Randall CTC, Paterson J. Plasma levels of morphine and morphine glucuronides in the treatment of cancer pain: relationship to renal function and route of administration. *Eur J Clin Pharmacol* 1990; 38:121–124.

68. Milne RW, Nation RL, Somogyi AA, Bochner F, Griggs WM. The influence of renal function on the renal clearance of morphine and its glucuronide metabolites in intensive care patients. *Br J Clin Pharmacol* 1992; 34:53–59.

69. Osborne R, Joel S, Grebenik K, Trew D, Slevin M. The pharmacokinetics of morphine and morphine glucuronides in kidney failure. *Clin Pharmacol Ther* 1993; 54:158–167.

70. Laizure SC, Miller JH, Stevens RC, et al. The disposition and cerebrospinal fluid penetration of morphine and its two major glucuronidated metabolites in adults undergoing lumbar myelography. *Pharmacotherapy* 1993; 13:471–475.

9

The Emerging Role of the Fentanyl Series in the Treatment of Chronic Cancer Pain

MICHAEL E. GAUTHIER AND PERRY G. FINE

Historically, the fentanyl series of opioid analgesics was not developed with chronic pain indications in mind. The driving force for synthetic opioid research and development during the past three decades has centered around surgical anesthesia needs. Fentanyl only recently emerged in a formal manner outside the operating theater.

In the Netherlands, Janssen began investigations to develop an opioid more potent that morphine in 1953. By 1960, his research led to the synthesis of fentanyl. The impetus behind this work was the overly long duration of action and hemodynamic instability associated with high-dose morphine anesthesia. In the ensuing years up to the present, the goal has been to develop opioids with high therapeutic indices (TI), consistent pharmacodynamics, and predictable pharmacokinetics.[1]

Once fentanyl was synthesized and approved for clinical trials, it was heavily studied in the area of cardiovascular anesthesia. It was found that its TI was four times greater than morphine and large doses could be used safely and very effectively in cardiovascular anesthesia. Doses of 50 to 100 μg/kg provided excellent operative conditions with few adverse hemodynamic effects.

With the success of fentanyl, the search for other opioids with even safer profiles continued. Sufentanil, an even more potent congener of fentanyl, was developed and approved for clinical use by the FDA in 1984. Alfentanil, a somewhat less potent but shorter-acting congener of fentanyl, was also approved for use in the 1980s (see Table 9.1).

Table 9.1. Comparison of properties of morphine, meperidine, and fentanyl class of opioids[2,3]

	Relative potency	Relative solubility	TI
Morphine	1	1	70
Meperidine	1/10	30	5
Fentanyl	50–100	500	277
Alfentanil	25	100	1080*
Sufentanil	500–1000	1100	25,000*

TI = therapeutic indices.

*In rats.

Pharmacokinetics and Routes of Administration

In order to utilize the fentanyl opioids in an effective, sensible, and safe manner, it is of paramount importance to comprehend their pharmacokinetics. In this, computer modeling has been an invaluable tool.[4,5] By way of quick review,[6] the essential pharmacokinetic parameters (i.e., what the body does to the drug) are volume of distribution (Vd); concentration in the plasma at steady state, which gives the desired effect (e.g., analgesia) (Cpss); clearance (Cl); and elimination half-life ($t_{1/2}$). For intravenous administration, these values are used to calculate the loading dose (a function of Vd and Cpss) and the maintenance dose (a function of Cpss and Cl).

Volume of distribution refers to how widely the drug is distributed within the body, based on inferences drawn from plasma levels. This is a mathematical value, not a literal tissue volume per se. Volume of distribution is influenced by the drug's solubility, ionization state, molecular size, and amount of protein binding (see Fig. 9.1).

Clearance refers to the decrease in concentration of the drug in the plasma through elimination and biotransformation. This parameter is commonly derived from integrating area under the curve (AUC) from the plot of drug concentration versus time, with clearance inversely related to the magnitude of this value (see Fig. 9.2).

The elimination half-life is used to describe the rate at which a drug concentration falls after administration. It occurs in two general phases. The distribution phase occurs immediately after drug enters the bloodstream and begins to circulate. This is the initial drop in blood drug concentration secondary to redistribution into other compartments. The elimination phase results from clearance mechanisms. Typically, the distribution phase is rapid and the elimination phase is slower (see Fig. 9.3).

Many studies have addressed the pharmacokinetics of continuous intravenous infusion of fentanyl[7–14] and alternative routes (see Table 9.2).[15,16] However, few studies have compared the intravenous route with other routes

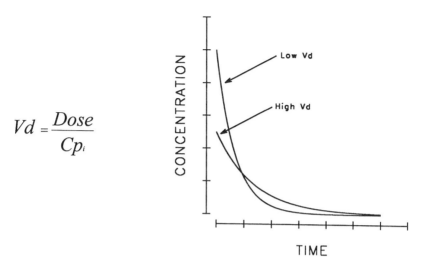

$$Vd = \frac{Dose}{Cp_i}$$

Figure 9.1. An equation and graphic defining the concept of volume of distribution. The graphic contrasts the concentration vs. time profiles that result after intravenous bolus administration of identical doses of a drug in a one-compartment model in which clearance has been held constant and volume of distribution has been altered. Volume of distribution is greater when the initial peak concentration is low. An increase in volume of distribution results in a longer half-life and a slower drop in drug concentration. VD = volume of distribution; Cp_1 = initial drug concentration in the plasma. (Reprinted with permission from Egan TD.[6])

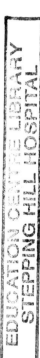

of fentanyl administration in the same patient. This is particularly important to determine comparative drug bioavailability, which affects the clinical utility of any potential delivery route. Along these lines, Varvel and coworkers[17] described the systemic absorption characteristics of transdermal fentanyl by determining the plasma bioavailability and rate of absorption of transdermal fentanyl and intravenous fentanyl.

Fentanyl was administered intravenously (IV) and transdermally (TDS) to eight surgical patients to determine the systemic bioavailability and rate of absorption of the transdermally administered drug. Prior to induction of general anesthesia, the patients received an infusion of fentanyl, 150 μg/min for 5 minutes. Blood samples were drawn before and at frequent intervals after administration up to 1440 minutes after the start of the infusion. No further fentanyl was administered until 24 hours after the infusion, at which time a transdermal system of 100 μg/hr was applied. Blood sampling was performed repeatedly up to 72 hours after TDS placement, although the TDS patch was removed after 24 hours.

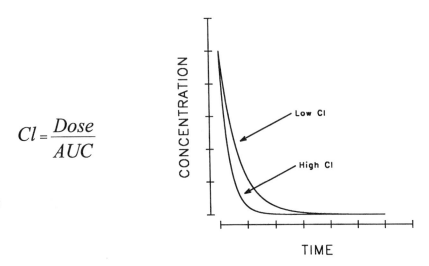

$$Cl = \frac{Dose}{AUC}$$

Figure 9.2. An equation and graphic defining the concept of clearance. The graphic contrasts the concentration vs. time profiles that result after intravenous bolus administration of identical doses of a drug in a one-compartment model in which volume of distribution has been held constant and clearance has been altered. Clearance is greater when the area under the concentration vs. time curve (AUC) is small. An increase in clearance results in a shorter half-life and a more rapid drop in drug conception. Cl = clearance; AUC = area under the curve. (Reprinted with permission from Egan TD.[4])

Pharmacokinetic analysis involved plotting the serum concentration of fentanyl for both intravenous and transdermal routes versus time. The serum concentration was extrapolated to 0 ng/ml to allow calculation of the AUC. The AUC was calculated for each route of delivery (AUC_{IV} and AUC_{TDS}). Next, the clearance (Cl_{IV}) was calculated as the ratio of the intravenous dose and AUC_{IV}. The amount of fentanyl delivered by the transdermal route was the difference between the initial content and residual content after removal. The amount absorbed (dose) from the transdermal system was calculated by the product of Cl_{IV} and AUC_{TDS}. Finally the bioavailability of the transdermal system is calculated as the ratio of the total absorbed (dose) to the amount delivered. The mean bioavailability was 0.92 (see Figs. 9.4, 9.5 and Table 9.3). The almost threefold increase in the half-life of the TDS compared to the IV route is explained by deposition and retention in the skin.

Streisand and coworkers[20] looked at the bioavailability and absorption of fentanyl from oral transmucosal fentanyl citrate (OTFC) in 12 volunteers. The investigators examined and determined the pharmacokinetic parameters for intravenous, OTFC (buccal), and oral (enteral) routes. (OTFC consists of a

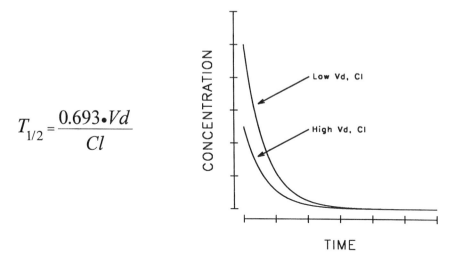

$$T_{1/2} = \frac{0.693 \cdot Vd}{Cl}$$

Figure 9.3. An equation and graphic defining the concept of half-life. The graphic contrasts the concentration vs. time profiles that result after intravenous bolus administration of identical doses of a drug in a one-compartment model in which half-life has been held constant but clearance and volume of distribution have been altered. Note that despite the same half-lives and identical doses, the concentration vs. time profiles are significantly different. Without knowledge of how clearance and volume of distribution have been altered, it is difficult to predict how the concentration vs. time profile will change. $T_{1/2}$ = half-life; Cl = clearance; Vd = volume of distribution. (Reprinted with permission from Egan TD.)[6]

Table 9.2. Absorption of transdermally administered fentanyl: IV fentanyl pharmacokinetic parameters (mean ± SD) with two previously published parameter sets for comparison[17]

	Present study	*Scott and Stanski*[18]	*McClain and Hug*[19]
Rapid distributional half-life (min)	1.35* ± 0.77	1.0* ± 0.6	1.65* ± 0.22
Slow distributional half-life (min)	24.7* ± 27.7	18.5* ± 11.9	12.7* ± 3.1
Elimination half-life (min)	428* ± 239	475* ± 193	241* ± 66
Vc (l)	15.9 ± 8.9	12.7 ± 5.9	26.6 ± 9.8
Vdss (l)	398 ± 163	339 ± 139	311 ± 36
Clearance (l/min)	0.77 ± 0.33	0.57 ± 0.21	0.88 ± 0.17

*Harmonic mean.

181

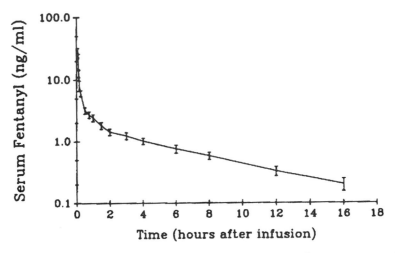

Figure 9.4. Mean and SEM of the study group's serum fentanyl concentrations after the intravenous fentanyl infusion. (Reprinted with permission from Varvel JR et al.[17])

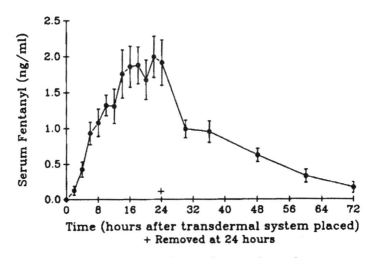

Figure 9.5. Mean and SEM of the study group's serum fentanyl concentrations measured during the transdermal pharmacokinetic study. (Reprinted with permission from Varvel JR et al.[17])

Table 9.3. Comparative pharmacokinetics of intravenous and transdermal fentanyl[17]

Fentanyl	Peak (hr)	Vdss (l)	$t_{1/2}$ (hr)	Cl (l/min)	Cpss (ng/mL)
IV	1.35 (min)	398 ± 163	6.1 ± 2	0.77 ± 0.33	1.9
TDS	14	*	17 ± 2.3	*	1.8 ± 0.8

Vdss = volume of distribution at steady state.

$t_{1/2}$ = elimination half-life.

Cl = clearance.

Cpss = concentration in the plasma at steady state.

*Data not available.

lozenge containing fentanyl citrate and sucrose with a handle and it can be prepared in differing concentrations.) The subjects received a 15 μg/kg unit dose during each 24-hour study session, either by the intravenous or oral transmucosal route. Eight subjects returned for the third session, which involved swallowing an oral solution (see Fig. 9.6).

Their study determined clearance (Cl_{IV}) of the intravenous route from the

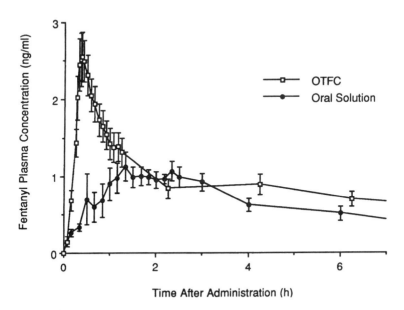

Figure 9.6. Plasma concentrations of fentanyl (mean ± SEM) after OTFC or oral administration for the eight subjects who completed these sections of the study. OTFC was consumed in 15 min, and the oral solution was swallowed within 10 s. (Reprinted with permission from Streisand JB et al.[20])

AUC_{IV} and dose and used them to calculate the OTFC and oral dosages similar to the methods used by Varvel and coworkers.[17] The terminal elimination for each route of administered drug was the same. As expected, the initial plasma concentration of fentanyl was 10 times greater after the intravenous administration (Fig. 9.7 and Table 9.4).

Ashburn and coworkers[21] performed iontophoresis with fentanyl on five volunteers. This preliminary study demonstrated that iontophoresis could be used to deliver clinically significant plasma levels of fentanyl. (Iontophoresis is a method of enhanced transdermal administration of drugs using an external

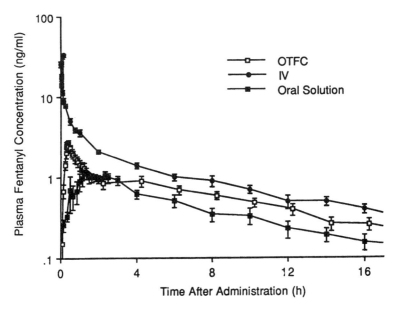

Figure 9.7. Plasma concentrations of fentanyl (mean ± SEM) after intravenous (n = 10), OTFC (n = 10), or oral (n = 8) administration of fentanyl 15 μg/kg. Intravenous fentanyl was infused at a rate of 150 μg/kg; OTFC was consumed in 15 min; and the oral solution was swallowed within 10 s. (Reprinted with permission from Streisand JB et al.[16])

Table 9.4. Comparison of pharmacokinetic values for different routes of fentanyl[20] administration

Fentanyl route	Cmax (ng/mL)	Time to Cmax (min)	Peak abs. rate (μg/mL)	Time to peak abs. rate (min)	Bioavailability
OTFC	3.0 ± 1.0	22 ± 2.5	11.1 ± 4.3	19 ± 2.6	0.52 ± 0.1
Oral	1.6 ± 0.6	101 ± 48.8	3.6 ± 2.1	87.5 ± 38.1	0.32 ± 1

OTFC = oral transmucosal fentanyl citrate.

electrical field.) Each volunteer was tested three times on separate days. Serially, they received passive treatment of 0.0 mA for 2 hours (0 mA · min), iontophoresis using 1.0 mA for 2 hours (120 mA · min), and iontophoresis using 2.0 mA for 2 hours (240 mA · min). Plasma fentanyl levels were determined before, during, and 10 hours after administration. No fentanyl was detected after passive fentanyl delivery. The maximum fentanyl concentration for the 1.0 mA group was 0.726 ng/mL and 1.586 ng/mL for the 2.0 mA group. They also used extrapolation and linear regression to estimate AUC. Doubling the mA · min dose doubled the AUC and peak plasma concentration. The time to plasma fentanyl concentration of 0.5 ng/mL was twice as fast at 2.0 mA · min than at 1.0 mA · min. An intravenous arm was not performed in this study, so comparative bioavailability could not be determined (see Figs. 9.8, 9.9).

Intranasal sufentanil has been studied as a preoperative premedication in pediatric[22] and adult patients.[23] Pharmacokinetic values were not reported. Although children treated with nasal sufentanil more readily accepted separation from their parents, crying with administration was common. The intraoperative and postoperative requirements for anesthesia and analgesia were reduced in both children and adults. Both of these clinical end points suggest appreciable uptake of sufentanil into the systemic circulation by this route of administration.

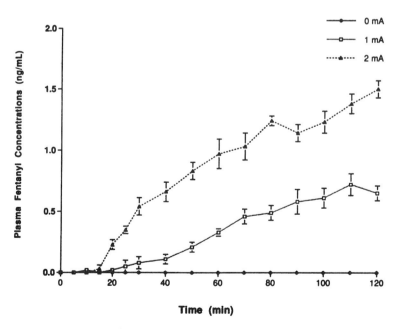

Figure 9.8. Mean±SEM plasma fentanyl concentration versus time (0 – 120 min) after 120-min iontophoretic delivery. (Reprinted with permission from Ashburn MA et al.[17])

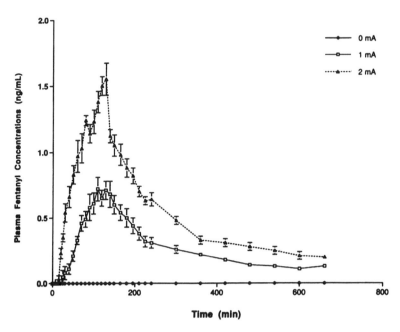

Figure 9.9. Mean ± SEM plasma fentanyl concentration versus time (0–660 min) after 120-min iontophoretic delivery. (Reprinted with permission from Ashburn MA et al.[21])

Although subcutaneous administration of opioids is commonly applied in palliative care, we are unable to find any human pharmacokinetic studies involving this technique with fentanyl. Indications for using fentanyl in this manner might derive from several possible clinical scenarios. These include sensitivities to other available opioids, toxicity from metabolites of high-dose infusions of other opioids, and the need for a high-potency opioid when severe pain and opioid tolerance have developed. Notwithstanding these circumstances, there are no formal studies with which to establish a scientific basis of practice beyond knowledge gleaned from the aforementioned intravenous pharmacokinetic studies in (noncancer) volunteers and surgical patients. The latter information must be interpreted cautiously in patients with malignant disease because of the possibility of metabolic changes (e.g., alterations in serum proteins and in hepatic and renal function), the potential impact on phamacokinetics of long-term and high-dose administration of opioids, and the limited relevance of data obtained in opioid-naive study populations.

The same holds true at this time for neuraxial (spinal opioid analgesia) administration of fentanyl or similar compounds. There is a paucity of information available for fentanyl in cancer patients using the epidural or intrathecal route, either through bolus or continuous infusion. Sadler and coworkers[24] demonstrated nearly equivalent pharmacodynamic effects and plasma pharmacokinetics in thoracotomy patients when fentanyl was delivered by either IV or epidural routes. There is little reason to suspect that these findings would be different in cancer patients, taking into account the caveats already discussed. This is due to the extensive metabolism of fentanyl by the liver to norfentanyl, 4-N-anilinopiperidine, and propionic acid. In normal subjects, less than 10% of fentanyl is excreted unchanged in the urine. The activity of the fentanyl metabolites is unknown.[25] Yaksh and coworkers[26] reported preliminary pharmacological findings using neuraxial alfentanil in animals, but applicability in humans is unclear.

Chronic Cancer Pain Therapy

Parenteral and neuraxial routes

Controlled clinical trials investigating fentanyl in the treatment of chronic cancer pain are limited. Extrapolating from other clinical settings is about the best that can be accomplished at the present time. For instance, Duthie[9] describes fentanyl plasma concentrations and pain relief remaining relatively stable with a postoperative intravenous infusion for up to 24 hours. Whether this bears any relation to the more chronic situation of continuous pain due to cancer remains to be determined. As previously mentioned, there are descriptive and clinical reports of fentanyl and sufentanil use via epidural and intrathecal catheters in cancer patients. Credible sources acknowledge the current objective limitations in defining the indications for and risk/benefit of this family of drugs in the neuraxis. Practically speaking, these sources can serve as a reference guide for thought and clinical care in hard-to-manage situations.[27–31]

Transdermal route

Transdermal fentanyl has been the modality most extensively investigated for this indication.[32–39] In 1989, Simmonds and coworkers[40] studied the efficacy and safety of transdermal fentanyl in 39 cancer patients. They found patient acceptance and compliance to be excellent with use as long as 1 year. Zech and colleagues[41] performed an open study involving 20 cancer patients. These patients were placed on IV patient-controlled analgesia (PCA) using fentanyl 50 μg/cm^3. After 24 hours, the IV dose was converted to transdermal fentanyl equivalents (see Table 9.5), and a TDS was applied to the patient. The PCA was continued another 48 hours and this dose was also converted to patch equivalents. This additional patch dose was added to the original patch dose to

Table 9.5. Conversion table for daily parenteral fentanyl dose to TTS fentanyl*

Total daily parenteral fentanyl (mg/day) (range)	TTS fentanyl delivery rate (mg/day)
0.1–0.8	0.6
0.9	0.6/1.2
1.0–1.4	1.2
1.5	1.2/1.8
1.6–2.0	1.8
2.1	1.8/2.4
2.2–2.6	2.4
2.7	2.4/3.0
2.8–3.2	3.0
3.3	3.0/3.6

Source: Reprinted with permission from Zech et al.[41]

*In doses higher than 3.3 mg of IV fentanyl the same conversion ratio was continued.

determine the total TDS that was applied at the 72-hour mark. The investigators reported very rapid and effective pain control using this technique. There were no serious side effects such as respiratory depression or somnolence. While they found this a very valuable way to determine a safe and effective transdermal fentanyl dose for patients' basal level of pain, they (as well as others they referenced) were troubled by breakthrough pain when using fentanyl patches alone. Our experience is similar.

Payne and colleagues[42] recently published guidelines for the use of transdermal fentanyl. The first and most important step is patient selection. The patient's pain syndrome should be responsive to opioid treatment and the character of pain should be stable with only modest amounts of incident or breakthrough pain. Usually the patient is stabilized with oral morphine for 24 to 48 hours. The dose consumed for a 24-hour period is then converted to fentanyl patch equivalents, which are applied. The transdermal fentanyl takes 12 to 24 hours to reach steady-state plasma levels. If a sustained-release formulation of morphine has been in use, this should be discontinued and a more rapidly peaking formulation of an opioid such as immediate-release morphine, oxycodone, or hydrocodone should be given. The patient is instructed to take this on an as-needed basis (prn). Payne reports that approximately 50% of patients will experience breakthrough pain. After the original patch has been in place for 72 hours, it may be replaced with a greater dose if the patient is requiring frequent dosing of the prn opioid. Payne recommends increasing patch doses by 25 µg/hr increments. The frequency of TDS changes can be advanced to every 48 hours and the prn dosing of oral opioids should be used as a guide to dosage increases.

Lehmann and Zech[43] recently reviewed the transdermal system and associated clinical pharmacology. The amount of fentanyl released from each system per hour is proportional to the surface area. Essentially the fentanyl must diffuse through the skin to gain access into the general circulation, a process that takes approximately 14 hours to obtain clinically relevant plasma levels. The rate-limiting step of absorption is the passive diffusion through the keratinized and oily stratum corneum. The patch is changed every 48 to 72 hours based on clinical effect. The commercial transdermal system containing fentanyl is currently available in 25, 50, 75, and 100 μg/h delivery rates.

One of the difficulties with the transdermal system is that it does not lend itself well to rapid titration of drug effect. To deal with this in a practical manner, Korte[44] reports using the TDS for dose titration in 20 cancer patients. This author's patients changed the patches every 24 hours and had a visual analogue scale (VAS 0 to 100 mm) of less than 35 mm within 48 hours. Why this would accelerate the process of reaching steady-state basal analgesia (and presumably steady-state levels of blood levels) is not readily evident. Others, including our own observations, find that many patients do not obtain a full 72 hours of analgesia, despite plasma level studies that do not show appreciable decline.

There are four case reports of withdrawal symptoms[45,46] in patients who were switched from oral opioids to a transdermal fentanyl system. The patients experienced opioid withdrawal due to physical dependence despite good pain relief. Symptoms included diarrhea, abdominal cramps, nausea, sweating, restlessness, crawling sensations in the extremities, headache, freezing sensations, and shivering. The withdrawal symptoms were relieved with morphine. Higgs and Vella-Brinant[45] postulate these observations may be accounted for by known differences between morphine and fentanyl affinity to opioid receptors in the gut.

Portenoy and coworkers[38] performed repeat dose pharmacokinetic analyses using the recommended dosing schedule of changing the patch every 72 hours. They found steady-state serum concentrations were approached by the end of the second dose and remained stable thereafter. The elimination half-life was slightly longer at 21.9 hours than in Varvel's[17] study at 17.0 hours. In a postoperative pain study, Gourlay and coworkers[47] found results similar to Varvel. Again, we would postulate that these variations are most likely a function of population differences; that is, altered clearance in cancer patients versus postoperative patients versus volunteers.

Oral transmucosal route

Oral transmucosal fentanyl citrate was originally introduced as a premedication prior to general anesthesia for pediatric patients.[48,49] The first case report for its use to treat cancer pain was in 1989: a patient who was experiencing intractable episodes of breakthrough pain associated with metastatic carcinoma of the lung.[50] In addition to methadone 20 mg every 6 hours, diflunisal 500 mg every 8 hours, and amitriptyline 25 mg at bedtime, he sucked a 700 µg OTFC on an as-needed basis. He eventually needed to increase the dose to 1000 µg, requiring 2 to 3 doses per day. His pain ratings decreased from 5 out of 10 to 1 out of 10 (VAS) within a few minutes after OTFC administration.

Fine and coworkers[51] performed an open-label study of OTFC for the treatment of cancer pain. Ten patients were given OTFC 10 to 15 µg/kg 4 or 5 times each over 2 days. There were no complications or clinically significant side effects. Pain scores were dramatically reduced, with a mean onset time of 9.5 minutes. Methodologically sound multicenter trials are currently under way to determine the safety and efficacy of this delivery system for the control of cancer pain, especially the common symptom of breakthrough pain (Shoemaker S, MD, personal communication).

Most recently, OTFC has been successfully used in children to treat procedure-related pain.[52] The noninvasive nature of OTFC with relatively rapid onset of potent analgesia allows for reduction of pain and fear in the physically and psychologically noxious environment that attends lumbar punctures and bone marrow aspirates, without adding to it.

Iontophoresis

"Iontophoresis is the transfer of ionic solutes through biologic membranes under the influence of an electric field"[53] (see Fig. 9.10). Iontophoresis provides an alternative route to enteral, buccal, parenteral, or passive transdermal drug delivery and allows for comparatively rapid achievement of therapeutic plasma levels of fentanyl.[21] In this study, it was demonstrated that therapeutic levels of fentanyl could be achieved very quickly in healthy volunteers. Unlike TDS, evaluation of the elimination half-life revealed that there is no depot effect in the skin. Iontophoresis more closely resembles parenteral administration. Further studies are necessary to determine if this technique can be used for prolonged periods and if it has applicability in cancer pain control.

The new fentanyls

Egan[54] points out that although fentanyl, sufentanil, and alfentanil have virtually replaced morphine and meperidine for surgical anesthesia, these synthetic opioids still possess troublesome side effects in surgical patients. These include respiratory depression, nausea, vomiting, muscle rigidity, and bradycardia. There is inadequate experience to determine whether side effect profiles of these drugs are less, the same, or more than the conventionally used opioids (e.g., morphine) when used in equivalent analgesic doses on a long-term basis in cancer patients. The additional issue of tolerance development or incomplete cross-tolerance is also unresolved.

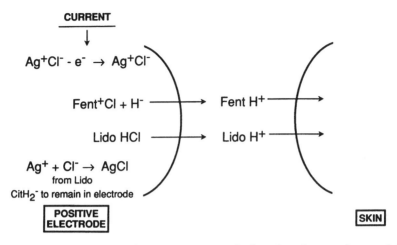

Figure 9.10. When positive direct current is applied to the silver conductor of the drug electrode, negative ions in the drug reservoir are thought to accumulate at the positively charged conductor surface, forming a capacitive electric double layer. As the electric potential in the double layer rises, the silver becomes sacrificial and oxidizes, forming free silver ions in solution. Current then begins to flow across the drug reservoir and into the skin in the form of solvated ions, including fentanyl (Fent H^+) and lidocaine (Lido H^+) ions. Silver ions are removed by precipitation of insoluble silver chloride from solution. The chloride ions used to precipitate silver ions are derived from the dissolution of lidocaine hydrochloride (Lido) in the solution. $CitH_2^-$ = citrate ion. (Reprinted with permission from Ashburn MA et al.[21])

Meanwhile, two new members of the fentanyl family are on the horizon. Remifentanil is unique among the fentanyl series in that it possesses an ester linkage that is susceptible to hydrolysis in blood.[55] This results in a very short-acting analgesic effect and also a very brief respiratory depressant effect. Trefentanil is also a very short-acting agent undergoing clinical trials. The potential use of these agents in chronic pain is unclear at this time. Their unique physicochemical properties may be efficacious for rapid determination of opioid responsiveness and dose titration in the outpatient setting. In addition, these new fentanyl derivatives may prove beneficial in treating incidental pain or breakthrough pain syndromes.

Conclusion

The fentanyl class of opioids has proved invaluable in the realm of surgical anesthesia. Only recently has there been interest, experience, and a slowly developing body of literature related to use of these drugs in patients with chronic pain. The landscape of methodologically sound clinical studies is sparse. Such studies are difficult and quite expensive. However, increasing awareness of the heretofore poorly addressed public health problem of cancer pain has taken root. Recognition of difficult-to-treat, limited, or costly options for the treatment of breakthrough pain in cancer is currently a driving force for the instigation of well-designed controlled studies, with OTFC as the current paradigm. Time alone will tell if the crossover of fentanyl to this new clinical territory has merit.

References

1. Stanley TH. The history and development of the fentanyl series. *J Pain Symptom Manage* 1992; 7(3)S:S3–S7.
2. Janssen PAJ. In: Estafanous FG, ed. The development of new synthetic narcotics. Boston: Butterworth; 1984:40.
3. Bailey PL, Stanley TH. Narcotic intravenous anesthetics. In: Miller RD, ed. *Anesthesia*, 3rd ed. New York: Churchill Livingstone; 1990:283.
4. Hughes MA, Glass PSA, Jacobs JR. Context-sensitive half-time in multicompartment pharmacokinetic models for intravenous anesthetic drugs. *Anesthesiology* 1992; 76:334–341.
5. Shafer SL, Varvel JR. Phasrmacokinetics, pharmacodynamics, and rational opioid selection. *Anesthesiology* 1991; 74:53–63.
6. Egan TD. Pharmacokinetics and rational intravenous drug selection and administration in anesthesia. *Advances in Anesthesia, Year Book*. St. Louis: Mosby; 1995:363–387.
7. Alvis JM, Reves JG, Govier AV, et al. Computer-assisted continuous infusions of fentanyl during cardiac anesthesia: comparison with manual method. *Anesthesiology* 1985; 63:41–49.
8. Andrews CJH, Prys-Roberts C. Intravenous infusions of fentanyl. *Clin Anesthesiol* 1984; 2(1):139–143.
9. Duthie DJR, McLaren AD, Nimmo WS. Pharmacokinetics of fentanyl during constant rate I.V. infusion for the relief of pain after surgery. *Br J Anaesth* 1986; 58:950–956.
10. Hoffman P. Continuous infusion of fentanyl and alfentanil in intensive care. *Eur J Anaesthesiol* 1987; (1):71–75.
11. Hynynen M, Takkunen M, Salmenpera M, Haataja H, Heinonen J. Continuous infusion of fentanyl or alfentanil for coronary artery surgery. *Br J Anaesth* 1986; 58:1252–1259.
12. Nimmo WS, Todd JG. Fentanyl by constant rate I.V. infusions for postoperative analgesia. *Br J Anaesth* 1985; 57:250–254.
13. Shafer A, White PF, Schuttler J, Rosenthal MH. Use of a fentanyl infusion in the intensive care unit: tolerance to its anesthetic effects? *Anesthesiology* 1983; 59(3):245–248.
14. White PF. Clinical uses of intravenous anesthetic and analgesic infusions. *Anesth Analg* 1989; 68:161–171.
15. Loper KA, Ready BL, Downey M, et al. Epidural and intravenous fentanyl infu-

sions are clinically equivalent after knee surgery. *Anesth Analg* 1990; 70:72–75.

16. Holley FO, Van Steennis C. Postoperative analgesia with fentanyl: pharmacokinetics and pharmacodynamics of constant-rate I.V. and transdermal delivery. *Br J Anaesth* 1988; 60:608–613.

17. Varvel JR, Shafer SL, Hwang SS, Coen BS, Stanski DR. Absorption characteristics of transdermally administered fentanyl. *Anesthesiology* 1989; 70:928–934.

18. Scott JC, Stanski DR. Decreased fentanyl and alfentanil requirements with age: A simultaneous pharmacokinetic and pharmacodynamic evaluation. *J Pharmacol Exp Ther* 1987; 240:159–166.

19. McClain DA, Hug CC. Intravenous fentanyl kinetics. *Clin Pharmacol Ther* 1980; 28:106–114.

20. Streisand JB, Varvel JR, Stanski DR, et al. Absorption and bioavailability of oral transmucosal fentanyl citrate. *Anesthesiology* 1991; 75:(2):223–229.

21. Ashburn MA, Streisand J, Zhang J, et al. The iontophoresis of fentanyl citrate in humans. *Anesthesiology* 1995; 1995:1146–1153.

22. Henderson JM, Brodsky DA, Fisher DM, Brett CM, Hertzka RE. Pre-induction of anesthesia in pediatric patients with nasally administered sufentanil. *Anesthesiology* 1988; 68:671–675.

23. Vercauteren M, Boeckx E, Hanegreefs G, Noorduin H, Vanden Bussche G. Intranasal sufentanil for pre-operative sedation. *Anaesthesia* 1988; 43:270–273.

24. Sandler AN, Stringer D, Panos L, et al. A randomized, double-blind comparison of lumbar epidural and intravenous fentanyl infusions for postthoracotomy pain relief. *Anesthesiology* 1992; 77:626–634.

25. McEvoy G, ed. *American Hospital Formulary Service Drug Information.* Bethesda: American Society of Health System Pharmacists, 1995:1371.

26. Yaksh TL, Noueihed R, Durant PA. In: Estafanous FG, ed. *Opioids in Anesthesia.* Boston: Butterworth, 1984:161–166.

27. Cousins MJ, Mather LE. Intrathecal and epidural administration of opioids. *Anesthesiology* 1984; 61:276–310.

28. Fine PG, Stanley TH. Spinal opioid analgesia: present status and future developments. In: Rawal N, Coombs DW, eds. *Spinal Narcotics.* Boston: Kluwer Academic Publishers; 1990:129–143.

29. Glass PSA, Estok P, Ginsberg B, Goldberg JS, Sladen RN. Use of patient-controlled analgesia to compare the efficacy of epidural to intravenous fentanyl administration. *Anesth Analg* 1992; 74:345–351.

30. Hogan Q, Haddox D, Abram S, Weissman D, Taylor ML, Janjan N. Epidural opiates and local anesthetics for the management of cancer pain. *Pain* 1991; 46:271–279.

31. Yaksh TL. The spinal pharmacology of acutely and chronically administered opioids. *J Pain Symptom Manage* 1992; 7(6):356–360.

32. Ahmedzai S, Allen E, Fallon M, et al. Transdermal fentanyl in cancer pain. *J Drug Dev* 1994; 6(3):93–97.

33. Calis KA, Kohler DR, Corso DM. Transdermally administered fentanyl for pain management. *Clin Pharm* 1992; 11:22–36.

34. Cherny NI, Portenoy RK. Cancer pain management: current strategy. *Cancer* 1993; 72(11):3393–3415.

35. Levy MH, Rosen SM, Kedziera P. Transdermal fentanyl: seeding trial in patients with chronic cancer pain. *J Pain Symptom Manage* 1992; 7(3):S48–S50.

36. Miser AW, Narang PK, Dothage JA, Young RC, Sindelar W, Miser JS. Transdermal fentanyl for pain control in patients with cancer. *Pain* 1989; 37:15–21.
37. Payne R. Experience with transdermal fentanyl in advanced cancer pain. *Eur J Pain* 1990; 11:98–101.
38. Portenoy RK, Southam MA, Gupta SK, et al. Transdermal fentanyl for cancer pain. *Anesthesiology* 1993; 78:36–43.
39. Simmonds MA, Richenbacher J. Transdermal fentanyl: long-term analgesic studies. *J Pain Symptom Manage* 1992; 7(3):S36–S39.
40. Simmonds MA, Payne R, Richenbacher J, Moran K, Southam MS. TTS (fentanyl) in the management of pain in patients with cancer. *Proc Am Soc Oncol* 1989; 8:324. Abstract 1260.
41. Zech DFJ, Grond SUA, Lynch J, Dauer HG, Stollenwerk B, Lehmann KA. Transdermal fentanyl and initial dose-finding with patient-controlled analgesia in cancer pain: a pilot study with 20 terminally ill cancer patients. *Pain* 1992; 50:293–301.
42. Payne R, Chandler S, Elnhaus M. Guidelines for the clinical use of transdermal fentanyl. *Anticancer Drugs* 1995; 6(3):S50–S53.
43. Lehmann KA, Zech D. Transdermal fentanyl: clinical pharmacology. *J Pain Symptom Manage* 1992; 7(3):S8–S16.
44. Korte W. Titration with TTS fentanyl systems for previously uncontrolled cancer pain. *Anesth Analg* 1994; 79:612–613.
45. Higgs CMB, Vella-Brincat J. Withdrawal with transdermal fentanyl. *J Pain Symptom Manage* 1995; 10(1):4–5.
46. Zenz M, Donner B, Strumpf M. Withdrawal symptoms during therapy with transdermal fentanyl (fentanyl TTS)? *J Pain Symptom Manage* 1994; 9(1):54–55.
47. Gourlay GK, Kowalski SP, Plummer JL, Cherry DA, Gaukroger P, Cousins MJ. The transdermal administration of fentanyl in the treatment of postoperative pain: pharmacokinetics and pharmacodynamic effect. *Pain* 1989; 37:193–202.
48. Nelson PS, Streisand JB, Mulder SM, Pace NL, Stanley TH. Comparison of oral transmucosal fentanyl citrate and an oral solution of meperidine, diazepam, and atropine for premedication in children. *Anesthesiology* 1989; 70:616–621.
49. Ashburn MA, Streisand JB, Traver SD, et al. Oral transmucosal fentanyl citrate of premedication in paediatric outpatients. *Can J Anaesth* 1990; 37(8):857–866.
50. Ashburn MA, Fine PG, Stanley TH. Oral transmucosal fentanyl citrate for the treatment of breakthrough cancer pain: a case report. *Anesthesiology* 1989; 71: 615–617.
51. Fine PG, Marcus M, De Boer AJ, Van der Oord B. An open label study of oral transmucosal fentanyl citrate (OTFC) for the treatment of breakthrough cancer pain. *Pain* 1991; 45:149–153.
52. Schechter NL, Weisman SJ, Rosenblum MK, Bernstein B, Conard PL. The use of oral transmucosal fentanyl citrate for painful procedures in children. *Pediatrics* 1995; 95(3):335–339.
53. Nimmo WS. Novel delivery systems: electrotransport. *J Pain Symptom Manage* 1992; 7(3):160–162.
54. Egan TD. New intravenous opioids. *Exp Opin Invest Drugs* 1994; 3(10):997–1003.
55. Dershwitz M, Randal GI, Rosow CE, et al. Initial clinical experience with remefentanil, a new opioid metabolized by esterases. *Anesth Analg* 1995; 81:619–623.

10

Intraindividual Variability in Opioid Response: A Role for Sequential Opioid Trials in Patient Care

SHARON WATANABE

Intraindividual variability in response to different opioids, or to the same opioid over time, is a commonly appreciated clinical phenomenon. Variability may be manifested in the relative intensity of analgesic and nonanalgesic effects, and in the spectrum of nonanalgesic effects experienced. Recent literature has suggested a role for sequential opioid trials when the balance between analgesia and adverse effects is unfavorable. This chapter will review the evidence for the existence of this phenomenon, the possible underlying mechanisms, and implications for clinical practice.

Evidence for Variability in Opioid Response

Evidence for differential response to opioids consists largely of case reports and retrospective studies. Galer and coworkers[1] formally recognized this phenomenon in their description of five patients with malignant and nonmalignant pain who experienced inadequate analgesia on morphine despite escalation to doses that produced a variety of side effects. Sequential drug trials ultimately identified an opioid that provided an acceptable balance between analgesia and toxicity. Improved response was achieved with hydromorphone in one case, levorphanol in one, and methadone in three.

A series of three cancer patients was reported who had poor pain control on morphine, in one case associated with sedation and myoclonus; all improved with a switch to methadone.[2] Four cancer patients were described with hyper-algesia, allodynia, and myoclonus on morphine; satisfactory analgesia with resolution of toxicity was achieved on methadone, sufentanil, and keto-bemidone.[3] Intractable pain was reported in six cancer patients on morphine, hydromorphone, and fentanyl, in some cases accompanied by somnolence and nausea; improved pain control without side effects was obtained with metha-done.[4] Uncontrolled pain, delirium, and myoclonus were described in three cancer patients on hydromorphone; a more favorable balance between anal-gesia and toxicity occurred with a switch to morphine.[5] In a retrospective review of intravenous opioid infusions for cancer pain, it was noted that of six patients who underwent a trial of alternative opioids because of inadequate analgesia in the presence of dose-limiting toxicity, four demonstrated an im-proved response.[6]

Bruera and coworkers[7] reported a retrospective study examining the im-pact of opioid rotation on the incidence of agitated delirium on a palliative care unit. Two consecutive series of 117 and 162 patients each were compared. The latter group differed in that they were subjected to regular cognitive screen-ing, with initiation of hydration and opioid rotation upon detection of cognitive failure. Twenty-one percent of patients in the former group underwent an opioid switch versus 41% percent in the latter group; correspondingly, the incidence of agitated delirium declined from 26% to 10%. However, the rela-tive contributions of the cognitive monitoring and hydration to this improve-ment could not be determined.

De Stoutz and coworkers[8] retrospectively described 80 patients admitted to a palliative care unit who underwent opioid rotation for indications such as uncontrolled pain, cognitive failure, hallucinations, myoclonus, and nausea. Morphine, hydromorphone, and methadone were involved in 90% of the switches. Leading symptoms improved in 73% of cases, and pain intensity scores declined significantly on a lower equivalent dose of opioid.

Mechanisms of Variability of Opioid Response

The mechanisms underlying differential response to opioids are not well un-derstood, but the following explanations have been proposed:

Genetic factors

Animal studies suggest that genetic factors may be important in determining patterns of opioid sensitivity. For example, some mouse strains are deficient in their expression of μ receptors,[9] and are correspondingly insensitive to the analgesic effects of morphine.[10] Sensitivity to μ and κ analgesia has been demonstrated to vary independently across mouse strains, suggesting that each receptor subtype is under independent genetic control.[11] It may be postulated, therefore, that analgesic and nonanalgesic response to an opioid in humans may depend on a genetically determined pattern of expression of receptor subtypes for which that opioid is selective. This, however, does not explain differential sensitivity to opioids with similar receptor subtype affinities. The effect of genetic factors on opioid response has not yet been studied in humans.

Tolerance

Individual variability in response to opioids has also been postulated to reflect the development of tolerance and the existence of incomplete cross-tolerance between opioids. Tolerance refers to a decrease in the effect of a drug due to prior exposure.[12] This phenomenon has been demonstrated experimentally in both animals and humans. Houde and coworkers,[13] for example, demonstrated in seven chronic pain patients that after they received morphine for 7 days at a mean daily dose of 77.3 mg intramuscularly, morphine 16.8 mg was required to achieve the same analgesic effect as 10 mg prior to exposure. The mechanisms underlying tolerance have not been conclusively established, although studies using rat brains[14] and guinea pig ilea[15] suggest a reduction in the number of coupled opiate receptors.

Tolerance to different opioid effects has been shown in rat models to occur at varying rates corresponding to mediation of these effects by different receptor subtypes.[16] If tolerance for analgesia develops more rapidly than for toxicity, this could manifest clinically as an imbalance between analgesic and toxic effects.

Switching opioids could be advantageous if cross-tolerance for analgesia was incomplete, and less than that for toxicity. Incomplete cross-tolerance between opioids for analgesia has been documented experimentally in animals[17] and humans. In the aforementioned study by Houde and coworkers,[13] patients also required a higher dose of metopon to achieve equivalent analgesia after (6.4 mg), as compared to before (5.1 mg), morphine exposure, but the magnitude of increase was less than that for morphine.

This phenomenon of incomplete cross-tolerance may occur as a result of differential affinity for receptor subtypes. For example, rats exposed to morphine, a μ agonist, develop analgesic tolerance to morphine but not to levorphanol, which binds to κ and δ as well as μ receptors.[18] Incomplete cross-tolerance among opioids selective for the same receptor subtype may be explained by differences in efficacy. That is, opioids differ in the fraction of receptors they need to occupy in order to achieve an equivalent effect. Experiments with guinea pig ilea, for example, have demonstrated a greater spare receptor fraction for methadone than for morphine.[19] Replacing a less efficacious opioid with a more efficacious one in the setting of tolerance should, in theory, result in improved pain control.

Although tolerance has been shown to occur experimentally, its importance in the clinical setting is controversial. Assessment of clinical tolerance is complicated by lack of control over intensity of the pain stimulus. One prospective study in cancer patients with pain demonstrated that of 25 patients who required increased morphine doses over time, 24 showed objective tumor progression, whereas of 4 patients who did not require a dose increase, all had stable or improved disease status.[20]

Opioid metabolites

Opioid metabolites have been postulated to affect the balance between analgesic and toxic effects of opioids. This phenomenon has been best described for morphine, which is metabolized mainly to 6- and 3-glucuronide forms. Morphine-6-glucuronide binds to the μ opiate receptor.[21] In animal models, its analgesic potency exceeds that of morphine by up to 200-fold.[22] Analgesic properties have also been reported in humans. Open administration of intravenous M-6-G to 6 cancer patients resulted in decreased visual analogue scores for pain intensity in 5.[23] A single-blind crossover study comparing equivalent intrathecal doses of morphine and M-6-G in 3 cancer patients demonstrated no differences in verbal rating scores for pain intensity or sedation, although rescue dose requirements were greater with morphine.[24] In a study of 14 chronic pain patients treated with intravenous morphine infusions, the plasma M-6-G:morphine ratio was significantly correlated with visual analogue measurements of pain relief.[25]

M-6-G has also been linked to opioid toxicities. In dogs, it is a more potent ventilatory depressant than morphine.[26] Three cases have been described of patients with renal failure who developed respiratory depression on morphine that persisted for days after discontinuation of the drug; although no morphine was detectable in plasma, M-6-G levels were very high.[27] One case has been reported of a morphine-treated cancer patient in whom nausea and confusion correlated more closely with plasma M-6-G rather than morphine levels.[28] However, a survey of 109 cancer patients on morphine did not find a correlation between the plasma M-6-G:morphine ratio and the presence of cognitive failure or myoclonus, although very high M-6-G levels in the setting of metabolic dysfunction were associated with respiratory depression and obtundation; other potentially neurotoxic metabolites such as morphine-3-glucuronide were not measured.[29]

Morphine-3-glucuronide (M-3-G) has low affinity for the opiate receptor; its site of action is currently unknown.[30] Intracerebroventricular administration in rats produces generalized neuroexcitatory effects at much lower doses than does morphine.[31] Intrathecal administration results in localized hyperalgesia and allodynia.[32] Studies using rat behavioral models suggest that M-3-G attenuates the analgesic effects of morphine and M-6-G.[33,34] However, electrophysiological studies in rats have not confirmed that M-3-G antagonizes morphine inhibition of C-fiber evoked responses.[35] It may be that the rat pain behavior interpreted as antagonism of analgesia actually represents central neuroexcitatory activity.

The effects of M-3-G in humans have not been well documented. One patient who developed myoclonus and seizures on morphine in the setting of renal failure was found to have high plasma and CSF levels of M-3-G.[36] Some authors have suggested that clinical analgesic effect is determined by the ratio of M-3-G to M-6-G.[37,38] In a study of cancer patients who had uncontrolled pain on maximally tolerated doses of morphine, plasma and CSF M-3-G:M-6-G ratios were not different from those reported in the literature in patients with good pain control; however, other factors potentially contributing to pain severity were not assessed.[39]

Individual variability in metabolite levels may be determined by several factors. Metabolite levels increase in proportion to morphine dose. However, metabolites accumulate relative to morphine in the presence of renal failure.[40–42] One study has suggested an effect of age, gender, and other drugs on the metabolite:morphine ratio.[43] Genetic variability in drug glucuronidation has also been proposed to explain individual differences in metabolite levels.[44]

Normorphine is another metabolite that has been suggested to have toxic effects. Normorphine was detected in the plasma of two patients with renal failure who developed myoclonus on morphine; however, M-3-G and M-6-G levels were also elevated.[45] Other morphine metabolites may have effects that have not yet been described.

Metabolite effects have been reported for other opioids. In a prospective study of 67 patients receiving meperidine for cancer pain or postoperative pain, neuroexcitatory effects were identified in 48, the severity of which correlated with plasma normeperidine but not meperidine levels.[46] Hydromorphone-3-glucuronide has been shown in one patient to accumulate with renal failure.[47] Although neuroexcitatory phenomena have been described in patients on hydromorphone,[5] correlation with metabolite levels is lacking.

If opioid metabolites are able to negatively influence the balance between analgesia and toxicity, then an opioid switch may allow a more favorable balance to be established by allowing clearance of the offending metabolites. However, similar metabolites may eventually accumulate with the new opioid. Theoretically opioids without known active metabolites, such as methadone, may be associated with fewer side effects.

Pain mechanism

Individual variability in opioid response has also been suggested to reflect mediation of analgesia by receptor subtypes specific to the pain mechanism. For example, it has been demonstrated in rats that thermal nociception is antagonized by μ and δ agonists, but not κ or ε agonists; in contrast, chemical nociception is preferentially antagonized by μ and κ agonists.[48] Pain mechanism–specific response to different opioids has not been reported clinically, although this may be due to the fact that the vast majority of available opioids are μ agonists.

Conclusion

Currently, there is a lack of prospective studies documenting the occurrence of individual variability in response to different opioids, the determinants of this variability, and the effects of sequential opioid trials. However, it can be argued that the weight of anecdotal evidence and theoretical considerations is sufficient to justify the use of alternative opioids when the balance between analgesia and toxicity is unfavorable.

The selection of an alternative opioid is largely empirical. Limited data exist to support the use of opioids that act at different receptor subtypes, have greater intrinsic efficacy, or lack active metabolites. Multiple opioid trials may be necessary before a suitable drug is identified.

The appropriate starting dose of the alternative opioid is uncertain. However, clinical experience suggests that the improved response is often achieved at doses that are significantly lower than would be predicted from standard equianalgesic ratios.[1–5] Some authors, therefore, recommend that the initial dose be reduced by as much as 50% to account for this observation.[5,6]

Over time, the balance of effects may again shift toward toxicity, at which point a further opioid switch would be indicated. In our experience, previous unfavorable response to a particular opioid does not preclude later usefulness of that drug in the same patient. Possible explanations include loss of analgesic tolerance or elimination of toxic metabolites with interruption in drug exposure, or intercurrent change in other clinical factors that may influence opioid response.

References

1. Galer B, Coyle N, Pasternak W, Portenoy R. Individual variability in the response to different opioids: report of five cases. *Pain* 1992; 49:87–91.
2. Leng G, Finnegan MJ. Successful use of methadone in nociceptive cancer pain unresponsive to morphine. *Palliat Med* 1994; 8:153–155.
3. Sjøgren P, Jensen N, Jensen T. Disappearance of morphine-induced hyperalgesia after discontinuing or substituting morphine with other agonists. *Pain* 1994; 59:313–316.
4. Crews JC, Sweeney NJ, Denson DD. Clinical efficacy of methadone in patients refractory to other μ-opioid receptor agonist analgesics for management of terminal cancer pain. *Cancer* 1993; 72:2266–2272.

5. MacDonald N, Der L, Allan S, Champion P. Opioid hyperexcitability: the application of alternate opioid therapy. *Pain* 1993; 53:353–355.

6. Portenoy R, Moulin D, Rogers A, Inturrisi C, Foley K. IV infusions of opioids for cancer pain: clinical review and guidelines for use. *Cancer Treat Rep* 1986; 70 (5):575–581.

7. Bruera E, Franco J, Maltoni M, Watanabe S, Suarez-Almazor M. Changing pattern of agitated impaired mental status in patients with advanced cancer: association and cognitive monitoring, hydration, and opioid rotation. *J Pain Symptom Manage* 1995; 10(4):287–291.

8. de Stoutz N, Bruera E, Suarez-Almazor M. Opioid rotation for toxicity reduction in terminal cancer patients. *J Pain Symptom Manage* 1995; 10(5):378–384.

9. Moskowitz AS, Goodman RR. Autoradiographic analysis of Mu_1 Mu_2 , and delta opioid binding in the central nervous system of C57BL/6BY and CXBK (opioid receptor-deficient) mice. *Brain Res* 1985; 360:108–116.

10. Vaught JL, Mathiasen JR, Raffa RB. Examination of the involvement of supraspinal and spinal mu and delta opioid receptors in analgesia using the mu receptor deficient CXBT mouse. *J Pharmacol Exp Ther* 1988; 245:13–16.

11. Pick CG, Cheng J, Paul D, Pasternak GW. Genetic influences in opioid analgesic sensitivity in mice. *Brain Res* 1991; 566:295–298.

12. Foley KM. Clinical tolerance to opioids. In: Basbaum A, Besson JM, eds. *Towards a New Pharmacotherapy of Pain*. New York: John Wiley & Sons; 1991:181–203.

13. Houde R, Wallenstein S, Beaver W. Evaluation of analgesics in patients with cancer pain. *Clin Pharmacol* 1966; 59–97.

14. Rogers NF, El-Fakahany E. Morphine-induced opioid receptor down-regulation detected in intact adult rat brain cells. *Eur J Pharmacol* 1986; 124:221–230.

15. Chavkin C, Goldstein A. Opioid receptor reserve in normal and morphine-tolerant guinea pig ileum myenteric plexus. *Proc Natl Acad Sci USA* 1984; 81:7253–7257.

16. Ling G, Paul D, Simantov R, Pasternak G. Differential development of acute tolerance to analgesia, respiratory depression, gastrointestinal transit and hormone release in a morphine infusion model. *Life Sci* 1989; 45(18):1627–1636.

17. Sosnowski M, Yaksh T. Differential cross-tolerance between intrathecal morphine and sufentanil in the rat. *Anesthesiology* 1990; 73:1141–1147.

18. Moulin DE, Ling G, Pasternak GW. Unidirectional analgesic cross-tolerance between morphine and levorphanol in the rat. *Pain* 1988; 33:233–239.

19. Ivarsson M, Neil A. Differences in efficacies between morphine and methadone demonstrated in the guinea pig ileum: a possible explanation for previous observations on incomplete opioid cross-tolerance. *Pharmacol Toxicol* 1989; 65:368–371.

20. Collin E, Poulain P, Gauvain-Piquard A, Pichard-Leandri P, Pichard-Leandri E. Is disease progression the major factor in morphine 'tolerance' in cancer pain treatment. *Pain* 1993; 55:319–326.

21. Pasternak GW, Bodnar RJ, Clark JA, Inturrisi CE. Morphine-6-glucuronide, a potent mu agonist. *Life Sci* 1987; 41:2845–2849.

22. Abbott FV, Palmour RM. Morphine-6-glucuronide: analgesic effects and receptor binding profile in rats. *Life Sci* 1988; 43:1685–1695.

23. Osborne RJ, Joel S, Trew D, Slevin M. Analgesic activity of morphine-6-glucuronide. *Lancet* 1988; 1:828.

24. Hanna MH, Peat SJ, Woodham M, Knibb A, Fung C. Analgesic efficacy and CSF pharmacokinetics of intrathecal morphine-6-glucuronide: comparison with morphine. *Br J Anaesth* 1990; 64:547–550.

25. Portenoy RK, Thaler HT, Inturrisi CE, Friedlander-Klar H, Foley KM. The metabolite morphine-6-glucuronide contributes to the analgesia produced by morphine infusion in patients with pain and normal renal function. *Clin Pharmacol Ther* 1992; 51(4):422–431.

26. Pelligrino DA, Riegler FX, Albrecht RF. Ventilatory effects of fourth cerebroventricular infusions of morphine-6- or morphine-3-glucuronide in the awake dog. *Anesthesiology* 1989; 71:936–940.

27. Osborne RJ, Joel SP, Slevin ML. Morphine intoxication in renal failure: the role of morphine-6-glucuronide. *Br Med J* 1986; 292:1548–1549.

28. Hagen NA, Foley KM, Cerbone DJ, Portenoy RK, Inturrisi CE. Chronic nausea and morphine-6-glucuronide. *J Pain Symptom Manage* 1991; 6(3):125–128.

29. Tiseo PJ, Thaler HT, Lapin J, Inturrisi CE, Portenoy RK, Foley KM. Morphine-6-glucuronide concentrations and opioid-related side effects: a survey in cancer patients. *Pain* 1995; 61:47–54.

30. Bartlett SE, Dodd PR, Smith MT. Pharmacology of morphine and morphine-3-glucuronide at opioid, excitatory amino acid, GABA and glycine binding sites. *Pharmacol Toxicol* 1994; 75:73–81.

31. Labella FS, Pinsky C, Havlicek V. Morphine derivatives with diminished opiate receptor potency show enhanced central excitatory activity. *Brain Res* 1979; 174:263–271.

32. Woolf CJ. Intrathecal high dose morphine produces hyperalgesia in the rat. *Brain Res* 1981; 209:491–495.

33. Smith MT, Watt JA, Cramond T. Morphine-3-glucuronide—a potent antagonist of morphine analgesia. *Life Sci* 1990; 47:579–585.

34. Gong QL, Hedner J, Bjorkman R, Hedner T. Morphine-3-glucuronide may functionally antagonize morphine-6-glucuronide induced antinociception and ventilatory depression in the rat. *Pain* 1992; 48:249–255.

35. Hewett K, Dickenson AH, McQuay HJ. Lack of effect of morphine-3-glucuronide on the spinal antinociceptive actions of morphine in the rat: an electrophysiological study. *Pain* 1993; 53:59–63.

36. Sjøgren P, Dragsted L, Christensen CB. Myoclonic spasms during treatment with high doses of intravenous morphine in renal failure. *Acta Anaesthesiol Scand* 1993; 37:780–782.

37. Bowsher D. Paradoxical pain. *Br Med J* 1993; 306:473–474.

38. Morley JS, Watt JWG, Wells JC, Miles JB, Finnegan MJ, Leng G. Methadone in pain uncontrolled by morphine. *Lancet* 1993; 342:1243.

39. Goucke CR, Hackett LP, Ilett KF. Concentrations of morphine, morphine-6-glucuronide and morphine-3-glucuronide in serum and cerebrospinal fluid following morphine administration to patients with morphine-resistant pain. *Pain* 1994; 56:145–149.

40. Sawe J. Morphine and its 3- and 6- glucuronides in plasma and urine during chronic oral administration in cancer patients. In: Foley KM, Inturrisi CE, eds. *Advances in Pain Research and Therapy*; vol. 8. New York: Raven Press; 1986: 45–55.

41. Peterson GM, Randall CTC, Paterson J. Plasma levels of morphine and morphine

glucuronides in the treatment of cancer pain: relationship to renal function and route of administration. *Eur J Clin Pharmacol* 1990; 38:121–124.

42. Portenoy RK, Foley KM, Stulman J, et al. Plasma morphine and morphine-6-glucuronide during chronic morphine therapy for cancer pain: plasma profiles, steady-state concentrations and the consequences of renal failure. *Pain* 1991; 47:13–19.

43. McQuay HJ, Carroll D, Faura CC, Gavaghan DJ, Hand CW, Moore RA. Oral morphine in cancer pain: influences on morphine and metabolite concentration. *Clin Pharmacol Ther* 1990; 48(3):236–244.

44. Burchell B, Coughtrie WH. UDP-glucuronosyltransferases. *Pharmacol Ther* 1989; 43:261–289.

45. Glare PA, Walsh TD, Pippenger CE. Normorphine, a neurotoxic metabolite? *Lancet* 1990; 335:725–726.

46. Kaiko RF, Foley KM, Grabinski PY, et al. Central nervous system excitatory effects of meperidine in cancer patients. *Ann Neurol* 1983; 13(2):180–185.

47. Babul N, Darke AC, Hagen N. Hydromorphone metabolite accumulation in renal failure. *J Pain Symptom Manage* 1995; 10:184–186.

48. Schmauss C, Yaksh TL. In vivo studies on spinal opiate receptor systems mediating antinociception. II. Pharmacological profiles suggesting a differential association of mu, delta and kappa receptors with visceral chemical and cutaneous thermal stimuli in the rat. *J Pharm Exp Ther* 1984; 228:1–12.

IV

PSYCHOSOCIAL ADAPTATION TO CANCER

Introduction: Psychopathology in Patients with Progressive Medical Disorders: What Is "Normal"?

MARY JANE MASSIE

Normal Patient Responses to Crisis Points in Progressive Medical Illness

> A 34-year-old professional woman says to her psychiatrist: "I'm behaving in ways not characteristic for me; I'm indecisive, I can't sleep, I'm anxious, and I act like a terrified little animal in front of my doctors. I don't know if what I'm feeling, thinking and doing is normal. Tell me, what is normal when you have just been told that you have metastatic breast cancer and maybe you are going to die—and you have four little kids and your husband works half a world away?"

The normal responses of individuals to crisis points (diagnosis or the diagnosis of disease recurrence or progression) in progressive medical illness have been described as being similar to the responses of any individual to overwhelming stress.[1] Patients who have just learned that they have a life-threatening or progressive medical illness describe first feeling terrified, shocked, stunned, dazed, or emotionally numb. These initial feelings are often accompanied by a sense of disbelief ("This can't be happening to me; I'm going to wake up and realize this is just a horrible dream. I'm young and healthy; other people depend on me and I have so much left to accomplish. Illness happens to other people; it doesn't happen to me.") This initial response, which lasts several days, is often followed by mixed symptoms of anxiety and depression such as insomnia, crying, nervousness, emotional lability, fluctuating levels of awareness of the seriousness of the diagnosis and emotional reactions such as fear, hope, sadness, despair. These normal emotional responses to a catastrophic life event, in this case the diagnosis of progressive and possibly or likely terminal medical illness, are diagnosed in our current psychiatric terminology as an "Adjustment Disorder with Depressed Mood or Anxiety" (or both).[2] Usually, they gradually resolve as patients collect and intellectually integrate information, ally themselves with the medical staff to fight the illness, bargain for more time (i.e., to accomplish life goals or to see their children mature), orient themselves to the real or the perceived positive aspects of their condition ("I had 17 out of 20 positive lymph nodes; but that means I had three good nodes" or "My doctor says they have new things coming down the road all the time for this disease; by the time things get really bad with me, they will probably have all sorts of new treatments available"), and find reasons to be optimistic ("I know of a woman who has had metastatic breast cancer for 17 years; in 17 years my kids will be out of college and, God willing, I'll be a grandmother" or "This treatment my doctor has planned for me is nothing in comparison to what other people have to go through").

When Responses Are Not Normal

> Thirty-year-old nurse to a psychiatrist: "You have got to come do something to this woman. She does this every time she is admitted. She cries, yells, refuses routine tests, and questions everything the house officers do to the point they are so nervous that they start to make mistakes and are afraid to talk with her. I know she is only 30 years old and is going to die of breast cancer and that her mother says that this behavior is normal for her when she's scared. But it's not normal to us anymore. Somebody has got to get her to see that this isn't helping her and it's making us *nuts*."

There is a wide spectrum of normal behavior, and medical and nursing staff members know that normal personality traits are magnified under stress. It is *not* normal, however, to make treating staff feel so frustrated or intimidated that they are unable to provide care to patients. When behavior becomes maladaptive (as it was in the case described above), it is beyond the range of normal and needs to be addressed.

Feeling "out of control" is unpleasant for the patient. Acting "out of control" is unpleasant for both the patient and staff members and is humiliating when recalled by the patient. "Overlooking" the regressed or maladaptive behavior of the patient who is a "Very Important Person," or of the hospitalized health professional, does not do the patient a favor. Patients are often reluctant to report emotional symptoms to their doctor ("It's not my doctor's main interest" or "He would be so disappointed in my lack of will, he's trying so hard to keep me alive"). Many patients have read or heard that emotional strength affects disease outcome and are worried that mood symptoms such as depression will negatively affect their prognosis if left unchecked. It is better to openly acknowledge that an emotional disturbance exists, reassure them that a mood state alone does not alter prognosis, and let them know that they will fare better while undergoing medical treatments if they are not battling preexisting or new "demons" (depression, panic disorder, alcoholism). When referred, some patients pursue psychiatric evaluation, ostensibly to get relief from intolerable symptoms. After symptoms are controlled, many choose to continue psychiatric treatment to maximize opportunities to spend quality time with their loved ones, to "put their affairs in order," to prepare advance directives, to review life's satisfactions, or to come to terms with life's disappointments.

An ongoing effort of psychiatrists and palliative care experts who work with the medically ill has been to obtain objective information about the prevalence of psychiatric disorders and pain syndromes in patients with medical illness.[3,4] These prevalence data should encourage greater recognition of emotional problems. As the effectiveness of psychotherapeutic and behavioral interventions has been established by controlled trials and newer drugs with fewer side effects have been developed, physicians now are more willing to refer patients for evaluation, and there are more well-trained professionals available to treat those who are referred.

Clinicians and hospitals are utilizing daily nursing assessment scales, admission checklists (which include questions about the adequacy of pain control or the presence of symptoms of anxiety or depressed mood or suicidal thought), or validated screening instruments[4] to detect symptoms and syndromes that warrant clinical evaluation. These tools can rapidly identify the "at-risk" population and make staff aware that those who are suffering and those at risk for developing psychiatric symptoms require special and ongoing assessment and attention. It is best for the clinician to assume that everyone is "at risk"—all patients should be asked about their adaptation—and we should have the mechanisms in place to refer for further psychiatric assessment those whose mood, behavior, or adaptation is beyond the realm of normal.

Teaching Staff How to Identify Patients
with Distress Beyond the Range of Normal

> First-year medical oncology fellow after 6 months of service to an attending physician: "After you have been here awhile, do you begin to see all this emotional suffering as normal? I don't want it to become normal; but every person here suffers so much—after a while, do you just not see it? How do you know someone has a psychiatric problem when everyone is suffering so much?"
>
> Fifth-year plastic surgery resident to a psychiatrist at 3:00 A.M.: "I have sewn up a lot of people who have made suicide attempts, but this one was definitely not normal. When we found him, there was blood everywhere—almost like he did it on purpose. He may lose his arm; and the irony is, he could have 2 more good years before he dies of colon cancer."

The medical oncology fellow asks, "Can a health care provider become so philosophical about misery or so accustomed to treating individuals who are suffering that one doesn't notice?" The exhausted plastic surgery resident begins to see some suicide attempts as "routine" and doesn't question why someone with a terminal illness would give up "2 good years." Learning how to identify and manage behaviors and mood states that are beyond the range of "normal" in patients with progressive medical illness is a challenging task for the beginner of any discipline but is an essential skill for the veteran clinician who works with patients with progressive medical illness.

Only a small percentage of patients with any progressive medical disorder will have a chronic psychiatric disorder (i.e., mental retardation, schizophrenia, bipolar disorder) that antedates the diagnosis of their medical condition. These individuals will require special attention by the medical staff as they undergo evaluation and treatment for any medical condition. Special consideration—such as communication with family members or the psychiatric staff members previously involved in the patient's care; modifications in the patient's psychotropic medication schedule in the peri-operative period, during episodes of sepsis or electrolyte imbalance, or during terminal periods; collaborative monitoring by medical, palliative care, and psychiatric staff members; and a realistic appraisal of the dual-diagnosis patient's ability to participate in his or her care—facilitates the adaptation of the chronically mentally ill to medical illness.

A challenge for all medical staff members are patients with substance abuse or personality disorders. Medical staff members may offer little compassion, forgiveness, or flexibility to those who are not likable; those whose "bad behavior" appears willful; those who are unable to acknowledge their chemical dependency or get help for their drug abuse or alcoholism; and those who, because of a core character stance of paranoid thinking and distrust, are unable or unwilling to follow through with evaluation and treatment recommendations.

Many medical school curricula include courses for first- and second-year students in "human behavior in medical illness." Often co-taught by psychiatrists and internists, these courses help the beginner conceptualize the distinction between normal and abnormal responses to stress. Inability to concentrate when a doctor delivers bad news is normal; inability to concentrate accompanied by agitation and hallucinations is not. Momentarily forgetting the date of your first chemotherapy treatment is normal; anomia is not. Disappointment or anger when a procedure is postponed is normal; rage attacks, suicide attempts, or 30 days of binge drinking are not.

The beginner learns that patients not only "don't mind" but also appreciate questions about their adaptation. The more the patient perceives questions about behavior and mental status as part of the routine medical exam, the more likely the patient will give "honest" responses. Saying "This is stressful for everyone; how is this stress manifesting in you?" and asking patients about their management of other stressful life events provides an easy entrée to a discussion about adaptation. Older patients may have had numerous previous stressful life events and may have insight into how they react to stress.

Those individuals who need to be in control of themselves and their surroundings to contain anxiety or maintain self-esteem have greater problems with declining health than those who do not have such needs. Those whose sense of themselves is closely tied to their perception of their physical strength or attractiveness are often the least able to tolerate deteriorating illnesses.

Conclusion

There is a spectrum of normal behavior. Our task is to identify maladaptive behavior, frankly psychotic symptoms, or persistent dysphoric mood states, and to distinguish psychopathology from "the afternoon blahs." Asking "Would I react this way if I were in the same boat?" isn't the best test for "normal" behavior. Instead, considering the patient's current behavior and mood state, defense mechanisms (healthy vs. less healthy), and the pervasiveness and the intensity of emotional symptoms permits accurate assessment of comfort, behavior, and mood.

References

1. Massie MJ, Holland JC. Overview of normal reactions and prevalence of psychiatric disorders. In: Holland JC, Rowland JR, eds. *Handbook of Psychooncology: Psychological Care of the Patient with Cancer*. New York: Oxford University Press; 1989:273–282.
2. American Psychiatric Association. *Diagnostic and Statistical Manual of Mental Disorders*. 4th ed. Washington, D.C.: American Psychiatric Association; 1994.
3. Derogatis LR, Morrow GR, Fetting J, et al. The prevalence of psychiatric disorders among cancer patients. *JAMA* 1983; 249:251–257.
4. Portenoy RK, Thaler HT, Kornblith AB, et al. The Memorial symptom assessment scale: an instrument for the evaluation of symptom prevalence, characteristics and distress. *Eur J Cancer* 1994; 30A:1326–1336.

11

"Normal" Adjustment to Cancer: Characteristics and Assessment

LINDA J. BEENEY, PHYLLIS N. BUTOW, AND STEWART M. DUNN

Until the latter half of the twentieth century, neoplastic diseases manifested as relatively acute, usually fatal illnesses for which there were few effective treatments. Thus, adjustment to cancer was largely irrelevant—the high and rapid mortality restricted the tasks of normal adjustment to coping with short-term survival or the prospect of an early death. Patients were seldom aware of the diagnosis, as it was infrequently disclosed,[1-3] and when they were, distress was often severe because cancer was perceived to be a dirty, unclean disease and the diagnosis equivalent to a death sentence. In the 1990s, adjustment to cancer has become a major issue for a wider population. Technical advances have dramatically prolonged survival and offered cure for some types of cancer.[4] For example, the diagnosis of Hodgkin's disease is a very different experience today—with 90% 5-year survival rates and a significant cure rate—than before the 1970s when the prognosis was seen as uniformly dismal.[5] Cure rates for testicular cancer are cited as 70% to 80%,[6] and expectations of longer-term survival in cancer generally have vastly improved.[7] Furthermore, disclosure of a cancer disgnosis is now the norm, at least in the United States and northern Europe.[8,9]

The issues of adjustment to cancer extend beyond the patient population to the wider community because of the emphasis on earlier detection and screening programs for at-risk groups and the symptom-free population. Those who never experience cancer directly are likely to be part of a family in which someone will receive a cancer diagnosis. In addition, coping with prolonged exposure to cancer and death, and avoiding burnout, are two burgeoning issues for health professionals in the medical oncology field.

In this chapter we investigate the meaning of normal adjustment for individuals who receive the diagnosis, as well as their families and their health professionals. Identification of the normal course of adjustment will not only allow the development of realistic expectations, but also facilitate accurate detection of psychological morbidity that will benefit from intervention. The detection and understanding of people who experience significant morbidity when diagnosed with cancer is important because of the detrimental effects of such distress on quality of life, decision making, and ultimately survival.[10] Excellent reviews of these topics are available, particularly as they pertain to adults with specific tumor types (e.g., breast cancer) or treatments,[11-13] and to children with cancer.[14]

Changing Social Concepts of Cancer

Before addressing the question of normal adjustment on an individual level, there are several reasons to first consider the broader social and medical context in which these individuals operate. An individual's first response to, and subsequent adjustment to, cancer will be strongly influenced by his or her own attitudes and perceptions, as well as a myriad of external factors. These factors include broad societal attitudes to illness, death, and cancer; perceived success rates for cancer therapy; and the attitudes and behaviors of health professionals.

Historically, cancer has been stigmatized as an unclean disease. In an interview study of 60 people with mixed cancers at the Massachusetts General Hospital in 1953, patients commonly felt they were perceived by others as unclean and repellent.[15] Guilt feelings were also common. Two years later, a study of women with breast cancer treated by radical mastectomy identified a deep concern that people in the community would discover the fact of their surgery.[16]

In 1926, Charles Mayo wrote, "While there are several chronic diseases more destructive to life than cancer, none is more feared" (*Annals of Surgery* 1926 83:357). Despite the vast improvements in objective outcomes of cancer since the 1920s (for example, the 5-year survival rate for all sites combined exceeded 50% in 1984[17]), and the fact that other diseases carry equally serious or worse prognoses, data from recent studies in different countries show that public attitudes toward cancer are still colored by fears and misconceptions. Cancer was by far the most feared illness in an Australian survey population in 1993, with more than twice the mentions of the next most feared disease.[18] Similar results were noted by Eisinger and coworkers,[19] who surveyed a random sample of the French population aged 18 to 75 years and found that cancer remains the most highly feared disease. The majority of Murray and McMillan's[20] sample of 700 adults also identified cancer as the most fearful disease; women reported being more frightened of cancer than did men, and the greatest fear of cancer was related to its perceived incurability and the associated suffering.

These fears and misconceptions persist despite the increased emphasis on improving cancer awareness among the general public. Evidence that earlier diagnosis of cancer combined with improved treatments would improve prognosis was the impetus for public education campaigns in America in the early 1950s. These gave wide publicity to the symptoms and signs of cancer to encourage the public to seek medical advice early and to influence the fatalistic attitudes of both doctors and patients.[21] To evaluate the impact of education campaigns, Samp and Curreri[22] asked a mixed sample of 560 cancer patients, family members, and randomly selected members of the general public about their awareness of cancer and their responses to cancer public education efforts. Education was seen as provoking fear; however, information was seen as helping to decrease this fear.

Cancer, particularly breast cancer, has acquired a high media profile. In the Western world, popular magazines and electronic media regularly feature stories about high-profile people who have cancer. We might therefore expect that with nearly 40 years of continuing public education regarding symptom awareness and detection practices, the public in the 1990s would now be more knowledgeable and less subject to misconceptions. However, Fallowfield and coworkers[23] showed that many misconceptions and myths about breast cancer remain. One reason may be that cancer was typically not discussed when older women, who are now being diagnosed with breast cancer, were growing up.

Medical Attitudes and Behavior Affect Patient Adjustment

To understand the origins of this fear, we need to focus on the medical profession's attitudes to communication with cancer patients. Whether doctors disclose the diagnosis to patients, the details they communicate concerning the prognosis, and the manner in which this information is conveyed will influence patient evaluation of that information and may affect subsequent adjustment.[24] Current evidence suggests that providing information is beneficial to the majority of patients who prefer full information, but may be detrimental to those who cope by avoiding information.[24-26] The way information is delivered also appears to be important. For example, Shapiro and coworkers[27] reported that 20 women at risk of breast cancer, randomized to receiving mammogram results from a worried physician, recalled significantly less information, had higher anxiety and pulse rates, and perceived their clinical situation as more severe than 20 women who received identical mammogram results from a nonworried physician.

Until the 1970s, most physicians did not disclose a cancer diagnosis to the patient (Table 11.1), although even back in the 1940s opinion was divided.[1-3] Seelig,[2] for example, stressed the great mental shock this sudden knowledge

Table 11.1. Physicians' views on disclosing a
cancer diagnosis[154]

Year	Country	Sample (N)	Always/Usually (%)
1953	USA	444	30
1961	USA	219	10
1979	USA	264	98
1980	Japan	72	66
1987	England	548	81
1989	Japan	116	31

might induce in the patient. This viewpoint reflected the trend in medicine to withhold any information that might severely upset patients.[21,28] In contrast, other clinicians stressed the importance of education and truth telling.[29,30]

Oken[28] recognized that physicians' covert attitudes can have a profound influence on patients' well-being. He argued that "the medical profession plays a pivotal role in cancer control far beyond its direct functions in diagnosis and treatment. When doctors lose hope their patients know it. If doctors communicate the feeling that cancer is dreadful and irremediable, how can patients fail to despair? And frightened and despairing, how can they deal with the possibility they have cancer?" Oken investigated current practice in a study of 219 cancer physicians in 1961. Ninety percent of physicians in this study reported that they never told the patient the diagnosis. Specific words, such as cancer and malignancy, were almost never used; euphemisms were the general rule. The majority of these doctors believed that most patients really do not want to know their diagnoses, regardless of what they say. The argument against telling centered on the anticipation of profoundly disturbing psychological effects and the need to maintain hope.

This rationale was still being cited in the 1970s. Following a survey of consecutive admissions to a Scottish teaching hospital in 1976, McIntosh[31] concluded ". . . there will always be anxiety associated with cancer, whether it is grounded in uncertainty or in patients' knowledge of their condition." He suggested that many patients chose the anxiety resulting from uncertainty, as it allowed them hope. Patients who were not told directly had other ways of finding out. This information was accessible, for example, through the tangible evidence of treatment in a setting commonly connected with cancer patients. A policy of routinely informing all patients was considered distressing to most and largely unnecessary to the remainder.

A contrary view suggested that euphemisms and prevarication often leave patients and families with an enormous barrier of deceit and the removal of this "web of deception" is met with great relief. Smith[32] said "the malignant reputation of cancer is enhanced by the secrecy surrounding it." This view has now gained precedence, at least in the United States. Using the same questions Oken[28] had employed, Novack and coworkers[8] found that the number of doctors revealing the diagnosis had increased from 10% in 1961 to 97% in 1979.

In Europe the pace of change has been variable, with use of the word "cancer" being considerably higher in Scandinavian than in Latin countries.[33] A 1991 study of gastroenterologists in all parts of Europe showed considerable variability across Europe in the attitudes and behavior of the sampled doctors.[9] It is not known whether this variation reflects attitudes among the doctors or the doctors' response to attitudes among their patients. A recent survey of Japanese physicians from teaching hospitals, including all cancer centers in the country, reported that 56% of physicians do not inform patients of a diagnosis of cancer, partly due to a fear of harming their relationships with their patients.[34] Certainly, there is considerable cross-cultural variability in patients' reported preferences for disclosing the cancer diagnosis (Table 11.2). Additional comparative studies of patients' expectations and information preferences and their relationships with family patterns, religious convictions, and cultural attitudes are needed.

In conclusion, the prognoses of many cancers and the attitudes of doctors and the community have all changed radically over the past 50 years. What would have been a normal (and realistic) response to cancer in the 1940s may not be normal or adaptive now. It is important to remember that adjustment to cancer will depend to some extent on the cultural and medical context of an individual. Interpretation of research findings must take this into account.

The Individual's Adjustment to Cancer

The dictionary defines adjustment as "the act of adapting to a new environment." In this case, the new environment would be the fact, implications, and

Table 11.2. Patients' views on disclosing a cancer diagnosis[154]

Year	Country	Sample (N)	Definitely/Preferably (%)
1955	USA	560	81
1959	USA	231	66
1962	USA	278	82
1976	UK	74	68
1978	Denmark	640	54
1981	UK	200	49
1989	Germany	147	90
1990	USSR	280	94
1993	Australia	142	90

consequences of having cancer. While these would vary depending on the site and severity of the cancer, major themes have emerged from the literature on coping with cancer, such as dependence, disability, disfigurement, distance in relationships, and death.[5] Cohen and Lazarus[35] described five main adaptive tasks required in coping with these stresses:

1. To reduce harmful environmental conditions and enhance prospects of recovery.
2. To tolerate or adjust to negative events and realities.
3. To maintain a positive self-image.
4. To maintain emotional equilibrium.
5. To continue satisfying relationships with others.

The strong desire, especially in younger patients, for more information and greater involvement in treatment decisions[25,36] suggests that a sixth important function is:

6. To maintain a sense of personal control over one's life.

These tasks require behavioral, emotional, and practical effort in complying with treatment regimens, dealing with negative emotions, and learning to handle post-treatment changes, such as a prosthesis or colostomy.[37] Clearly, it will take time for these adaptations to occur, and there will be variation in how well and how consistently they are maintained.

The concept of "normal" is an important adjunct to the word "adjustment," because it implies that there is an expected or standard way of responding to cancer, against which an individual may be measured. A certain amount of distress and difficulty is to be expected; indeed the absence of distress strikes warning bells. Furthermore, the concept of normality has implications for intervention. Some have argued that in the context of minimal resources, it is important to identify those people who have "abnormal adjustment" and to concentrate scarce resources on this group. The empirical data supporting the efficacy of interventions are scarce, and some argue that those who provide such interventions should act to demonstrate their "incremental efficacy."[38] Patients who are going through a predictable sequence of responses leading to a satisfactory, or at least average, conclusion may not need assistance. Others have argued that a person receiving a diagnosis of cancer is in crisis and would benefit, as in any other crisis, from psychosocial assistance.[39]

What is the "normal" process of adjusting to cancer? As there is a relative dearth of research involving patients other than those with breast cancer, it is difficult to comment on a general, or even site-specific, process of adjustment. A Medline literature search for the years 1990 to 1994, using as keywords "psychological adjustment" together with "breast cancer," "melanoma," "lung cancer," "colo-rectal cancer," and other cancer types, found 102 references for breast cancer, but fewer than 10 for most other cancer types and none for several of these. Furthermore, many of the studies investigating the clinical course and prognosis of psychological adjustment to breast cancer lack methodological rigor,[11] with small sample sizes and noncomparable, idiosyncratic measurement instruments. Nevertheless, current information is largely derived from the breast cancer literature, and therefore conclusions must be viewed as tentative, and generalization to other cancer sites uncertain.

Anxiety and depression are common mood disorders among cancer patients. The frequency of depression has been frequently studied in the cancer setting, with prevalence varying from a low of 4.5%[40] to a high of 58%.[41] The variability is no doubt partly due to different measures and sampling frames. Derogatis and coworkers[42] found that 47% of a randomly selected set of 215 cancer patients studied with traditional structured psychiatric interviews and patient self-report scales had sufficient psychiatric symptoms to warrant the diagnosis of a psychiatric disorder, mostly reactive depression, anxiety, or both. Their data provide a helpful estimate of the range of psychological responses among a large group of ambulatory cancer patients. They suggest that 50% experience normal responses in coping with cancer, which include heightened levels of anxiety and depression at transition or crisis points. These points usually occur in relation to a change in the disease or treatments. Symptoms abate as the crisis resolves and the individual returns to both normal mood and function. The remaining 50% experience more severe distress, mainly reactive anxiety and depression. Preexisting psychiatric problems that worsen during treatment and complicate care constitute only a minority of the cases; by far the majority of problems relate to the efforts of psychologically stable individuals to adjust to cancer and its treatment.

Time Course of Adjustment—The Hurdles of Cancer

Prediagnosis

Delays in seeking help

Lay populations consistently overestimate the mortality figures for cancer in all sites.[39] A worrisome symptom suggests the worst-case scenario. Excessive fear can lead to a delay in seeking help, sometimes to the point of compromising survival. Eddy and Eddy[43] reviewed studies of delay and its effects on survival and found that long-term survival of patients who had delayed seeking help by more than 3 months was reduced by 10% to 20%. Some workers have estimated that approximately 20% of women with symptoms of breast cancer delay seeking help for 3 months or more,[44,45] and figures of 35% to 50% have been quoted for heterogeneous cancer groups.[46–48]

Interestingly, a study by Hackett and coworkers[49] showed that delay rates of cancer patients treated at Massachusetts General Hospital showed no change over a 30-year period between the 1940s and 1970s. The authors concluded that because education and knowledge of cancer had improved in this time, psychological factors were likely to be responsible. Fallowfield and

Clark[39] note that many myths about the causality and treatment of cancer are still commonly held and must be partially responsible for treatment delay.

Some characteristics of "delayers" have been identified (Table 11.3). These include demographic factors such as older age and lower socioeconomic status; psychological factors such as preexisting emotional difficulties; knowledge and attitudes such as ignorance of the significance of symptoms; fear of doctors, hospitals, and cancer in particular; and a feeling of "it couldn't happen to me."[45,50–56] Clearly, this is an area that deserves further research attention.

Waiting for results
After seeking help, waiting for results is the next hurdle. Many patients describe the period between the detection of symptoms and the confirmation of cancer as the most stressful time of the entire cancer experience.[57] One woman in a retrospective study of the experiences and preferences of patients with breast cancer or melanoma commented that "the waiting was the worst: not knowing whether my life would be in total chaos next week or back to normal. I tried to put it at the back of my mind, but all I could think about was cancer, cancer, cancer. In the end, finding out that I did have cancer was almost a relief."[57]

Table 11.3. Factors associated with delay in seeking care for a cancer symptom

Factors	Specific characteristics
Sociodemographic variables	Older age
	Lower educational level
	Lower social class
Psychological and coping factors	More anxiety and depression
	Preexisting psychiatric diagnosis
	Tendency to deny or repress disturbing information
	Sense of invulnerability
	External locus of control
Knowledge, attitudes, and beliefs about cancer	Excessive fears of cancer, surgery, and hospitals
	Ignorance of the significance of symptoms
	Pessimism about treatment
	Low perceived susceptibility to cancer
	Emotional meaning and beliefs about cancer (e.g., shame, guilt)
	Previous experience with someone who had severe treatment side effects or a poor outcome
Poor or absent relationship with doctors	

The longer the wait, the harder it is. In the study of Butow and co-workers,[59] most patients were told their diagnosis within 1 week of seeking medical help and coped with that quite well. However, cancer was not confirmed for more than 1 month in 16% of cases and 96% of these patients felt that this was too long. Similarly, although the majority of patients learned the extent of their cancer within 1 week of diagnosis, 26% waited more than 1 week. Of the latter group, 63% felt that this time period was too long. While some delays may be unavoidable, an explanation of the reasons for delay, provision of support, and maintenance of contact with the patient during the waiting period may assist some people in getting through this difficult time.

With the increasing availability of cancer-screening programs, the effect of attendance and recall on people who do not have cancer is also an important area of inquiry. Breast cancer screening programs, although still relatively new, have been most extensively studied. Increased emotional distress has been noted in women who have recently attended a breast cancer screening program or who have had a benign breast lump, although this had dissipated by 8-month follow-up.[58] This anxiety may be translated into positive health practices. In one study, benign breast biopsies were associated with increased breast cancer detection practices (breast self-examination, mammogram, clinical breast examination) compared with a sample of women with no history of breast disease.[59] However, excessive anxiety may be an iatrogenic effect of screening.

The diagnosis

People react to the diagnosis of cancer in a variety of ways. For most, it is the cause of great distress and disruption. Some people experience a great sense of shock, and it is not uncommon to hear patients say "I did not hear a thing after the doctor said the word cancer." In a retrospective study, 40% of breast cancer patients and 34% of melanoma patients reported that their cancer diagnosis was a complete surprise.[57] Such a response suggests that the patient had not been adequately prepared for the possibility that the diagnosis could be cancer.

Morris and her colleagues[60] interviewed a large number of women with breast cancer about their responses to diagnosis and categorized their responses into five coping styles: denial, fighting spirit, stoic acceptance, fatalism, and anxious/depressed acceptance. These categories have been used extensively in research into the relationship between initial coping response and outcome in breast cancer.

Typical responses to a cancer diagnosis in men and in other cancer types have been less well studied. Ginsburg and coworkers[61] used interviews to assess psychiatric illness and psychosocial concerns in 52 newly diagnosed lung cancer patients. Reactions varied, with 44% reporting sadness, 8% guilt, and 29% fear, but only 13% seemed to be coping poorly. However, it is difficult to untangle the influence of gender and the site-specific issues involved in breast and lung cancer. As it is estimated that 83% (85% in men, 75% in women) of lung cancer is related to smoking, the emotional impact of this diagnosis may be quite different from that of breast cancer.

Can we influence how a person responds initially to the diagnosis of cancer? Relatively unchangeable features of the patient and his or her social milieu have been shown to influence patient adjustment to cancer, including patient education,[62] premorbid psychologic factors,[63] and level of social support.[64] However, even when these factors have been taken into account, modifiable factors such as doctor–patient communication have been shown to influence adjustment. Indeed, a recent prospective study reported that the most significant factor contributing to long-term maladjustment in breast cancer was the patient's perception of the way in which the diagnosis of cancer was communicated.[65] Roberts and coworkers[24] showed that patient ratings of physician behavior in the diagnostic interview accounted for 21% of the variance in psychological adjustment for 100 women with breast cancer.

Recent studies have identified considerable variability in the way the diagnosis of cancer is communicated and in patients' preferences. They also show discrepancies between patients' experiences and preferred characteristics of communication. For example, only 11% of patients in the study of Lind and coworkers[66] were told their cancer diagnosis by their general practitioner (GP), whereas 86% of the sample of Sardell and coworkers[67] preferred the GP to tell. Most (84%) patients preferred to have a relative present,[67] whereas only 38% of the sample of Peteet and coworkers[68] were accompanied by a relative when told their diagnosis.

In the study of Butow and coworkers,[57] the majority of patients dissatisfied with the diagnostic interview wanted more information, better emotional support, and a shorter time period between seeking help and confirmation of cancer. Seventy percent of patients endorsed the idea of a question prompt sheet providing sample questions commonly asked by patients facing a cancer diagnosis. These patient-preferred procedures would be inexpensive additions to clinical practice and merit introduction and review.

Information transfer and treatment decision making

Acquisition of information and involvement in decision making are thought to be important contributors to the process of adjusting to a cancer diagnosis. Available research offers conflicting evidence regarding the majority preference for involvement in decision making:[25,36,69,70] the trend is for most people to prefer maximum information and an active role, but it is well worth noting that a significant number of patients prefer minimal information and/or a passive role. One explanation for this diversity in preferences is that patients cope with cancer in different ways. Miller[71] categorizes people into two groups, depending on the behavioral strategy they use to deal with information about an aversive event. "Monitors" actively seek information, whereas "blunters" avoid or distract themselves from the information. Steptoe and coworkers[72] found that patients who reported the highest amount of satisfaction with the information they had received were more avoidant in their coping style (i.e., blunters). Monitors were least satisfied, but actually possessed greater factual knowledge than the blunters. Miller suggested that "forcing" information on a blunter may be as injurious as withholding it from a monitor.

Others have suggested that information and involvement preferences may change when a person becomes ill. Degner[70] found that while the majority of well people preferred an active role in decision making, the majority of sick people preferred the doctor to make the decisions. At a time when they may feel physically unwell and overwhelmed with anxiety, many patients appear to sanction a degree of paternalism in decision making, opting to exercise their "autonomous choice of dependency."[73] For example, the late Dr. Franz Ingelfinger, for many years the editor of the *New England Journal of Medicine*, wrote these words after being diagnosed with cancer:

> I received from physician friends throughout the country a barrage of well-intentioned but contradictory advice . . . as a result not only I but my wife, my son and daughter-in-law (all doctors) and other family members became increasingly confused and emotionally distraught. Finally when the pangs of indecision had become nearly intolerable, one wise physician friend said "what you need is a doctor." He was telling me to forget the information I already had . . . and seek instead a person who would tell me what to do, who would in a paternalistic manner assume responsibility for my care. When this excellent advice was followed, my family and I sensed immediate and immense relief.[74]

Poor communication about treatment decisions, which can result in a transitory state of dissatisfaction and confusion, may also have long-term effects. Fallowfield and coworkers[75] assessed patients who had a mastectomy or lumpectomy at 2 weeks, 3 months, and 12 months. The surgeons were divided into those who favored mastectomy, favored lumpectomy, or offered a choice. In contrast to the treatment received, which had no effect on anxiety or depression at any stage, there was a significant relationship, still present at 12 months, between surgeon type and anxiety ($p < .01$) and a trend toward significance for depression ($p = .06$). Patients whose surgeons offered choice coped significantly better than those who received a definite recommendation. This effect was still present at 3 years' followup (Fallowfield, personal communication).

In another study exploring psychological adjustment following surgery, 100 women newly diagnosed with breast cancer completed a questionnaire measuring their perceptions of doctor–patient communication during the consultation in which diagnosis and treatment options were discussed.[24] In a multiple regression adjusting for other possible predictors of adjustment (such as level of social support and previous psychiatric status), patient perceptions of physician communication were significantly related to psychological adjustment. A factor analysis of patients' responses indicated that the physician's caring attitude was perceived by the women as the most important dimension.

Treatment

Surgery, radiotherapy, and chemotherapy are common experiences for the majority of people diagnosed with cancer. There have been many largely anecdotal reports of the psychological responses of patients to these therapies.

Surgery

The universal reaction to an anticipated surgical procedure is fear and anxiety,[12] and there is considerable evidence that levels of preoperative anxiety are associated with postoperative adjustment and recovery in both adults and children. Adequate preparation beforehand and good postoperative pain control appear to be the major factors that assist patients in coping with the immediate stresses of surgery.[76-78] A small number of studies have examined psychological responses related to the specific site and functional loss experienced, such as head and neck surgery,[79] colostomy following colorectal cancer,[80] and genitourinary surgery.[81] However, the bulk of the literature by far deals with the comparison of responses to mastectomy and lumpectomy.[39]

The literature on mastectomy and lumpectomy exemplifies the need for data to evaluate popular expectations. The widely held assumption that replacing total mastectomy with lumpectomy would substantially alleviate the distress of women undergoing surgery for breast cancer has not been confirmed. Studies conducted in this area have shown very little difference in the numbers of women found to be anxious or depressed after either surgery. Some studies have shown a small advantage to women receiving a lumpectomy in terms of body image, but the main issue for women who undergo either type of surgery appears to be the cancer itself, with the accompanying potential risk of recurrence and death.[82]

Other studies have demonstrated that the impact of type of surgery and prognosis is modified by other factors. Taylor and coworkers[37] explored psychological adjustment to breast cancer in 78 women. While radical surgery was more likely to produce continuing disabilities after treatment, the effect of type of surgery on adjustment appeared to be mediated by the woman's sense of disfigurement and by changes in the sexual and affectional patterns in her marriage, rather than by prognosis or disability.

Radiotherapy and chemotherapy

Both radiotherapy and chemotherapy have been perceived as more frightening to patients than surgery.[83] In an interesting study of the effects of framing on decision making, McNeil and coworkers[84] asked radiologists, business school graduates, and patients to imagine that they had lung cancer and decide between two treatments, radiotherapy and surgery. Information about the outcomes of both treatments was provided to the subjects. When the treatments were assigned neutral labels (treatment A and treatment B), the three groups were significantly more likely to choose radiotherapy; however, when the treatments were identified, people expressed a strong preference for surgery. All subject groups appeared to be prejudiced against the notion of radiotherapy.

Many people are so concerned about the possible side effects of these treatments that they exhibit significant psychopathology even before treatment begins. Middleboe and coworkers[85] reported depressive states in 40% of a sample of 36 patients prior to chemotherapy. These distressed responses appear to be over and above those elicited by the fact of having cancer. Maguire and coworkers[86] compared the psychiatric morbidity of women who had received surgery alone with those receiving surgery plus chemotherapy and found that a significantly greater proportion of the women who received chemotherapy were anxious or depressed. Those women who had experienced the most severe side effects were most emotionally distressed.

In limbo—between treatment and 5-year survival

The specific reactions to the diagnosis of cancer and short-term adjustment constitute only one aspect of a continuous sequence of psychological attempts to integrate the threat of cancer and the possibility of disability and premature death. There are few longitudinal studies that track the progress from diagnosis through long-term survival or relapse. Studies that have employed prospective designs[60,87,88] have generally found that adjustment improves over time. Cross-sectional data also provide some evidence that patients' initial psychological distress diminishes over time. Three months after diagnosis, the psychological status and well-being of patients with cancer has been shown to be comparable to that of patients with other chronic illnesses and better than that of psychiatric patients.[89] Other cross-sectional studies indicate that the psychological status of cancer survivors 3 years or more after diagnosis is similar to that found in general population studies.[89,90]

However, the evidence suggests that there is a substantial minority of patients with severe psychological distress that persists long after the initial diagnosis. These findings have been replicated across a number of different cancer types, especially those whose treatment offers a good prognosis, but causes substantial long-term disability. A controlled German study of male patients indicated that 4 years after laryngectomy, approximately 50% of patients suffered from depressive states that impaired their interpersonal relationships and work capacity.[91]

The data from laryngectomy patients might suggest that other disfiguring surgeries would be accompanied by psychological distress in a high proportion of patients. Data are very limited, however. Several studies report relatively impaired social life and sexual activity as well as depression among patients who have had a colostomy for colon cancer.[92-94] Devlin and coworkers[92] compared patients having permanent colostomies with those who had their bowel continuity restored; depression, social isolation, and severe impairment of sexual function were found to be associated with permanent colostomy, and 23% of patients developed depressive states of sufficient severity to warrant psychiatric help. Patients who had a colostomy 8 to 9 years previously reported significantly more social impairment—for example, greater loneliness (27%) and reduced frequency of cinema visits (61%)—compared with those who had colonic resection without colostomy.[93] Overall, 75% of men reported significantly decreased sexual activity.

The long-term adaptation to breast cancer has been relatively well studied. Morris[95] observed that approximately three of four married or older women will recover from the experience of mastectomy within 12 months; however, a substantial minority (25% to 33%) will be left with feelings of personal inadequacy, anxiety, and depression. This conclusion was partially based on two well-designed studies of mastectomized patients that suggested that 1 to 2 years after surgery 22% to 25% had depression severe enough to require treatment, compared with 8% to 10% of women with benign breast disease, and that 18% to 33% had serious sexual problems compared with 6% to 8% of controls.[96,97]

Omne-Ponten and coworkers[98] compared psychosocial adjustment in women with breast cancer who had had either a mastectomy or breast-conserving surgery at 13 months and 6 years follow-up. Levels of maladjustment were lower after 6 years than at 13 months post-treatment; however, 10% of the women still exhibited poor adjustment. There were no significant differences between the two groups on psychosocial adjustment at either time point, suggesting that differences in patient psychosocial adjustment could not be ascribed to the type of surgery.

A somewhat paradoxical finding is that completion of chemotherapy is sometimes accompanied by a heightened sense of anxiety about the cancer recurring, rather than a sense of relief that treatment is over.[99] This anxiety is normally greater for several weeks to months after therapy is discontinued. However, the data of Meyerowitz and coworkers[100] showed that even as long as 2 years after adjuvant therapy for breast cancer ceased, 37% of women were still experiencing significant anxiety about the possibility of recurrence. Decreased medical surveillance during this time can cause a heightened fear of recurrence for some patients; these patients may benefit from a tighter schedule of follow-up consultations than would normally be offered. However, Kiebert and coworkers[101] found that for the majority of patients, follow-up visits were a time of particular stress during this period; regular follow-up visits were welcomed but psychological distress was significantly higher 1 month before the appointment and on the day of the appointment compared with 2 weeks after the appointment.

Some treatment-related symptoms persist in the long term. Cella and Tross[102] have reported that episodes of nausea and anxiety can persist for as long as 10 years after chemotherapy. These episodes are precipitated by exposure to specific cues, such as sights and sounds, that evoke memories of the treatment experience.

Relapse

Is the diagnosis of recurrent disease more or less distressing than the initial cancer diagnosis? Weisman and Worden[103] showed that 30% of 102 mixed-cancer patients perceived recurrence as less traumatic than the original diagnosis. Fallowfield and Clark[39] reported that reactions to recurrent breast cancer are very mixed and include relief at ending the uncertainty and anxiety about recurrence; worry about the distress the diagnosis may have on their families; and extreme distress, fear, and anger. There is also some evidence that psychological morbidity is worse for patients with recurrent disease than those with advanced disease.[104]

Advanced disease and death

Available research suggests that between 25% and 50% of patients with advanced cancer are depressed and anxious at some time. For example, Plumb and Holland[63] reported that 20% to 30% of patients with advanced cancer experienced moderate to severe depression. The degree of physical disability that accompanies advanced disease may contribute to these rates of depression—patients who are physically exhausted become emotionally exhausted as well.[105] Not surprisingly, when a person has reached the stage of advanced disease, this also has particular influence on significant relationships. Couples reported an increased need for physical and verbal expressions of affection when one person was dying; at the same time, however, the illness interfered with sexual aspects of the relationship.[106]

The prospect of death provokes profound emotions and quite variable reactions. Patients usually approach death in a manner consistent with their style of adjustment during the course of the illness. Bereavement is extremely painful but it is a universal and, therefore, normal life experience, and it is important not to expect a single optimal pattern of response.[107] Denial is often maintained together with hope in the last months of life; a positive outlook in the setting of advanced disease is possible.[108]

Adjustment to survival from cancer

Improved cancer therapy options now mean that more people will survive long past the 5-year checkpoint and can consider themselves to be cured, especially those diagnosed with Hodgkin's disease, testicular cancer, and other neoplasms. Recurrence of most tumors is rare after the 5-year survival point, but other difficulties can occur in longer-term adjustment. Tross and Holland[109] suggest that there are five major sources of psychological adjustment for cancer survivors:

1. Late or delayed effects of medical treatment.
2. Sexual complications of treatment.
3. Central nervous system complications of treatment, resulting in neuropsychological late effects.
4. Psychological responses to having had a life-threatening illness.
5. Practical and social complications of reentry into normal activities and work.

Despite the message of cure after 5 years' cancer-free survival, there is evidence that aggressive therapy is associated with an increased risk of morbidity and mortality from secondary malignancy, organ failure, or infection. For example, 20-year survival rates for 5-year survivors of childhood malignancies (79% to 83%) are lower than rates for children in the general population (97%)[110] and sterility and secondary sexual impairment are evident in survivors of Hodgkin's disease.[111]

Cella and Tross[102] identified three types of stressors to which cancer survivors are prone: anticipatory, residual, and current psychological consequences after cure. Anticipatory consequences, also referred to as the Damocles syndrome,[112] are similar to the anticipatory grief reaction reported in the families of patients dying from prolonged illness.[113]

Most of the survival literature has focused on the adult survivor of childhood cancer and breast cancer patients. Positive effects of cancer adjustment are not emphasized in this literature, as measurement instruments tend to detect the negative aspects of adjustment to cancer. While there is no doubt that significant problems in the sense of well-being, employment, and marital and family relationships are the legacy of cancer survival for many people (for example, Fobair et al.[114]), there may be positive outcomes for cancer survivors. There is some evidence to suggest that survivors have adaptive advantages in everyday life, reflecting their difficult yet interpersonally rewarding experiences during illness. Kennedy and colleagues[115] documented a dramatic rise in optimism and appreciation of life as a benefit of having survived the experience of cancer. Gray and coworkers[116] reported that adult survivors of childhood cancer were found to be at least as well adjusted when compared with their peers. A summary of the sequence of likely hurdles cancer patients will face in their process of adjustment, realistic expectations for responses to these acute distress points, and suggestions for possible avenues to assist or intervene are presented in Table 11.4.

The literature suggests that the "normal" process of adjustment is not a fixed and inflexible process. Patients vary in both their responses and their coping and adaptive resources. While the literature shows that the majority of people respond to the hurdles cancer presents with initially high levels of

Table 11.4. Acute distress points in adjustment to cancer

Hurdles of adjustment	Expectations for response	Possible interventions
Pre-diagnosis	Anticipatory anxiety: "worst-case scenario"	Provide diagnosis as quickly as possible
		Keep patient informed of progress
		Provide interim support
	Delay in seeking diagnosis	Educate the community about cancer
		Provide culturally appropriate services
The diagnosis	Shock	Facilitate patient–doctor communication
	Denial	Provide information and emotional support
	Stoic acceptance	
	Fighting spirit	
	Fatalism	
	Anxiety and depression	
	Guilt	
Treatment	Fear and anxiety before surgery	Tell patients what they will experience beforehand
	Sense of body and sexual disfigurement	Provide good postoperative pain control
	Anxiety and depression	Provide counseling and support
		Involve patient in treatment decisions
		Minimize side effects
Post-treatment	Ongoing anxiety and depression in 20%–40% of patients	Establish individualized follow-up schedules
		Inform patients about support services
Relapse	Fear and depression	Provide information and emotional support
	Anger	
	Worry about effect on family	
	Relief that the waiting is over	
Advanced disease	Depression in 20%–50% of patients	Provide individual and group support
	Denial	
	Acceptance	
Survival	Anxiety about secondary effects	Offer participation in group support
	Residual grief	
	Practical social/personal problems	
	Enhanced sense of well-being	

distress but go on to adjust well over time, there is a significant subpopulation whose severe psychosocial morbidity is persistent and does not resolve without intervention. These are likely to be the patients in greatest need of effective interventions.

Assessment and Intervention Instruments

A variety of tools have been used to assess the impact of cancer on social, physical, emotional, and other factors. Cella and coworkers[117] summarized the instruments that have been used frequently and are most appropriately used in research. For clinical purposes, these instruments can be impractical and often unnecessary. Asking the patient if nausea and vomiting are serious problems is more efficient than using a questionnaire. Screening instruments are more valuable in clinical settings and could identify the minority whose morbidity is persistent and may benefit from referral or interventions. Well-researched instruments like the Hospital Anxiety and Depression Scale (HADS)[118] and the Symptom Checklist-90 (SCL-90-R)[119] provide a screening test that can quickly and reliably identify patients at serious risk. Ibbotson and coworkers[120] compared these questionnaires against the gold standard of psychiatric diagnosis by DSM III criteria in a sample of 513 cancer patients. Both the HADS and the SCL were successful in detecting patients in treatment, but the Mental Adjustment to Cancer Scale (MAC)[121] was not a useful predictor. Razavi and coworkers[122] also supported the usefulness of the HADS as a simple, sensitive, and specific screening tool for psychiatric disorders in an oncology population. It is to be expected that patients will exhibit a certain level of distress in response to the hurdles of cancer and that these measures can be used to identify those at the more extreme end of the distribution. It is also important to remember that the absence of distress is itself a warning sign and may be considered an abnormal response.

Most of the scales used to measure the impact of cancer on the individual are generic; there are few cancer-specific scales. Although it is costly and time-consuming to develop new questionnaires, there is a strong argument for disease-specific tools. Cancer stands out as the most feared disease and it is likely that the central concerns of cancer patients will differ from those with diabetes, for example, or a mixed group of general medical patients. Measures for cancer patients should focus on those issues that are especially important for them and avoid irrelevancies that cloud the picture. For example, indicators of depression, anxiety, energy, and positive well-being in the general population that are included in the Beck Depression Inventory[123] are likely to be confounded with symptoms and side effects of chemotherapy or radiotherapy in people with cancer.

Several cancer-specific scales have been developed to measure coping and psychological adjustment: most notably the MAC Scale[121] and the more recently developed Psychological Adjustment to Cancer Scale (PAC).[124] The MAC has emerged as a psychometrically validated cancer-specific measure of cognitive coping, and the PAC is a reliable and valid measure of emotional adjustment. These scales are not designed to screen for psychiatric disorders but rather to assess variability in adjustment to cancer for research and clinical purposes. They may have an important role in detecting the more subtle impact of psychiatric or psychological interventions.

Family Adjustment to Cancer

A common perception about the impact of cancer on a family is that the experience either draws people closer together or drives them apart. The media tend to show simplified resolution of family conflicts and happy endings when one member of a family or a partnership is diagnosed with cancer. The reality of the impact of cancer on family members is much more complex, and often more tragic. The literature presents an inconsistent picture: for example, childhood leukemia has been associated with increased divorce in one study[125] and with no impact on the marriage relationship.[126] There is some support for the expectation that family functioning is significantly worse with longer duration and greater severity of cancer.[112] Indeed, Rait and Lederberg[127] assert that family members should be considered second-order patients in their own right.

Not only does cancer present a huge emotional burden to families, but there is often a high financial cost in terms of employment and income. In one survey, one quarter of primary caregivers gave up or lost jobs following the diagnosis of cancer in a family member.[128]

The spouse or partner

As early as 1955, authors were discussing the need to facilitate the adjustment and coping of the spouse of a patient with cancer: ". . . husbands of mastectomy patients should have the opportunity of discussing their fears and misconceptions with the physician in order to minimize the disruptive effects on the marital relationship and on the patient herself. . . ."[16]

The partner or spouse of a person with cancer is subject to many conflicting emotions and adjustment tasks: conflict among feelings of loss, sadness, and sometimes guilt; difficulty in knowing how to talk to the person with cancer; worry about the possibility of death; and difficulty in adjusting to bodily changes in the partner (for example, the husbands of women who have had a mastectomy). There is often pressure to be strong and supportive for the patient, which may come from health professionals who expect that the family will automatically provide such support.

Some families are able to rise to the occasion, with few problems. For example, the majority of couples in Hughes' study[129] reported that their relationships were stable or enhanced in response to the wife's breast cancer diagnosis.

Other families have severe difficulties. Even when there are close family relationships, the spouse may be unable to cope with his or her own distress and find it difficult to provide the patient with strength and support. It is also possible that the extra strain will exacerbate underlying or existing conflict within a marriage.

Several studies show that the spouse of a cancer patient experiences levels of distress at least as severe as that of his or her partner following treatment and when the disease is advancing,[130–132] although one study of women with breast cancer reported significantly more role adjustment problems among the patients than their husbands, especially in work, domestic, and social roles.[130] Furthermore, spouse distress may persist for some time. Maguire[133] reported that 36% of husbands had symptoms of anxiety 1 year after their wives received treatment for breast cancer. The needs of spouses may not be adequately recognized or addressed: a small study that examined 36 partners of cancer patients for stress, coping, and appraisal before and after surgery found that the patients' distress decreased over time, but the spouse's level of distress remained elevated.[134] Much less is known about the factors associated with prolonged distress in spouses than in patients. There is also little family-oriented research outside of breast cancer and, accordingly, more about the reactions of husbands than wives to partners' cancer diagnosis.

Among the concerns of a woman undergoing surgery for breast cancer is the fear that mastectomy will threaten or diminish femininity and attractiveness, and that she will ber rejected by her partner.[13] This might suggest that the type of surgery would affect adjustment among the husbands of women treated for breast cancer. Omne-Ponten and coworkers[132] measured psychosocial adjustment among 56 husbands of women who underwent operation for breast cancer using either breast-conserving surgery (BCS) or mastectomy (MT). Almost half of the sample (48%) expressed some emotional distress, but the husbands of women with BCS were less distressed, anxious, and depressed after 4 months. The authors concluded that the type of surgery did not appear to be a major determinant of the psychosocial outcome for breast cancer patients' spouses.

Many husbands are willing to admit a high degree of distress in response to their wives' diagnosis; some conceal their emotional reactions in an attempt to adopt a protective role. Spouses may misinterpret the latter behavior as rejection.[135] Thus, there is a need to investigate possible interactional difficulties in response to a cancer diagnosis, as well as the individual adjustment of both patients and their spouses.

Parents of children with cancer

A child with cancer can produce a tremendous strain on the parents, both individually and in terms of the marriage relationship. In a longitudinal study,

Sawyer and coworkers[136] reported, not surprisingly, that soon after diagnosis, mothers of children with cancer reported significantly more anxiety and insomnia, somatic symptoms, and social dysfunction than control group mothers. After 12 months, this distress had declined, but mothers of cancer patients still reported significantly more symptoms of depression and somatic symptoms than the controls. Fathers had a similar pattern of adjustment, though generally at lower levels of distress. The authors also reported that after one year, families of children with cancer were functioning less effectively than control families in the community.

Cancer in a child can disturb marital functioning. Dahlquist and coworkers[137] reported that 25% of mothers and 28% of fathers of children with cancer reported significant marital distress. Factors associated with marital distress included general emotional distress, a discrepancy between partners' stated anxiety levels, and use of sensitizing coping strategies. However, this study did not include a control group of parents with healthy children to compare levels of marital distress.

The severity of the impact of childhood cancer on the parents may be mediated by other factors. Speechley and Noh[138] found an inverse relationship between social support and psychological distress among parents of children with cancer; this relationship was significantly stronger for the mothers.

Children of parents with terminal illness

Children who are in a family in which either an adult or child member has cancer can be in a very vulnerable position. They may have a range of difficult feelings to deal with, such as anger and jealousy at being neglected because of the extra attention paid to a sibling with cancer or because of a parent's illness.

Several recent studies have looked at children's adjustment and behavior when a parent has cancer or a fatal disease of another kind. In a recent study, Siegel and coworkers[139] reported that such children had significantly higher levels of self-reported depression and anxiety, and lower self-esteem than the control group. Parents also reported a significantly greater number of behavior problems and lower social competence in the children of a parent with a fatal illness. However, Christ and coworkers[140] found that most adolescent children of parents with terminal cancer coped with the stress without resorting to severe acting-out. Armsden and Lewis[141] reported that children of women with breast cancer tended to score significantly lower on self-esteem, using children's self-report on the Personal Attribute Inventory for Children, compared with children of women with biopsy-proven fibrocystic breast disease; children of women with breast cancer were also assessed by nurses to be better behaviorally adjusted than children in noncancer illness groups.

Compas and coworkers[142] explored predictors of child distress and found that both the patients' and family members' distress was related to subjective appraisals of the seriousness and stressfulness of the cancer, but was not related to objective characteristics of the disease. Symptoms of stress, including anxiety and depression, differed in children as a function of age, and the gender of the child and the parent. Adolescent girls whose mothers had cancer were the most significantly distressed.

Siblings of children with cancer

Both positive and negative effects of cancer on siblings have been reported. For example, Havermans and Eiser[143] used the Sibling Perception Questionnaire and found that siblings reported more empathy toward others and a perception that life had more value after a brother or sister was diagnosed with cancer. However, some also perceived that their interpersonal relations were negatively affected, especially with their parents, and others reported heightened concerns that their sibling might die. The authors suggest that siblings should have opportunities to talk about the implications of the disease, especially worries about death, and that more efforts should be made to prepare siblings for visiting the hospital and seeing the sick brother or sister. One recent study of 129 siblings of pediatric cancer patients[144] found that high levels of family cohesion and adaptability were associated with better adaptation for siblings.

Health Professional Adjustment to Cancer

Issues of staff stress became apparent in the high-technology, high-pressure environments of intensive care units and dialysis units in the 1960s and 1970s. There are complex factors contributing to stress among health workers: the responsibility of dealing with life-and-death situations, the strain of working in health systems where resources are stretched, the threat of being sued, unrealistic public expectations of what medicine can achieve, and long hours in often difficult working conditions. Lederberg[145] described sources of staff stress based on work by Cassem and Hackett:[146,147]

1. High morbidity, high mortality
2. Complex technology
3. High frequency of life–death decisions
4. Terminal care issues
5. Third-party conflicts
6. Interstaff conflicts
7. "Limelight" medicine
8. Response to severe debilitation and disfigurement
9. Response to "difficult" patients (excessive anger, dependency, uncooperativeness)
10. Response to suicidal ideation
11. Issue of inflicting pain as part of treatment.

These stresses can have a serious impact on the individual[148] and, therefore, it is important to be aware of potential problems.

Significant levels of depression and distress have been found in samples of general medical graduates. Almost 1 in 4 (23%) of 1805 Canadian doctors at all levels of training were found to have some degree of depression or distress.[149] Another study of 77 emergency physicians found 66% of the sample reported medium to high emotional exhaustion and depersonalization.[150] Data from oncology specifically is sparse, but Schmale and coworkers[151] showed that a random sample of 147 physician members of the American Society of Clinical Oncology identified a need for more emotional support for themselves to deal with the difficult issues of dying patients, ineffective treatments, and their pressured workload. Burnout is a burgeoning issue for health professionals in many areas of medicine, including oncology. Over half (56%) of a sample of 598 American oncologists reported experiencing symptoms of burnout in their professional lives, citing insufficient personal time (57%) and continuous exposure to fatal illness (53%) as two of the primary problems.[152] To alleviate burnout, 69% indicated the need for more personal time and 60% preferred to decrease the time they spent on patient care. While the response rate of 60% suggests that the population rate of burnout may be considerably lower than the 56% reported by the respondents, the problem is a relevant and disturbing one. More work is required to define the incidence and characteristics of burnout in oncology and identify strategies to manage or prevent the negative consequences.

Conclusion

Although clinicians must appreciate the range of normal adjustment to cancer, experience does not provide a reliable basis for accurate expectations. For example, physicians performed poorly in estimating psychological distress in cancer patients receiving bad news.[153] Other studies report that distress is related to subjective appraisals of the seriousness and stressfulness of cancer, rather than to medically defined disease severity. As a result, reality may be counterintuitive. Although it would be expected that mastectomy is more distressing than lumpectomy as treatment for breast cancer, Fallowfield and coworkers[75] reported that rates of anxiety and/or depression were equally high. Expectations need to be based on empirical data.

There is no single standard way in which people respond to or adapt to cancer, and normal adjustment encompasses a wide range of response patterns. Significant distress, often expressed as depression or anxiety, is typical at all stages. Indeed, the absence of distress is a likely indicator of poor adjustment. In the clinical setting, normalizing patient experiences and distress should be a high priority. Normal adjustment process can differ with cultural attitudes; the attitudes of the medical profession; wider society beliefs about death, illness, and cancer; and understanding of cancer morbidity and mortality. More information about these factors is needed.

A small proportion of people who experience significant morbidity that fails to recede over time require suitable interventions. Rather than offering interventions to all, or to people on a random basis, the judicious use of screening tools can be used to identify those people who are at long-term risk. The variety of ways in which people react and adjust to the threat of a cancer diagnosis is less important than whether the outcome is adaptive or maladaptive. When coping strategies reduce quality of life, jeopardize the possibility of positive outcomes by negatively influencing compliance with therapy, or lead to pychopathology, then assistance and intervention is appropriate.

The issues of adjustment to cancer extend beyond the patient who receives the diagnosis to their family members and also to health professionals. Research shows that family members are important sources of support to patients, but also that spouses, children, siblings, and parents can be severely distressed. More attention to their adjustment problems is warranted. There is still little understanding of the adaptive processes of families of patients with cancer, other than patients with breast cancer.

Although the literature appears biased in concentrating on the negative impact of a cancer diagnosis, it is heartening to see that occasionally good can arise from the experience of having cancer. Havermans and Eiser[143] showed that, along with the negative impact of having a brother or sister diagnosed with cancer, siblings reported more empathy toward others and that life had more value. It is also reassuring to see that although the diagnosis of cancer arouses deep-seated fears and profound distress, this distress does dissipate over time and the majority of people successfully adapt to having cancer in the long term.

References

1. Sachs B. Be an optimist. *J Mt Sinai Hosp* 1942; 8:323–325.
2. Seelig MG. Should cancer victims be told the truth? *J Miss State Med Assoc* 1943; 40:33–35.
3. Piatt LM. Physician and the cancer patient. *Ohio State M J* 1946; 42:371–372.
4. Schottenfeld D, Fraumeni JF, eds. *Cancer Epidemiology and Prevention.* Philadelphia: W. B. Saunders; 1982.
5. Rowland JH. Developmental stage and adaptation: Child and adolescent model. In: Holland JC, Rowland JH, eds. *Handbook of Psychooncology.* New York: Oxford University Press; 1989:519–543.
6. Bosl GJ. Status and prospects of the treatment of disseminated germ-cell tumors. *World J Urol* 1984; 2:38–42.
7. Silverberg E. Probabilities of eventually developing or dying of cancer. *Cancer Statistics* 1985; 35:36–56.
8. Novack DH, Plumer R, Smith RL, et al. Changes in physicians' attitudes towards telling the cancer patient. *JAMA* 1979; 241:897–900.

9. Thomsen OO, Wulff HR, Martin A, Singer PA. What do gastroenterologists in Europe tell cancer patients? *Lancet* 1993; 341:473–476.

10. Massie MJ, Holland JC. Overview of normal reactions and prevalence of psychiatric disorders. In: Holland JC, Rowland JH, eds. *Handbook of Psychooncology*. New York: Oxford University Press; 1989:273–282.

11. Irvine D, Brown B, Crooks D, Roberts J, Browne G. Psychosocial adjustment in women with breast cancer. *Cancer* 1991; 67:1097–1117.

12. Jacobsen P, Holland JC. Psychological reactions to cancer surgery. In: Holland JC, Rowland JH, eds. *Handbook of Psychooncology*. New York: Oxford University Press; 1989:117–133.

13. Rowland JH, Holland JC. Breast cancer. In: Holland JC, Rowland JH, eds. *Handbook of Psychooncology*. New York: Oxford University Press; 1989:188–207.

14. Holland JC, Rowland JH, eds. *Handbook of Psychooncology*. New York: Oxford University Press; 1989.

15. Abrams RD, Finesinger JE. Guilt reactions in patients with cancer. *Cancer* 1953; 6(3):474–482.

16. Bard M, Sutherland AM. Psychological impact of cancer and its treatment. *Cancer* 1955; 8(4):656–672.

17. National Cancer Institute. Surveillance, Epidemiology, and End Results Program (SEER) cancer patient survival statistics. *Update: Annu Cancer Stat Rev* 1984; 1–8.

18. Borland R, Donaghue N, Hill D. Illnesses that Australians feared in 1986 and 1993. *Aust J Public Health* 1994; 18(4):366–369.

19. Eisinger F, Moatti JP, Beja V, Obadia Y, Alias F, Dressen C. Attitude of the French female population to cancer screening. *Bull Cancer (Paris)* 1994; 81(8):683–690.

20. Murray M, McMillan C. Gender differences in perceptions of cancer. *J Cancer Educ* 1993; 8:53–62.

21. Fitts WT, Ravdin IS. What Philadelphia physicians tell patients with cancer. *JAMA* 1953; 153(10):901–904.

22. Samp RJ, Curreri AR. A questionnaire survey on public cancer education obtained from cancer patients and their families. *Cancer* 1957; 10:382–384.

23. Fallowfield LJ, Rodway A, Baum T. What are the psychological factors influencing attendance, non-attendance, and reattendance at a breast cancer screening centre? *J R Soc Med* 1990; 83:547–551.

24. Roberts CS, Cox CE, Reintgen MD, Baile WF, Gibertini M. Influence of doctor communication on newly diagnosed breast patients' psychologic adjustment and decision-making. *Cancer Suppl* 1994; 74:336–341.

25. Cassileth BR, Zupkis RV, Sutton-Smith K, March V. Information and participation preferences among cancer patients. *Ann Intern Med* 1980; 92:832–836.

26. Fallowfield LJ, Hall A, Maguire GP, Baum M. Psychological outcomes of different treatment policies in women with early breast cancer outside a clinical trial. *Br Med J* 1990; 301:575–580.

27. Shapiro DE, Boggs SR, Melamed BG, Graham-Pole J. The effect of varied physician affect on recall, anxiety and perceptions in women at risk for breast cancer: an analogue study. *Health Psychol* 1992; 11:61–66.

28. Oken D. What to tell cancer patients: a study of medical attitudes. *JAMA* 1961; 175(13):1120–1128.

29. Lund CC. Doctor, patient and the truth. *Ann Intern Med* 1946; 24:955–959.

30. Underwood FJ. Early cancer is curable. *Mississippi Doctor* 1949; 26:280–281.

31. McIntosh J. Patients' awareness and desire for information about diagnosed but undisclosed malignant disease. *Lancet* 1976; 3980:300–303.

32. Smith A. Should a doctor tell the truth when a patient has cancer? London: *The Times*, May, 1976.

33. Holland JC, Marchini A, Tross S. An international survey of physician practices in regard to revealing the diagnosis of cancer. Fourteenth Int Cancer Congr Abstr Lect Symp Free Commun. Vol 3. Basel: Karger; 1986. Abstract 3964.

34. Uchitomi Y, Sugihara J, Fukue M, Kuramoto Y, Akechi T, Oomori N, Yamawaki S. Psychiatric liaison issues in cancer care in Japan. *J Pain Symptom Manage* 1994; 9(5):319–324.

35. Cohen F, Lazarus R. Active coping processes, coping dispositions, and recovery from surgery. *Psychosom Med* 1973; 35:375–389.

36. Sutherland HJ, Llewellyn-Thomas HA, Lockwood GA, Tritchler DL, Till JE. Cancer patients: their desire for information and participation in treatment decisions. *J R Soc Med* 1989; 82:260–263.

37. Taylor SE, Lichtman RR, Wood JV, Bluming AZ, Dosik GM, Leibowitz RL. Illness-related and treatment-related factors in psychological adjustment to breast cancer. *Cancer* 1985; 55:2506–2513.

38. Derogatis LR, Spencer PM. Psychometric issues in the psychological assessment of the cancer patient. *Cancer* 1984; 53(10):2228–2232.

39. Fallowfield L, Clark A. *Breast Cancer*. London: Tavistock/Routledge, 1991.

40. Lansky SB, List MA, Herrmann CA, Ets-Hokin EG, DasGupta TK, Wilbanks GD, Hendrikson FR. Absence of major depressive disorder in female cancer patients. *J Clin Oncol* 1985; 3:1553–1560.

41. Hinton J. Psychiatric consultation in fatal illness. *Proc R Soc Med* 1972; 65:29–32.

42. Derogatis LR, Morrow GR, Fetting J, et al. The prevalence of psychiatric disorders among cancer patients. *JAMA* 1983; 249:751–757.

43. Eddy DM, Eddy JF. Delay factors in the detection of cancer. *Proc Am Cancer Soc Fourth Ntl Conf on Human Values and Cancer*. New York: American Cancer Society; 1984:32–40.

44. Cameron A, Hinton J. Delay in seeking treatment for mammary tumours. *Cancer* 1968; 21:1121–1126.

45. Williams EM, Baum M, Hughes LE. Delay in presentation of women with breast disease. *Clin Oncol* 1976; 2:327–331.

46. Kalmer H, ed. Reviews of research and studies related to delay in seeking if diagnosis is cancer. *Health Educ Monogr* 1974; 2(2).

47. DiClemente RJ, Temoshok L, Pickle LW, Barrow AR, Ehlke G. Patient delay in the diagnosis of cancer, emphasising malignant melanoma of the skin. *Prog Clin Biol Res* 1982; 83:185–194.

48. Feldman JG, Saunders M, Carter AC, Gardner G. The effects of patient delay and symptoms other than a lump on survival in breast cancer. *Cancer* 1983; 51:1226–1229.

49. Hackett TP, Cassem NH, Rake JW. Patient delay in cancer. *N Engl J Med* 1973; 289:14–20.

50. Antonovsky A, Hartman H. Delay in the detection of cancer: a review of the literature. *Health Educ Monogr* 1974; 2:98–128.

51. Green LW, Roberts BJ. The research literature on why women delay in seeking medical care for breast symptoms. *Health Educ Monogr* 1974; 2(2):129–177.

52. Green LW, Rimer ET, Elwood JM. Behavioural approaches to cancer prevention and detection. In: Weiss S, Herd A, Fox B, eds. *Perspectives on Behavioural Medicine.* New York: Academic Press; 1981:215–234.

53. Greer S. Psychological aspects: delay in the treatment of breast cancer. *Proc R Soc Med* 1974; 67:470–473.

54. Margarey CJ, Todd PB, Blizzard PJ. Psychosocial factors influencing delay and breast self-examination in women with symptoms of breast cancer. *Soc Sci Med* 1977; 11:229–232.

55. Buttlar CH, Templeton AC. The size of breast masses at presentation: the impact of prior medical training. *Cancer* 1983; 21:1121–1126.

56. Watson M, Pruyn J, Greer S, van den Borne B. Locus of control and adjustment to cancer. *Psychol Rep* 1990; 66(1):39–48.

57. Butow PN, Kazemi JN, Beeney LJ, Griffin AM, Dunn SM, Tattersall MHN. When the diagnosis is cancer: patient communication experiences and preferences. *Cancer.* In press.

58. Cockburn J, Staples M, Hurley SF, Luise TD. Psychological consequences of screening mammography. *J Med Screen* 1994; 1:7–12.

59. Benedict S, Williams RD, Baron PL. The effect of benign breast biopsy on subsequent breast cancer detection practices. *Oncol Nurs Forum* 1994; 21(9):1467–1475.

60. Morris J, Royle GT. Choice of surgery for early breast cancer: pre- and postoperative levels of clinical anxiety and depression in patients and their husbands. *Br J Surg* 1987; 74:1017–1019.

61. Ginsburg ML, Quirt C, Ginsburg AD, Mackillop WJ. Psychiatric illness and psychosocial concerns of patients with newly diagnosed lung cancer. *Can Med Assoc J* 1995; 152(5):701–708.

62. Ganz PA. Patient education as a moderator of psychological distress. *J Psychosoc Oncol* 1988; 6:181–197.

63. Plumb MM, Holland JC. Comparative studies of psychological function in patients with advanced cancer, II: interviewer-rated current and past psychological symptoms. *Psychosom Med* 1981; 43:243–254.

64. Northouse LL. Social support in patients' and husbands' adjustment to breast cancer. *Nurs Res* 1988; 37:91–95.

65. Omne-Ponten M. Psychosocial adjustment after breast cancer in stages I/II: a longitudinal study including assessments of women and husbands. Uppsala, Sweden: *Acta Universitatis Upsaliensis;* 1993.

66. Lind SE, Good MD, Seidel S, Csordas T, Good BJ. Telling the diagnosis of cancer. *J Clin Oncol* 1989; 7(5):583–589.

67. Sardell AN, Trierweiler SJ. Disclosing the cancer diagnosis. *Cancer* 1993; 72:3355–3365.

68. Peteet JR, Abrams HE, Murray Ross D, Stearns NM. Presenting a diagnosis of cancer: patients' views. *J Fam Pract* 1991; 32:577–581.

69. Blanchard CG, Labreque MS, Ruckdeschel JC, Blanchard EB. Information and decision-making preferences of hospitalized cancer patients. *Soc Sci Med* 1988; 27:1139–1145.

70. Degner LF, Sloan JA. Decision-making during serious illness: what role do patients really want to play? *J Clin Epidemiol* 1992; 45:941–950.

71. Miller SM. Monitoring and blunting: validation of a questionnaire to assess styles of information seeking under threat. *J Pers Soc Psychol* 1987; 52(2):345–353.

72. Steptoe A, Sutcliffe I, Allen B, Coombes C. Satisfaction with communication, medical knowledge, and coping style in patients with metastatic cancer. *Soc Sci Med* 1991; 32:627–632.

73. Williamson C. Whose standards? Consumer and professional standards in health care. Buckingham: Open University Press; 1992.

74. Ingelfinger FJ. Arrogance. *N Engl J Med* 1980; 301:1507–1511.

75. Fallowfield LJ, Baum M, Maguire GP. Effects of breast conservation on psychological morbidity associated with diagnosis and treatment of early breast cancer. *Br Med J* 1986; 293:1331–1334.

76. Mumford E, Schlesinger HJ, Glass GV. The effects of psychological intervention on recovery from surgery and heart attacks: an analysis of the literature. *Am J Public Health* 1982; 72:141–151.

77. Devine ED, Cook TD. Clinical and cost-saving effects of psychoeducational interventions with surgical patients: A meta-analysis. *Res Nurs Health* 1986; 9:89–105.

78. Massie MJ, Holland JC. The cancer patient with pain: psychiatric complications and their management. *Med Clin North Am* 1987; 71:243–258.

79. Scott DW, Oberst MT, Dropkin MJ. A stress-coping model. *Adv Nursing Sci* 1980; 3:9–23.

80. Oberst MT, James R. Going home: Patient and spouse adjustment following cancer surgery. *Top Clin Nurs* 1985; 7:46–57.

81. Schover LR, von Eschenbach AC, Smith DB, Gonzalez J. Sexual rehabilitation of urologic cancer patients: a practical approach. *CA Cancer J Clin* 1984; 34:66–74.

82. Hall A, Fallowfield LJ. Psychological outcome of treatment for early breast cancer: a review. *Stress Med* 1989; 5:167–175.

83. Holland JC, Lesko LM. Chemotherapy, endocrine therapy and immunotherapy. In: Holland JC, Rowland JH, eds. *Handbook of Psychooncology.* New York: Oxford University Press; 1989:146–162.

84. McNeil BJ, Pauker SG, Sox HC, Tversky A. On the elicitation of preferences for alternative therapies. *N Engl J Med* 1982; 306:1259–1262.

85. Middelboe T, Ovesen L, Mortensen EL, Bech P. Depressive symptoms in cancer patients undergoing chemotherapy. *Psychother Psychosom* 1994; 61(3–4):171–177.

86. Maguire GP, Tait A, Brooke M, et al. Psychiatric morbidity and physical toxicity associated with adjuvant chemotherapy after mastectomy. *Br Med J* 1980; 2:1179–1180.

87. Weisman AD, Worden JW. The emotional impact of recurrent cancer. *J Psychosoc Oncol* 1976; 3:5–16.

88. Gottschalk LA, Hoigaard-Martin J. The emotional impact of mastectomy. *Psychiatry Res* 1986; 17:153–167.

89. Cassileth BR, Lusk EJ, Strouse TB, et al. Psychosocial status of chronic illness: a comparative analysis of six diagnostic groups. *N Engl J Med* 1984; 311:506–511.

90. Schmale AH, Morrow GR, Schmitt MH, et al. Well-being of cancer survivors. *Psychosom Med* 1984; 45:163–169.

91. Wochnik M. Psychological inquiries in patients after laryngectomy in comparison with normal persons and teachers with hearing disorders. *Z Arztl Fortbild (Jena)* 1976; 70(23):1213–1218.

92. Devlin HB, Plant JA, Griffin M. Aftermath of surgery for anorectal cancer. *Br Med J* 1971; 3:413–418.

93. Wirsching M, Druner HU, Herrman G. Results of psychosocial adjustment to long-term colostomy. *Psychother Psychosom* 1975; 7(1):46–57.

94. Eardley A, George WD, Davis F, Schofield PF, Wilson MC, Wakefield J, Sellwood RA. Colostomy: the consequences of surgery. *Clin Oncol* 1976; 2:277–283.

95. Morris T. Psychological adjustment to mastectomy. *Cancer Treat Rev* 1979; 6:41–61.

96. Morris T, Greer HS, White P. Psychological and social adjustment to mastectomy. *CA Cancer J Clin* 1977; 40:2381–2387.

97. Maguire GP, Lee EG, Bevington DJ, et al. Psychiatric problems in the first year after mastectomy. *Br Med J* 1978; (1):963–965.

98. Omne-Ponten M, Holmberg L, Sjoden PO. Psychosocial adjustment among women with breast cancer stages I and II: six-year follow-up of consecutive patients. *J Clin Oncol* 1994; 12(9):1778–1782.

99. Hurt GJ, McQuellon RP, Barrett RJ. After treatment ends: neutral time. *Cancer Pract* 1994; 2(6):417–420.

100. Meyerowitz VW, Watkins IK, Sparks FC. Psychosocial implications of adjuvant chemotherapy: a two-year follow-up. *Cancer* 1983; 52:1541–1545.

101. Kiebert GM, Welvaart K, Kievit J. Psychological effects of routine follow-up on cancer patients after surgery. *Eur J Surg* 1993; 159(11–12):601–607.

102. Cella DF, Tross S. Psychological adjustment to survival from Hodgkin's disease. *J Consult Clin Psych* 1986; 54:618–622.

103. Weisman AD, Worden JW. The emotional impact of recurrent cancer. *J Psychosoc Oncol* 1986; 3:5–16.

104. Silberfarb PM, Philibert D, Levine PM. Psychosocial aspects of neoplastic disease: II. Affective and cognitive effects of chemotherapy in cancer patients. *Am J Psychiatry* 1980; 137(5):597–601.

105. Bukberg J, Penman D, Holland JC. Depression in hospitalized cancer patients. *Psychosom Med* 1984; 46:199–212.

106. Lieber L, Plumb M, Gerstenzang M, Holland J. The communication of affection between cancer patients and their spouses. *Psychosom Med* 1976; 38:379–389.

107. Koocher GP. Coping with a death from cancer. *J Consult Clin Psychol* 1986; 54:623–631.

108. Yates JW, McKegney FP, Kun LE. A comparative study of home nursing care of patients with advanced cancer. *Proc Am Cancer Soc Third Natl Conf on Human Values and Cancer.* 1981:207–218.

109. Tross S, Holland JC. Psychological sequelae in cancer survivors. In: Holland JC, Rowland JH, eds. *Handbook of Psychooncology.* New York: Oxford University Press; 1989:101–116.

110. Li FP, Myers MH, Heise HW, Jaffe N. The course of five-year survivors of cancer in childhood. *J Pediatr* 1978; 93:185–187.

111. Chapman R, Sutcliffe S, Malpas J. Male gonadal dysfunction in Hodgkin's disease. *JAMA* 1981; 245:1323–1328.

112. Koocher GP, O'Malley JE. *Damocles Syndrome: Psychological Consequences of Surviving Childhood Cancer.* New York: McGraw-Hill; 1981.
113. Futterman E, Hoffman I. Crisis and adaptation in the families of fatally ill children. In: Anthony EJ, Koupernik C, eds. *The Child in His Family: The Impact of Disease and Death.* New York: Wiley; 1973:127–144.
114. Fobair P, Hoppe RT, Bloom J, Cox R, Varghese A, Spiegel D. Psychosocial problems among survivors of Hodgkin's disease. *J Clin Oncol* 1986; 4:805–814.
115. Kennedy BJ, Tellegen A, Kennedy S, Havernick N. Psychological response of patients cured of advanced cancer. *Cancer* 1976; 38:2184–2191.
116. Gray RE, Doan BD, Shermer P, et al. Psychologic adaptation of survivors of childhood cancer. *Cancer* 1992; 70(11):2713–2721.
117. Cella DF, Jacobsen PB, Lesko LM. Research methods in psychooncology. In: Holland JC, Rowland JH, eds. *Handbook of Psychooncology.* New York: Oxford University Press; 1989:737–749.
118. Zigmond AS, Snaith RP. The hospital anxiety and depression scale. *Acta Psychiatr Scand* 1983; 67:370–374.
119. Derogatis LR. *The SCL-90-R.* Baltimore: Clinical Psychometrics Research, 1975.
120. Ibbotson T, Maguire P, Selby P, Priestman T, Wallace L. Screening for anxiety and depression in cancer patients: the effects of disease and treatment. *Eur J Can* 1994; 30A:37–40.
121. Watson M, Greer S, Young J, Inayat Q, Burgess C, Robertson B. Development of a questionnaire measure of adjustment to cancer: the MAC scale. *Psychol Med* 1988; 18:203–209.
122. Razavi D, Delvaux N, Farvacques C, Robaye E. Screening for adjustment disorders and major depressive disorders in cancer in-patients. *Br J Psychiatry* 1990; 156:79–83.
123. Beck A, Ward C, Mendelson M, Mock J, Erbaugh J. An inventory for measuring depression. *Arch Gen Psychiatry* 1961; 4:561–571.
124. Dunn SM, Patterson PU, Butow PN, Smartt HH, McCarthy WH, Tattersall MHN. Cancer by another name: a randomized trial of the effects of euphemism and uncertainty in communicating with cancer patients. *J Clin Oncol* 1993; 11(5):989–996.
125. Kaplan DM, Grobstein R, Smith A. Predicting the impact of severe illness in families. *Health Soc Work* 1976; 1(3):71–82.
126. Lansky SB, Cairns NU, Hassanein R, Weir J, Lowman JT. Childhood cancer: parental discord and divorce. *Pediatrics* 1978; 62(2):184–188.
127. Rait D, Lederberg M. The family of the cancer patient. In: Holland JC, Rowland JH, eds. *Handbook of Psychooncology.* New York: Oxford University Press; 1989:585–597.
128. Murinen JM. The economics of informal care: labor market effects in the national hospice study. *Med Care* 1986; 24:1007–1017.
129. Hughes J. *Cancer and Emotion. Psychological Preludes and Reactions to Cancer.* Chichester: John Wiley; 1987.
130. Plumb M, Holland J. Comparative studies of psychological function in patients with advanced cancer—self-reported depressive symptoms. *Psychosom Med* 1977; 39(4):264–276.
131. Northouse LL, Swain MA. Adjustment of patients and husbands to the initial impact of breast cancer. *Nurs Res* 1987; 36:221–225.

132. Omne-Ponten M, Holmberg L, Bergstrom R, Sjoden PO, Burns T. Psychosocial adjustment among husbands of women treated for breast cancer; mastectomy vs. breast-conserving surgery. *Eur J Cancer* 1993; 29A (10):1393–1397.

133. Maguire P. The repercussions of mastectomy on the family. *Int J Family Psychiatry* 1981; 1:485–503.

134. Keitel MA, Zevon MA, Rounds JB, Petrelli NJ, Karakousis C. Spouse adjustment to cancer surgery: distress and coping responses. *J Surg Oncol* 1990; 43(3):148–153.

135. Sabo D, Brown J, Smith C. The male role and mastectomy: support groups and men's adjustment. *J Psychosoc Oncol* 1986; 4:19–31.

136. Sawyer MG, Antoniou G, Toogood I, Rice M, Baghurst PA. A prospective study of the psychological adjustment of parents and families of children with cancer. *J Paediatr Child Health* 1993; 29(5):352–356.

137. Dahlquist LM, Czyzewski DI, Copeland KG, Jones CL, Taub E, Vaughan JK. Parents of children newly diagnosed with cancer: anxiety, coping, and marital distress. *J Pediatr Psychol* 1993; 18(3):365–376.

138. Speechley KN, Noh S. Surviving childhood cancer, social support, and parents' psychological adjustment. *J Pediatr Psychol* 1992; 17(1):15–31.

139. Siegel K, Mesagno FP, Karus D, Christ G, Banks K, Moynihan R. Psychological adjustment of children with a terminally ill parent. *J Am Acad Child Adolesc Psychiatry* 1992; 31(2):327–333.

140. Christ GH, Siegel K, Sperber D. Impact of parental terminal cancer on adolescents. *Am J Orthopsychiatry* 1994; 64(4):604–613.

141. Armsden GC, Lewis FM. Behavioural adjustment and self-esteem of school-age children of women with breast cancer. *Oncol Nurs Forum* 1994; 21(1):39–45.

142. Compas BE, Worsham NL, Epping-Jordan JE, et al. When Mom or Dad has cancer: markers of psychological distress in cancer patients, spouses and children. *Health Psychol* 1994; 13(6):507–515.

143. Havermans T, Eiser C. Siblings of a child with cancer. *Child Care Health Dev* 1994; 20(5):309–322.

144. Cohen DS, Friedrich WN, Jaworski TM, Copeland D, Pendergrass T. Pediatric cancer: predicting sibling adjustment. *J Clin Psychol* 1994; 50(3):303–319.

145. Lederberg M. Psychological problems of staff and their management. In: Holland JC, Rowland JH, eds. *Handbook of Psychooncology.* New York: Oxford University Press; 1989:631–646.

146. Cassem NH, Hackett TP. Stress in the nurse and therapist in the intensive-care unit and the coronary care unit. *Heart Lung* 1975; 4:252–259.

147. Cassem N, Hackett TP. Psychiatric medicine in intensive care settings. In: Manschrek T, ed. *Psychiatry Medicine Update: MGH Reviews for Physicians.* New York: Elsevier; 1979:135–161.

148. Cartwright LK. Sources and effects of stress in health careers. In: Stone GC, Cohen F, Adler NE, eds. *Health Psychology.* San Francisco: Jossey-Bass; 1979.

149. Hsu K, Marshall V. Prevalence of depression and distress in a large sample of Canadian residents, interns and fellows. *Am J Psychiatry* 1987; 144:1561–1566.

150. Orlowki JP, Bulledge AD. Critical care stress and burnout. *Crit Care Clin* 1986; 2:173–181.

151. Schmale J, Weinberg N, Pieper S. Satisfactions, stresses, and coping mechanisms

of oncologists in clinical practice (summary). *Proc Am Soc Clin Oncol* 1987; 6:255.

152. Whippen DA, Canellos GP. Burnout syndrome in the practice of oncology: results of a random survey of 1,000 oncologists. *J Clin Oncol* 1991; 9(10):1916–1920.

153. Ford S, Fallowfield L, Lewis S. Can oncologists detect distress in their outpatients and how satisfied are they with their performance during bad news consultations? *Br J Cancer* 1994; 70:767–770.

154. Charlton RC. Breaking bad news. *Med J Aust* 1992; 157:615–621.

12

The Family as a Unit of Treatment

LINDA J. KRISTJANSON

Families of terminally ill cancer patients are not neutral bystanders to the illness experience. The literature documents the stressful nature of a family member's terminal illness on family members and recommends that health professionals view the family as the unit of treatment. But just how reliable, valid, and useful is the research supporting the family as a unit of treatment?

This chapter is a synthesis and critique of approximately 100 empirical studies published between 1970 and 1995 addressing the family's cancer experience during advanced stages of the disease. A search of both Medline and CINAHL using the keywords "family," "cancer," and "palliative/hospice" was undertaken to retrieve relevant literature. In reviewing the literature, three questions were posed: (1) How do families respond to advanced cancer in a member? (2) How can health care providers assess/identify functional family responses? and (3) What interventions are most helpful in supporting families through the terminal cancer illness of a loved one? The chapter follows these divisions, with comments in each major section related to the consistency of findings emerging from this work, the level of maturity of the science, and issues that warrant further attention.

How Do Families Respond to Advanced Cancer in a Member?

The literature describing family responses to advanced cancer fall into three themes: illness-related needs, alterations in family functioning, and health changes of family mambers. As this represents by far the largest body of literature, the comments and critique on its overall relevance follow in each division.

Illness-related needs

Considerable work has been undertaken to document the needs of family members of advanced cancer patients. These family care needs separate into two general categories: patient care needs that family members identify[1-3] and family members' own needs for support and assistance.[1-6]

The priority patient care need that family members identify consistently is patient comfort.[1,2,7-12] Family caregivers in home settings also identify needs for information about how to provide comfort and manage pain medications.[2,13] Family members report fears of drug addiction, respiratory depression, or drug tolerance, and may undermedicate patients even though patients are experiencing unrelieved pain.[7] The challenges of administering narcotics, managing infusion pumps, and delivering multiple medications have been reported to be anxiety producing for family members.[7,14,15]

Indeed, the most consistent care need reported in the literature is the need for information.[1,2,12,16] In addition to the need for information about pain management, family members identify needs for information and assistance with physical care management, treatment regimens, household management, and finances.[4,6,17-19]

There is mounting evidence that patients and families have different care needs and different perceptions of each other's care needs.[4,17,20,21] Hileman and Lackey[17] compared need statements from patient and family caregiver dyads and found that both groups underestimated each other's physical, psychological, information, household, financial, and spiritual needs. Grobe, Ahmann, and Ilstrup[20] studied 87 cancer patients and their family members and reported that patients underestimated the number and types of needs that family members indicated they required.

Higginson and colleagues[22] also reported incongruity between members' and patients' perceptions of symptom control, pain control, and anxiety. Family members who participated in this study rated the patient's distress as worse than the patient's ratings. Similar results have also been reported by Lobchuk.[23] These inconsistent findings raise questions about the direction of patient–family incongruity (do family members over- or underestimate patient distress?) and about the wisdom of using patients or family members as proxies for each other.

Certain times during the illness may create different or more needs for family members. For example, the end stage of the illness has been described as particularly difficult.[24-26] Stetz[6] documented that the strain of "standing by" or being continuously on duty during the care of the patient was stressful ($N = 65$). Hays[27] undertook a descriptive study of 50 patients and caregivers in a home hospice program. Family caregivers exhibited increased anxiety and fatigue in response to uncontrolled patient symptoms in the 10 days before the patient's death. Families also had slightly higher demands for home-based services during this period.

The literature indicates that families find changes in the patient's mental status the most distressing part of caregiving, and increased support from health professionals is particularly helpful at this time.[28,29] Bruera[30] reported that the incidence of conflict between health care providers and the family increased dramatically in patients with agitated delirium compared to the expected 5% conflict usually observed. Education of the family regarding the patient's mental changes and inclusion of the family in managing this symptom were reported to be useful strategies to reduce health professional–family conflict.

The work in this area is, for the most part, based on descriptive, cross-sectional studies. Although limited by small sizes, the findings are consistent. Patient comfort, information about treatment and care, and assistance with practical caregiving tasks are priority family needs. Family members' and patients' perceptions of each other's needs may be quite incongruent. It is also clear that the end stage of the patient's illness and changes in the patient's level of mentation are particularly difficult for families. These findings suggest directions for intervention research and timing of interventions. Longitudinal studies are also required to examine changes in family care needs over time.

Research is needed to clarify inconsistent reports of family's estimates of patient distress, identify factors/cues patients and family members use to determine each other's needs, and identify communication methods to reconcile needs assessment differences in the clinical setting. Researchers and clinicians are cautioned not to accept hastily the conclusion that family members overestimate the patient's distress. Patients may underestimate their distress in efforts to be "good patients" or as a coping mechanism (i.e., form of denial). This area warrants attention because of serious clinical and ethical questions about how to appropriately respond to patient suffering and family concerns.

Alterations in family functioning

The functioning of the family is at least temporarily affected by the terminal illness experience.[31–33] Family communication patterns, roles, and coping methods are components of family functioning affected by the cancer illness.[34–37]

However, results of studies of communication within families when a member has cancer are inconsistent. A number of studies[34,37–41] report that in an effort to protect each other, family members do not share their thoughts or concerns with one another.[34] Thorne's results[42] are consistent with these findings. She found that for some families, choosing not to discuss emotionally upsetting issues is consistent with prior family communication patterns and may help maintain their sense of normalcy and dignity.

In contrast, a family communication strategy documented in the literature as helpful is the ability to talk openly about the illness.[43] Spiegel and colleagues[44] studied 54 families of women with metastatic breast cancer and reported that in families where cancer was not discussed, these "conspiracies of silence" may have impeded coping.

Prior family communication patterns[33,42,45,46] have also been shown to influence family functioning during the cancer illness. Families who communicated effectively prior to the illness cope more effectively during the illness than those with histories of less functional communication.[47,48]

The role that the patient plays in the family (e.g., mother, adolescent)[49,50] imposes changes in family functioning. In families where the mother is the patient, communication may be strained if the mother was the primary "family communicator" and can no longer play that role.[49] Problems may also occur when children are asked to assume roles beyond their developmental abilities or when spouses are expected to assume too many additional roles.[51] Adolescents frequently turn to peers for support when a parent has cancer and report feeling isolated.[52]

Some families report improvements in family communication, family relationships, and feelings of closeness as a consquence of dealing with the cancer illness.[48,53,54] Yang and Kirschling[29] reported that regardless of the length of time the family caregivers spent with the patient, or how many tasks the family member performed for the patient, these tasks were reported as not difficult, upsetting, or tiring. Holing[25] also reported that one of the most positive aspects of the caregiving relationship was closeness to the patient.

A handful of studies[49,55,56] suggest that gender of the patient and caregiver may affect family functioning. Women (often between 40 and 70 years of age) most frequently act as caregiver to the patient.[2,17,55] These women may have health problems of their own, responsibilities for younger generations, and work commitments outside the home.[57–59] Caregiver fatigue, isolation, and family strain have been reported by these individuals as they cope with demands of caregiving.[17,28,40,60]

Cognitive coping strategies used by family members have been reported.[31,36,61] For example, Martens and Davies[36] interviewed spouses between 45 and 66 years of age to identify cognitive processes these individuals used to cope with the cancer illness. Spouses described four types of "work" that helped them cope: (a) hoping (to have a desirable outcome for the patient), (b) surviving (to protect and care for the patient and family), (c) persevering (to "hang on" or "carry on" during the situation), and (d) taking stock (to assess the previous life with the patient). The researchers also found that spouses relied more on family and friends for support than did patients and reported more uncertainty than patients.

The use of social support as a coping strategy by families is not straightforward. Some studies report benefits of social support to families as they cope with advanced phases of the illness.[62–64] Schumacher and colleagues[65] found social support had a weak, but significant, effect on depression among family caregivers (n = 75), accounting for 5% of the variance.

Kirschling and colleagues[66] studied perceptions of social support held by family members (N = 70) whose loved one was receiving care through a home hospice program. Size of support networks ranged considerably (4 to 150 people) and the extent of support perceived by family members was not related to size of the network.

Literature related to alterations in family functioning is limited and inconclusive, raising four issues: (a) questions about benefits of open versus less open communication, (b) uncertainty about how to help families prevent caregiver burden and receive rewards of caregiving, (c) immaturity of the science related to cognitive coping strategies of family members, and (d) questions about what constitutes a therapeutic dose of social support.

It appears that more open communication is helpful. However, further research is needed to investigate the extent to which families are helped by more open communication strategies and which families (if any) may benefit from less open communication.

The caregiving role may be experienced by family members as both stressful and satisfying. Research to identify family members at risk for caregiver fatigue and isolation must be pursued.

Research that identifies cognitive coping mechanisms used by families to help them integrate the cancer illness experience is limited by the cross-sectional, exploratory, descriptive designs. Samples are usually small and findings tenuous. Further work is needed to pursue this line of research using more rigorous designs and larger, representative samples.

Appropriate social support may help families to buffer stressful effects of the illness. However, the amount and quality of this social support must be more carefully studied to help families make optimal use of this coping strategy. There may be a curvilinear relationship between size of the support network and the family's sense of being supported, with families feeling less benefits from networks with too few or too many members. As well, the reciprocity of relationships in the network may influence the quality of the support received.[67]

Family health changes

Health changes experienced by family members during and following the patient's cancer illness have been documented.[52,68–72] Descriptions of health changes have been based on self-reports by family members of symptoms such as fatigue,[27,52,69] sleep disorders,[73,74] and mental health changes including depression and anxiety.[27,72,75] Exacerbations of chronic health problems have also been reported.[70,73] Kristjanson[73] found that children as young as 8 years of age experienced health changes during the time of their mothers' terminal cancer illnesses. Children described stomachaches, headaches, sleeping problems, and increased accidents (e.g., falls). Parents verified these symptoms and noted that some children also experienced "night terrors" following the deaths of their mothers.

This empirical work describing the impact of the cancer illness on family members' health is consistent, but fragmented and limited in volume. For the most part, findings are based on descriptive field studies and self-report methods. No research has been undertaken to determine the mechanism(s) by which the strain of the patient's illness contributes to health changs in family members, although an implicit assumption underlying the work is that stress is the mediating factor contributing to family health changes. This area of family research requires further attention, strengthened by longitudinal designs, use of control groups, and more precise measurement tools. To date, no intervention work in this area has been undertaken.

How Can Health Care Providers Identify/Assess Functional Family Responses?

Research in response to this question falls into two categories: instrument development and testing work and research delineating variables associated with indicators of family functioning.

Instrument development and testing research

There is a paucity of reliable and valid assessment tools with which to assess family functioning during the cancer illness experience. Instruments have been developed in the field of family therapy to assess family functioning and family structure.[76] Many of these tools are lengthy and require special expertise on the part of the practitioner who is assessing the family. Most family assessment tools have been developed and tested with families experiencing a psychological or family relationship problem (e.g., anorexia in a member, alcoholism, marital conflict). The extent to which these tools index the phenomena of concern to families of advanced cancer patients is unknown.

Some instruments have been tested with family members of advanced cancer patients and have evidenced sound psychometric properties. For example, the General Functioning Scale of the Family Assessment Device (FAD)[77] has been used to index family problem solving, communication, roles, affective responses, affective involvement, and behavior control. It is brief (12 items), has achieved acceptable reliability and validity estimates when tested with family members of advanced cancer patients, and can be completed by members as young as 10 years of age.

A few tools have been developed specifically for use with this population. For example, the FAMCARE[78] measures family satisfaction with advanced cancer care. It is also brief (20 items) and has met preset reliability and validity criteria. However, further instrumentation research is needed to refine and test other tools for use with this population. Subsequent hypothesis testing and experimental research relies on the existence of appropriate measurement tools.

Variables associated with indicators of family functioning

Correlational, descriptive studies undertaken to identify families at risk for dysfunction have produced some tentative results. Four categories of variables are apparent: family structure and resources, sociodemographic factors, quality-of-care variables, and illness characteristics. Indicators of family functioning vary across studies. These variables and associated indicators are summarized in Table 12.1.

Aspects of the family's internal family structure and function may affect the extent to which families cope well. Vess and colleagues[38,39] studied family role functioning in 54 married cancer patients, and their spouses and 14 children. Researchers found that families who used "achieved role assignment methods" (roles based on the person's own efforts and abilities) experienced less disrup-

Table 12.1 Variables associated with indicators of family functioning

Variable category	Variables	Indicators of family functioning
Structure and resources	Family composition Communication history Social support Coping efficacy	Family disruption Role conflict Role strain Caregiving stress Depression
Sociodemographic factors	Education Socioeconomic status Gender Age	Caregiver strain Depression Family care needs level
Quality-of-care factors	Unmet needs Satisfaction with care Pain management "Death surround"	Mental health Complicated grief Anxiety Helplessness Guilt Increased needs
Illness-related variables	Speed of illness Duration of illness Functional status of patient	Family care needs level Readiness for death Coping abilities Coping strain Depression Caregiver burden Role conflict

tion, less role conflict, and less role strain than did families who used "ascribed role assignment methods" (roles based on the person's age or sex). Families who had older children who could adopt expanded roles and those with more spousal communication also experienced less distress than families with younger children and those with histories of less spousal communication.

Schumacher and colleagues[65] studied strain and depression among family caregivers of persons receiving chemotherapy for cancer (N = 75). Two antecedent variables accounting for variance in caregiver strain and depression were perceived efficacy of coping strategies and perceived adequacy of social support. Caregivers with lower levels of perceived efficacy of coping were more strained and caregivers with less social support and coping efficacy were more depressed.

Researchers have also examined sociodemographic variables as predictors of family members at high risk. Oberst and colleagues[19] studied 47 family members of cancer patients and reported that family caregivers with less education and those in lower socioeconomic levels reported the highest stress scores on the Appraisal of Caregiving Scale (ACS). Mor and colleagues[79] also found that a greater degree of need was related to being older (the person with cancer and his or her family member). Family members who were female, had fewer years of education, and reported lower income levels also had higher degrees of need. Schumacher and coworkers[65] reported that caregivers of male patients and younger male patients were more strained and more depressed than caregivers of females. Only one other study reported that families of male cancer patients felt more overwhelmed with home care than families of female patients.[80] Further research is needed to examine the effect of gender on family caregiving experiences and the interactive nature of the caregiving relationships.

Factors associated with quality of patient care may affect family adjustment and coping. Kristjanson[81] studied 109 family members of advanced cancer patients to determine the extent to which their care needs were met, as measured by the Family Inventory of Needs (FIN).[82] Twenty percent of subjects rated their care needs as unimportant, indicated that their care needs had not been met, and reported low satisfaction with care (as measured by the FAMCARE described in Kristjanson[78]). A follow-up study[83] found that family members who rated their needs as less important and had fewer care needs met reported higher psychological distress, as measured by the Symptoms of Stress Scale.[84] A longitudinal study is under way to determine if family members who rate their needs as less important and those whose needs are not being met continue to experience distress and dysfunction.

Family members rate pain management as the most important quality-of-care factor. Ferrell and colleagues[7,8,85] have clearly documented the negative impact that the patient's pain has on the family. Family members report feelings of helplessness, anxiety, and even wishes for the patient's death when they feel unable to relieve the suffering of their loved one.[86] Kristjanson and

Avery[87] have termed these stressful responses of the family to pain in a loved one "vicarious suffering." Mor and colleagues[79] also reported that poor management of the patient's pain is associated with more family needs. As well, there is evidence[73] to suggest that family members who experience a "difficult death of the patient," or an illness trajectory characterized by unrelieved patient distress (e.g., poorly managed pain) may be at risk for more complicated grief reactions.

Rando,[88] Steele,[89] and Yancey and colleagues[90] studied the concept "death surround" as a predictor of grief responses of family members. The variable "death surround" refers to the factors associated with the death of the patient and includes the type of death, reason for death, and the extent to which the family members were prepared for the patient's death.[88] Inconsistent reports of the effect of location of death on the family have been reported. Steele[89] found location of death to have an effect on type of grief reactions. Family members of patients who died in a hospice program showed decreased feelings of guilt, dependency, loss of control, despair, numbness, shock, and disbelief. Survivors of patients who died at home had few guilt feelings and decreased death anxiety, but showed greater social isolation tendencies and were more apt to ruminate about the deceased. In contrast, Yancey and colleagues[90] reported no differences in family members' grief reactions associated with location of death. Methodological differences may have accounted for these inconsistent findings. For example, unlike subjects in the research of Yancey and colleagues, Steele's subjects did not have a choice regarding location of death.

Illness characteristics such as the speed and duration of the illness trajectory, and functional status of the patient may also affect family members' readiness for the patient's death, energy level, needs, and coping abilities.[65,79,91] Martocchio[92] reported that the extent to which the dying trajectory that the family expects matches the dying trajectory that occurs may influence the family's ability to cope in the bereavement period. Schumacher and colleagues[65] found that caregivers of patients with lower functional status reported more strain and more depression than caregivers of patients with higher functional status.

Buehler and Lee[91] undertook a qualitative study to explore the availability and perceived adequacy of formal resources to assist family caregivers of rural persons with cancer. The researchers found that the longer the dying trajectory and the greater the deterioration of the patient, the more resources became inadequate and the greater the caregiver burden. Oberst and colleagues[19] also reported that the acuity of the patient's illness and length of time of his or her illness were positively correlated with caregiver load. Yang and Kirschling[29] studied the amount of direct care and outcomes of caregiving experienced by family members of terminally ill older persons ($N = 55$). Long-term caregivers had higher mean scores for role conflict than did short-term caregivers.

Few tools exist to assess functional family responses during or following the illness of an advanced cancer patient. Although some have been developed and show promise, most are immature and require further refinement. There is also a lack of normative data based on these instruments against which study findings can be compared.

Families of advanced cancer patients experience extreme stress, interfering with their abilities to concentrate and complete lengthy assessment protocols. Therefore, the issue of subject burden is one that challenges researchers to select or construct brief, simple instruments for use with this population.[93]

Some speculative indicators of high-risk families (i.e., age, gender, duration of illness, family structure) have been generated, primarily based on cross-sectional, correlational designs. Empirical results are congruent with clinical observations. However, predictor and outcome variables are not consistently used or measured across the studies, clouding interpretation of results. Research is needed to more precisely identify ways of accurately, consistently, and systematically assessing the well-being and functioning of families. Without use of consistent tools that distinguish high-risk families, meaningful interventions cannot be offered to those most in need.

What Interventions or Therapeutic Approaches Are Most Helpful in Supporting Families Through the Terminal Illness of a Loved One?

Research related to this question was classified into three categories: studies describing health care provider behaviors important to families, intervention studies, and assessments of care facilities/programs.

Health care provider behaviors important to families

Health care provider behaviors that family members believe are important have been identified.[1,2,10,94,95] Behaviors reported by families to be most helpful match closely the priority care needs families identify. These behaviors include: attention to patient's comfort,[1,26,28,96] provision of specific information about the disease and treatment,[12,97,98] provision of information about side effects and changes in the patient's symptoms,[1,2] and assistance with how to provide physical care.[20] Stiles[99] also reported that families valued information shared by nurses regarding signs of impending death of the patient, as it helped them prepare psychologically for the death.

Intervention studies

Few intervention studies have been undertaken. One article reported use of a telephone counseling intervention to assist family caregivers to cope with the demands of caregiving, increase confidence in care management, help family identify supports and resources, and guide them in problem solving.[100] Unfortunately, the results of this intervention were not systematically evaluated and are reported in the form of four case studies. Nevertheless, this type of family support may provide a simple, cost-effective means of providing information, problem-solving advice, and support to family caregivers and should be systematically tested.

Walsh-Burke[101] undertook an intervention study to explore the role of communication in family coping and assess the impact of a weekend intervention designed to enhance communication in families experiencing cancer (N = 14 families). Families who communicated frequently and used a variety of coping strategies reported less difficulty coping with cancer than did those who used fewer strategies. Although these findings are limited by the small nonrepresentative sample and uncontrolled design, further testing of this intervention is warranted.

Ferrell and colleagues[85] implemented and tested a pain education program for family members of cancer patients (N = 40) using a stratified, random sampling method and experimental design. Patient and family members benefited from the intervention as indicated by improved scores on pain knowledge and attitude scales, medication compliance, a decrease in patients' pain intensity and severity ratings, decreased patient anxiety, and increased use of non-medication techniques (e.g., massage). This work must be replicated.

Assessments of care facilities-programs

A number of studies have been conducted to evaluate the effectiveness of hospice versus non-hospice services.[102–110] Brown and colleagues[111] reported that home care support to family caregivers facilitated the family's abilities to provide care in the home. Families whose loved ones receive care through a palliative care program report assurances regarding patient comfort, importance of respite care, decreased anxiety, and appreciation for spiritual support.[112–114] Higginson and colleagues investigated problems and needs of terminally ill cancer patients and their families and the extent to which patients anf family members were satisfied with the care provided by three different care services. Researchers found that palliative care support teams received the most praise, being rated by 89% of patients and 91% of family members as good or excellent. However, the researchers caution that results should be viewed tentatively because the study lacked a control group.

Interventions most helpful to many family members of advanced cancer patients focus on pain relief, education of family members about how to comfort the patient, information about treatment, and signs of impending death. The congruence of these findings with those reported in family needs assessment research is confirming and should be trusted. Researchers must now move beyond the descriptive design stage and undertake intervention research that builds on the existing body of knowledge. Specifically, a number of authors[15,18,114,115] have emphasized the need to pursue research aimed at educating and assisting family members to provide patient comfort. This work should become an immediate priority.

Although research comparing hospice versus non-hospice care setting outcomes has been important in testing hypotheses about differences in care models, absent from this work is a clear identification of the "active ingredients of supportive/palliative care" that are most beneficial to families. Some cues emerge from the literature related to health care provider behaviors helpful to family members. However, more exact testing is required to determine the components of supportive care services that are therapeutic for family members, and for different types of families.

As well, more rigorous research designs are required to test the effectiveness of hospice versus non-hospice interventions. Studies conducted to date purporting to compare the effectiveness of different care settings and care approaches may be clouded by selection bias problems. The types of patients and families cared for in the various care settings may be different. Without randomized prospective trials it is difficult to determine the extent to which a selection bias accounts for differences in care satisfaction.

Conclusion

The most substantial body of research has focused on the impact of the illness on the family and family responses to advanced cancer in a member. Less work has been undertaken to identify dysfunctional families and few intervention studies have been conducted.

Development of any research initiative must build logically and systematically upon the variable delineation/description phase, through the methodological and instrument development and testing phase, to hypothesis testing studies, intervention research, and evaluation projects. This area of supportive care science is still in the early phases of development, with most of the research at the variable delineation/description and methodological stages. This work has been necessary and will be the foundation for subsequent research. However, researchers are cautioned not to become stalled at this phase of knowledge development. Advances in supportive family care will depend on our willingness to take risks and pursue rigorous intervention studies.

Acknowledgments

This chapter is based, in part, on an earlier, broader literature review on the topic by L. J. Kristjanson and T. Ashcroft, published in 1994 (The family's cancer journey: A literature review, *Cancer Nursing* 17 (1):1–17). The author would like to acknowledge the career support funding provided by the Manitoba Health Research Council. As well, the assistance of Lynda Balneaves, Research Assistant, and Glennis Zilm is gratefully recognized.

References

1. Kristjanson LK. Indicators of quality of care from a family perspective. *J Palliat Care* 1986; 1(2):8–17.
2. Kristjanson LJ. Quality of terminal care: salient indicators identified by families. *J Palliat Care* 1989; 5(1):21–30.
3. Wingate AC, Lackey NR. A description of the needs of noninstitutionalized cancer patients and their primary caregivers. *Cancer Nurs* 1989; 12:216–225.
4. Blank JJ, Longman AJ, Atwood JR. Perceived home care needs of cancer patients and their caregivers. *Cancer Nurs* 1989; 12(2):78–84.
5. Grobe ME, Ahmann DL, Ilstrup DM. Needs assessment for advanced cancer patients and their families. *Oncol Nurs Forum* 1982; 9:26–30.
6. Stetz KM. Caregiving demands during advanced cancer: The spouse's needs. *Cancer Nurs* 1987; 10:260–268.
7. Ferrell BR, Ferrell BA, Rhiner M, Grant M. Family factors influencing cancer pain management. *Postgrad Med J* 1991b; 67(suppl 2):S64–S69.
8. Ferrell BR, Rhiner M, Grant M. Pain as a metaphor for illness. Part I: Impact of cancer pain on family caregivers. *Oncol Nurs Forum* 1991; 18:1303–1309.
9. Ferrell BR, Schneider C. Experience and management of cancer pain at home. *Cancer Nurs* 1988; 11(2):84–90.
10. Lewandowski W, Jones SL. The family with cancer. Nursing interventions throughout the course of living with cancer. *Cancer Nurs* 1988; 11:313–321.
11. Skorupka P, Bohnet N. Primary caregivers' perceptions of nursing behaviours that best meet their needs in a home care hospice setting. *Cancer Nurs* 1982; 5:371–374.
12. Wright K, Dyck S. Expressed concerns of adult cancer patients' family members. *Cancer Nurs* 1984; 6:371–374.
13. Taylor EJ, Ferrell BR, Grant M, Cheyney L. Managing cancer pain at home: The decisions and ethical conflicts of patients, family caregivers, and homecare nurses. *Oncol Nurs Forum* 1993; 20(6):919–927.
14. Ferrell BR, Cohen M, Rhiner M, Rozak A. Pain as a metaphor for illness. Part II: Family caregivers' management of pain. *Oncol Nurs Forum* 1991; 18:1315–1321.
15. Hays JC. High-technology and hospice home care: strange bedfellows. *Home Health Care* 1988; 23:329–340.
16. Tringali CA. The needs of family members of cancer patients. *Oncol Nurs Forum* 1986; 13(4):65–69.
17. Hileman JW, Lackey NR. Self-identified needs of patients with cancer at home and their home caregivers: a descriptive study. *Oncol Nurs Forum* 1990; 7:907–913.
18. Hinds C. The needs of families who care for patients with cancer at home: are we meeting them? *J Adv Nurs* 1985; 10:575–581.
19. Oberst MT, Thomas SE, Gass KA, Ward SE. Caregiving demands and appraisal of stress among family caregivers. *Cancer Nurs* 1989; 12:209–215.

20. Grobe ME, Ilstrup DM, Ahmann DL. Skills needed by family members to maintain the care of an advanced cancer patient. *Cancer Nurs* 1981; 4:371–375.

21. Longman AJ, Atwood JR, Sherman JB, Benedict J, Shang T. Care needs of home-based cancer patients and their caregivers. *Cancer Nurs* 1992; 15(3):182–190.

22. Higginson I, Wade A, McCarthy M. Palliative care: views of patients and their families. *Br Med J* 1990; 301:277–281.

23. Lobchuk MM. Perceptions of symptom distress in lung cancer patients: congruence among patients, primary caregivers and nurses. Unpublished master's thesis, University of Manitoba, Winnipeg, Manitoba, 1995.

24. Hays RD, Arnold S. Patient and family satisfaction with care for the terminally ill. *Hospice Journal* 1986; 2(3):129–150.

25. Holing EV. The primary caregiver's perception of the dying trajectory. *Cancer Nurs* 1986; 9(1):29–37.

26. Hull MM. Family needs and supportive nursing behaviors during terminal cancer: a review. *Oncol Nurs Forum* 1989; 16:787–792.

27. Hays JC. Patient symptoms and family coping: predictors of hospice utilization patterns. *Cancer Nurs* 1986; 9(6):317–325.

28. Hull MM. Sources of stress for hospice caring families. *Hospice Journal* 1990; 6(2):29–53.

29. Yang C, Kirschling JM. Exploration of factors related to direct care and outcomes of caregiving. *Cancer Nurs* 1992; 15(3):173–181.

30. Bruera E. Case report: severe organic brain syndrome. *J Palliat Care* 1991; 7(1):36–38.

31. Davies B, Reimer JC, Martens N. Family functioning and its implications for palliative care. *J Palliat Care* 1994; 10(1):29–36.

32. Matson CA. Families with a terminally ill member: a grounded theory of family relationships. *American Journal of Hospice Care* 1988; 5:38–41.

33. Pederson LM, Valanis BG. The effects of breast cancer on the family: a review of the literature. *Journal Psychosocial Oncology* 1988; 6:95–119.

34. Cooper ET. A pilot study on the effects of the diagnosis of lung cancer on family relationships. *Cancer Nurs* 1984; 7:301–308.

35. Gotay CC. The experience of cancer during early and advanced stages: the views of patients and their mates. *Soc Sci Med* 1984; 7:605–613.

36. Martens N, Davies B. The work of patients and spouses in managing advanced cancer at home. *Hospice Journal* 1990; 6(2):55–73.

37. Northouse PG, Northouse LL. Communication and cancer: issues confronting patients, health professionals and family members. *Journal Psychosocial Oncology* 1987; 5:17–46.

38. Vess JD, Moreland JR, Schwebel AI. An empirical assessment of the effects of cancer on family role functioning. *Journal Psychosocial Oncology* 1985; 3(2):1–16.

39. Vess JD, Moreland JR, Schwebel AI. A follow-up study of role functioning and the psychological environment of families of cancer patients. *Journal Psychosocial Oncology* 1989; 3(2):1–14.

40. Wellisch DK, et al. Evaluation of psychosocial problems of the home-bound cancer patient: the relationship of disease and the sociodemographic variables of patients to family problems. *Journal Psychosocial Oncology* 1983; 1(3):1–15.

41. Wortman CB, Dunkel-Schetter C. Interpersonal relationships and cancer: a theoretical analysis. *Journal Social Issues* 1979; 35:120–155.
42. Thorne S. The family cancer experience. *Cancer Nurs* 1985; October:285–291.
43. Koocher GP, O'Malley JE. Implications for patient care. In: Koocher GP, O'Malley JE, eds. *The Damocles Syndrome*. New York: McGraw-Hill; 1981.
44. Spiegel D, Bloom JR, Gottheil E. Family environment as a predictor of adjustment to metastatic breast carcinoma. *Journal Psychosocial Oncology* 1983; 1(1): 33–44.
45. Silberfarb PM. Psychiatric themes in the rehabilitation of mastectomy patients. *Int J Psychiatry Med* 1977–78; 8:159–167.
46. Wellisch DK. The psychologic impact of breast cancer on relationships. *Semin Oncol Nurs* 1985; 1:195–199.
47. Barbarin OA, Hughes D, Chesler MA. Stress, coping and marital functioning among parents of children with cancer. *Journal Marriage Family* 1985; 47:473–480.
48. Schover FR, von Eschenbach AC. Sexual and marital counseling with men treated for testicular cancer. *J Sex Marital Ther* 1984; 10(1):29–40.
49. Cohen P, Dizenhuz I, Winget C. Family adaptation to terminal illness and death of a parent. *Social Casework* 1977; 58:223–228.
50. Levenson PM, Pfefferbaum B, Silberberg Y, Copeland DR. Sources of information about cancer as perceived by adolescent patients, parents, and physicians. *Patient Counselling Health Education* 1981; Second Quarter:71–76.
51. Lloyd C, Coggles L. Psychological issues for people with cancer and their families. *Canadian Journal Occupational Therapy* 1990; 57:211–215.
52. Galloway SC. Young adults' reactions to the death of a parent. *Oncol Nurs Forum* 1990; 17(6):899–904.
53. Lichtman RR, Taylor SE, Wood JV. Social support and marital adjustment after breast cancer. *Journal Psychosocial Oncology* 1987; 5(3):47–74.
54. Walker CL. Siblings of children with cancer. *Oncol Nurs Forum* 1990; 3:355–360.
55. Nugent LS. The social support requirements of family caregivers of terminal cancer patients. *Canadian Journal Nursing Research* 1988; 20:45–58.
56. Sabo D, Brown J, Smith C. The male role and mastectomy: support groups and men's adjustment. *Journal Psychosocial Oncology* 1986; 4:19–31.
57. Brody EM. "Women in the middle" the family help to older people. *Gerontologist* 1981; 21(5):471–480.
58. Goldner SR. Generation and gender: normative and covert hierarchies. *Fam Process* 1988; 27:17–31.
59. Miller D. The "sandwich" generation: adult children of the aging. *Soc Work* 1981; 26:419–423.
60. Welch-McCaffrey D. Family issues in cancer care: current dilemmas and future directions. *Journal Psychosocial Oncology* 1988; 6:199–211.
61. Reimer JC, Davies B, Martens N. Palliative care: the nurse's role in helping families through the transition of "fading away." *Cancer Nurs* 1991; 14(6):321–327.
62. Friedman MM. Intervening with families of school-aged children with cancer. In: Leahey M, Wright LM, eds. *Families and Life-Threatening Illness*. Springhouse: Springhouse Corp.; 1987:219–234.

63. Hull MM. Coping strategies of family caregivers in hospice homecare. *Oncol Nurs Forum* 1992; 19(8):1179–1187.

64. Pesznecker BL, Zahlis E. Establishing mutual-help groups for family member care givers: a new role for community health nurses. *Public Health Nurs* 1986; 3: 29–37.

65. Schumacher KL, Dodd MJ, Paul SM. The stress process in family caregivers of persons receiving chemotherapy. *Res Nurs Health* 1993; 16:395–404.

66. Kirschling JM, Tilden VP, Butterfield PG. Social support: the experiences of hospice family caregivers . . . Reliability and validity of Tilden's (1986) cost and reciprocity index (CRI). *Hospice Journal* 1990; 6(2):75–93.

67. Kristjanson LJ, Ashcroft T. The family's cancer journey: a literature review. *Cancer Nurs* 1994; 17(1):1–17.

68. Koch A. "If only it could be me": the families of pediatric cancer patients. *Family Relations* 1985; 34:63–70.

69. Northouse L. The impact of cancer on the family: an overview. *Int J Psychiatry Med* 1984; 14:215–242.

70. Parkes CM. Terminal care: Home, hospital, or hospice? *Lancet* 1985; 1:115–117.

71. Poulshock SW, Deimling GT. Families caring for elders in residence: issues in the measurement of burden. *J Gerontol B Psychol Sci Soc Sci* 1984; 39(2):230–239.

72. Zisook S, Shuchter S. Depression through the first year after the death of a spouse. *Am J Psychiatry* 1991; 148:1346–1352.

73. Kristjanson LJ. Family decision making in terminal cancer: a descriptive study. Unpublished master's thesis, University of Manitoba, Winnipeg, Manitoba. 1983.

74. Rose MA. Problems families face in home care. *Am J Nurs* 1976; 16:416–418.

75. Goldberg RJ, Wool MS, Glicksman A, Tull R. Relationship of the social environment and patients' physical status to depression in lung cancer patients and their spouses. *Journal Psychosocial Oncology* 1985; 2(3/4):73–80.

76. Steinglass P. A systems view of family interaction and psychopathology. In: Jacob I, ed. *Family Interaction and Psychopathology*. New York: Plenum Press; 1987.

77. Miller IW, Kabacoff RI, Epstein NB, et al. The development of a clinical rating scale for the McMaster Model of Family Functioning. *Fam Process* 1994; 33: 53–69.

78. Kristjanson LJ. Validity and reliability testing of the FAMCARE Scale: measuring family satisfaction with advanced cancer care. *Soc Sci Med* 1993; 36(5): 693–701.

79. Mor V, Guadagnoli E, Wool M. An examination of the concrete service needs of advanced cancer patients. *Journal Psychosocial Oncology* 1987; 5:1–7.

80. Wellisch DK, Fawzy FI, Landsverk J, Pasnau RO, Wolcott DL. Evaluation of psychosocial problems of the homebound cancer patient: the relationship of disease and the sociodemographic variables of patients to family problems. *Journal Psychosocial Oncology* 1983; 1(3):1–15.

81. Kristjanson LJ. *Family satisfaction with palliative care: a test of four alternative theories*. Doctoral dissertation. Tucson:University of Arizona, 1991.

82. Kristjanson LJ, Atwood JR, Degner LF. Validity and reliability of the Family Inventory of Needs (FIN): measuring the care needs of families of advanced cancer patients. *J Nurs Meas* 1995; 3(2):109–126.

83. Kristjanson LJ. Family members' satisfaction with palliative care as a predictor of

family functioning and family members' health: a feasibility study. Unpublished NCIC research project, 1993–94.

84. Leckie E, Thompson M. *Symptoms of stress inventory: a self assessment.* Seattle: University of Washington, Dept. of Psychosocial Nursing, 1978.

85. Ferrell BR, Rhiner M, Ferrell BA. Development and implementation of a pain education program. *Cancer Supplement* 1993; 72(11):3426–3432.

86. Ferrell BR, Cohen M, Rhiner AM, Rozak A. Pain as a metaphor for illness, Part II: Family caregivers' management of pain. *Oncol Nurs Forum* 18(1/2):171–191.

87. Kristjanson LJ, Avery L. Vicarious pain: the family's perspective. *Pain Management Newsletter* 1994; 7(3):1–2.

88. Rando T. *Grief, dying and death: Clinical Interventions for Caregivers.* Champaign, Ill.: Research Press; 1984.

89. Steele LL. The death surround: factors influencing the grief experience of survivors. *Oncol Nurs Forum* 1990; 17:235–241.

90. Yancey D, Greger HA, Coburn P. Determinants of grief resolution in cancer death. *J Palliat Care* 1990; 6(4):24–31.

91. Buehler JA, Lee HJ. Exploration of home care resources for rural families with cancer. *Cancer Nurs* 1992; 15(4):299–308.

92. Martocchio BC. *Living While Dying.* Bowie: Robert J. Brady Co.; 1982.

93. Kristjanson LJ, Hanson EJ, Balneaves LG. Research with palliative care populations: ethical issues. *J Palliat Care* 1994; 10(3):10–15.

94. Hampe SO. Needs of the grieving spouse in a hospital setting. *Nurs Res* 1975; 24:113–120.

95. Freihofer P, Felton G. Nursing behaviours in bereavement: an exploratory study. *Nurs Res* 1976; 25:332–337.

96. Irwin B, Meier J. Supportive measures for evaluation of the fatally ill. *Community Nurs Res* 1973; 6:119–128.

97. Bond S. Communicating with families of cancer patients: 1. The relatives and doctors. *Nursing Times* 1982a; 78:962–965.

98. Bond S. Communicating with families of cancer patients: 2. The nurses. *Nursing Times* 1982; 78:1027–1029.

99. Stiles MK. The shining stranger: nurse-family spiritual relationship. *Cancer Nurs* 1994; 13(4):235–245.

100. Skipworth DH. Telephone counseling interventions with caregivers of elders. *J Psychosoc Nurs Ment Health Serv* 1994; 32(3):7–12.

101. Walsh-Burke K. Family communication and coping with cancer: impact of the We Can Weekend. *Journal Psychosocial Oncology* 1992; 10(1):63–81.

102. Buckingham RW, Lack SA, Mount MM, MacLean LD, Collins JT. Living with dying: use of the technique of participant observation. *Can Med Assoc J* 1976; 115:1211–1215.

103. Greer DS, Mor V. An overview of national hospice study findings. *J Chron Dis* 1986; 39:5–7.

104. Kane RL, Bernstein L, Wales J, Leibowitz A, Kaplan S. A randomized controlled trial of hospice care. *Lancet* 1984; April:890–894.

105. Lack SA, Buckingham RA. *First American Hospice: Three Years of Home Care.* New Haven: Hospice Inc.; 1978.

106. McGinnis SS. How can nurses improve the quality of life of the hospice client and family?: an exploratory study. *Hospice Journal* 1986; 2(1):23–36.

107. Mor D, Greer DS, Kastenbaum R. *The Hospice Experiment*. Baltimore: Johns Hopkins' University Press; 1988.
108. Royal Victoria Hospital. *Palliative Care Service, Report of the Pilot Project*. Montreal: Royal Victoria Hospital and McGill University; 1976.
109. St. Aubin M, Lund DA. A critical test of specific hospice objectives for family caregivers. *Hospice Journal* 1986; 2:1–19.
110. Smith CA, Hill PD. Grieving responses; a comparison after home or hospital care. *N Z Med J* 1978; 88:393–395.
111. Brown P, Davies B, Martens N. Families in supportive care: Part II: Palliative care at home. *J Palliat Care* 1990; 6(3):21–27.
112. Barzelai LP. Evaluation of a home based hospice. *J Fam Pract* 1981; 12:241–245.
113. Keizer MC. Primary care providers' perceptions of care. *J Palliat Care* 1992; 8(4):8–12.
114. Wakefield M, Ashby M. Attitudes of surviving relatives to terminal care in South Australia. *J Pain Symptom Manage* 1993; 8(8):529–538.
115. Austin C, Cody CP, Eyres PJ, Hefferin EA, Krasnow RW. Hospice home care pain management. *Cancer Nurs* 1986; 9:58–65.

13

Denial, Misinformation, and the "Assault of Truth"

PHYLLIS N. BUTOW, STEWART M. DUNN,
AND MARTIN H. N. TATTERSALL

Modern medical ethics emphasizes the patient's right to be fully informed of his or her medical condition, and to participate in decisions about treatment. Truth telling, once regarded as cruel and insensitive, is now thought by many to be morally obligatory.[1,2] Community attitudes have also shifted toward greater patient participation in and knowledge of medical matters.[3,4] The rationale for this approach is to safeguard the autonomy and integrity of the individual and to ensure that the patient plays an active role in decisions about his or her care.

At its extreme, patient autonomy means that each patient makes his or her own decisions about treatment on the basis of standard, comprehensive information provided by an otherwise passive doctor. Furthermore, the patient has the right, on the basis of proper and adequate information, to reach decisions that may seem wholly irrational by the standards of medicine or to the community in general.[5,6] In the United States, this approach has been at least partially embodied in legislation requiring fully informed consent for clinical trials.[7]

Some doctors have suggested that in the attempt to fulfill perceived moral or legal obligations, the individual patient's true wishes and best interests may be overlooked or poorly served.[8,9] This view has been expressed most commonly in the context of informed consent to clinical trials, but it is equally applicable to the standard clinical situation. Standards of disclosure are generally much higher in the clinical trial setting in comparison to the minimal documentation required when a patient receives the same treatment outside a trial. Indeed, some writers have argued against this current double standard.[8,10] Either agreement to standard treatment should be made more stringent[10] or the consent requirements for clinical trials should be subject to clinical judgment.[8] These and other issues pertaining to information provision are among the most hotly debated within the oncology literature. Some of the views expressed in this controversy are listed below:

> The malignant reputation of cancer is enhanced by the secrecy surrounding it.[11]

> An increasing degree of frankness on the part of the doctor, for the most part laudable and constructive, may cause considerable anxiety in those patients who would prefer to be directed rather than to participate as an equal partner.[8]

> The requirement to obtain informed consent is a rigid and somewhat brutal procedure, causing patients to be bombarded with technical details and complicated consent forms.[12]

> Truly informed consent allows the patient to make his or her own judgement about the impact of the various treatment options offered. . . . Risk is seen differently when it is your own. Doctors must not forget this.[13]

> An open, frank discussion of the relevant issues not only would promote trust in the doctor and enhance the doctor–patient relationship but would respect the patient's right to self-determination.[14,15]

Achieving the elusive balance between underinforming and overloading the patient is important. The outcomes of patient dissatisfaction with communication are noncompliance with medical advice,[16] "doctor shopping,"[17] exploration of alternative medicine treatments,[18] poorer coping,[19] and general dissatisfaction.[20] While the amount of information provided to patients has never been greater than at the present time, several of these outcomes have never been more prevalent.

The information debate ranges among issues of ethics and legal accountability, patient welfare, and the doctor–patient relationship. The arguments and evidence pertaining to each of these issues are discussed below.

The Ethics of Information Giving

Ethical decisions involve weighing up a number of ethical principles.[21] The traditional principles adopted by medicine have been beneficence (acting for the good of others) and paternalism, which requires the doctor to take responsibility for acting in their patients' presumed best interests. This model assumes that sickness makes the patient incompetent, and therefore places the responsibility for deciding what constitutes benefit or harm firmly upon the doctor. Providing information that portrays a gloomy prognosis or offering choice in treatments may cause psychological distress in some patients, albeit temporary; therefore it is advisable to "first, do no harm" and withhold information.

The principle of autonomy recognizes the need to respect the patient's integrity and right to self-determination. This model assumes that the patient wants information and involvement in decision making and is competent to assume this role.

Neither paternalism nor complete autonomy offers an ideal base for medical decisions. Paternalism is not ideal because the doctor cannot know all the patient's wishes, goals, and values. A patient may well choose not to disclose circumstances, objectives, and judgments that influence his or her information needs.[5] Several recent studies have reported that doctors are *not* very good at estimating the amount and sort of information patients want,[22,23] or how effective they have been in imparting accurate information.[24]

Autonomy, on the other hand, fails to acknowledge the differences between wellness and sickness. The sick person is not simply a well person with a disease, but rather is qualitatively different, not only physically but also socially, emotionally, and even cognitively.[25] Lantos[1] goes so far as to say that people who are ill and suffering, who know pain, and who perceive their own mortality, are in a different metaphysical state than healthy people. At a time when they may feel physically unwell and overwhelmed with anxiety, many patients appear to sanction a degree of paternalism in decision making, by opting to exercise their "autonomous choice of dependency."[26] Degner and Sloan[27] found that perceptions of the general public are often quite different from those of actual patients: 59% of patients versus 36% of the nonpatient public preferred to leave treatment decisions to the doctor.

Perhaps the ideal is a compromise between these two extremes. Both doctor and patient bring essential knowledge and values to the clinical decision, and a mutual, active, knowledge-sharing approach is best.[28,29] If information and involvement in decision making cause distress under some circumstances, then patients can be told of this risk, and decide on their preferred role accordingly.

The Legal View

Some have argued that ethical and philosophical debate about these issues has come too late; whether we like it or not, the law has already resolved the argument.[30] To some extent, this is true. The legal view pertaining to information provision is that the patient has a basic human right of self-determination that is protected by the written constitutions of Germany and the United States and by the common law of England.[5] This right has, however, been interpreted in various ways in different countries. Perhaps the most paternalistic interpretation is in English law, where informational requirements are based on the judgment of the individual *reasonable doctor*.[5] Discretion is allowed in weighing up the potential for causing harm by providing additional information, against the benefit of allowing the patient a totally antonomous choice. In Canada and several states of the United States, the standard of disclosure focuses on the informational needs of the *reasonable patient*, in the particular patient's position. This approach has been criticized because it may fail to protect those whose fears, apprehensions, religious beliefs, or superstitions (and therefore information needs) lie outside the mainstream of society. German law goes further still in declaring that "a doctor will be liable if he fails to supply such information regarding the proposed course of treatment, including the risks attendant thereupon, as he knew or ought to have known the *particular patient* would have required to reach his decision."[5] The ramifications of these laws are still being tested in court.

In addition to the law, many research councils have published guidelines that while not legally binding, may be consulted in disciplinary or civil proceedings. These attempt to take a more flexible, educational approach to influencing information provision. However, in attempting flexibility, the guidelines are often anything but clear. For example, the relevant document produced by the National Health and Medical Council of Australia states that information provided to patients should cover such aspects as known severe risks of treatment, even when occurrence is rare, the degree of uncertainty of any diagnosis or therapeutic outcome, and any significant long-term physical, emotional, mental, social, sexual, or other outcome that may be associated with a proposed intervention. However, the information should be "appropriate to the patient's circumstances, personality, expectations, fears, beliefs, values and cultural background" and may be influenced by "current accepted medical practice."[31] This leaves considerable latitude on the part of the doctor.

It has been argued that precisely because medical decision making raises issues of profound moral and ethical significance, the question of liability for insufficient disclosure should always be one of law, not to be circumvented by the exercise of medical discretion.[5] Individual patients are increasingly asserting their rights within the legal framework, as reflected in the growth of medical litigation.[32]

However, it has also been argued that using regulations to determine how much information to disclose can be problematic.[27,29] Some see legislation as too rigid, and incapable of covering the wide range of situations that might arise.[29] Others believe that legislation can be detrimental to the doctor–patient relationship.[27] Patients may ascribe unintended meanings to informed consent forms that erode their trust of the doctor. For example, one survey found that 80% of adult patients think that the main purpose of consent documents is to protect those conducting the study.[33] Furthermore, the doctor who relies on a legal formula may be less likely to explore individual patient preferences and needs. Most patients, it is argued, believe that *they* rather than the law should decide how much information they receive about their illness and its treatment.[34] They may deliberately not read consent documents because they see them as legalistic intrusions in a doctor/patient relationship that should be based on trust.[33]

Nevertheless the patient, the law, and the medical profession can work together in ensuring high standards of care. After all, as Mr. Justice Kirby, President of the New South Wales Court of Appeal, pointed out, "the fact that the patient gave an informed consent usually will not prevent him from suing: a warm relationship with a competent and caring physician will."[35] Even if the law proscribes standards of information provision, it will still be up to the individual doctor and patient to negotiate their own way forward.

Patient Preferences for Information

What do cancer patients want? A number of studies suggest that cancer patients place effective doctor communication high on their list of priorities for care. In an Australian study assessing the perceptions of 232 ambulatory cancer patients, doctor–patient communication dominated the top ten aspects of care regarded as important.[24] Over 99% of patients emphasized their need for information about their cancer and its progress and the opportunity to ask their doctor questions. Furthermore, there are data to suggest that these needs are not being met. While there is a pronounced positive skew in patient responses to satisfaction questionnaires generally,[36] dissatisfaction with communication is often quite high.[37,38] Fallowfield and coworkers[39] noted that even among breast cancer patients involved in treatment trials where a large amount of information had been provided, about 50% later said that the information they had received in hospital was inadequate.

Nevertheless, evidence regarding patient preferences for *amount* of information suggests that an inflexible standard would not serve all patients well. Although the majority of cancer patients (up to 85%) state that they want all information, good or bad,[3] a minority still prefers to receive minimal information only. When it comes to decision making, a larger percentage prefer to abdicate this role in favor of the doctor.[3,4] In a recently completed study of 80 cancer patients seeing a medical oncologist, we found that while 29 patients (36%) favored an equal and collaborative role in decision making, only 18 (23%) sought the dominant role. A sizable minority (41%) preferred to leave decision making in the hands of the doctor.[40]

In that study, we explored demographic, disease, and psychological predictors of information preferences. Cassileth[3] had earlier reported significant age differences in information preferences, but in this sample only locus of religious control, a subscale of the Cancer Locus of Control scale,[41] was significantly related to preference. Those who believed that God can influence the development and progression of their disease wanted less information ($p <$ .0001). This finding reflects the significant influence that religion and culture can have in determining attitudes not only to information, but to the role of the physician, the patient–physician interaction, and the role of the family when a member is ill.[42]

For example, Ali and coworkers[43] note that in Egypt the "patient must be dependent and nurtured, and is not to be involved in decision-making. . . . It is the family that makes decisions in Egypt because dignity, identity and security are bounded by belonging to the family." Therefore "disclosure of the exact serious diagnosis to a patient by the physician is a socially unacceptable behaviour and an untactful act. However the family is informed of the diagnosis and the plan of care." Egyptians also believe that physicians have enough education to treat their diseases; therefore "the patient cannot contradict or question the physician's orders because this would imply impolite behaviour, or interference in the physician's work or lack of respect from subordinate to superior." This approach is contrasted to the American culture of individualism, consumerism, and positive thinking, which generates quite different approaches to illness.

Charlton[44] collated a number of studies exploring patients' views on being told their diagnosis that revealed considerable cross-cultural diversity. For example, in studies spanning from 1978 to 1990, the percentage of cancer patients definitely wanting to be told their diagnosis varied from 49% in the United Kingdom and 54% in Denmark to 93.6% in the USSR and 90% in Germany. Such variation can make it extremely difficult in multicultural societies like Australia and America for doctors who are trying to negotiate between the dominant sociocultural attitude, the views of the patient and their family (sometimes expressed very forcefully), and the medico-legal environment.

The Role of Information

Variation in information and involvement preferences has led to speculation about the meaning and function of information for the patient. The legalistic view has been that the primary role of information is to allow the patient to make an informed decision. If this were so, one would expect that active decision-makers would seek and retain more information than those preferring a passive role. However, the data reveal a more complex picture. A recent study that explored the relationship between preferences for decisional control and illness information among women with breast cancer[45] showed that patients who desired an active role in decision making also desired significantly more detailed explanations of their illness (as expected). However, a substantial number of passive patients *also* desired detailed medical information. Information for this subgroup appeared to serve another need. One suggestion is that these patients want information so that they can understand the logic of their doctors' recommendations, not so they can synthesize and use the information themselves.[46] Once they feel confident that the right decision will be made, there is no longer any need to absorb or retain the facts, or indeed to contribute to the decision.

In another study, patients who desired maximum involvement performed no better on a stringent measure of recall than those wanting minimum information,[47] suggesting that they were not retaining additional information to aid their decision making. Indeed, recall for the whole group was poor. Patients recalled approximately one quarter of the information presented in the consultation and just under half of the points nominated as particularly significant by the oncologist. Furthermore, it appears that patients are forgetting or misreporting *important* information. Mackillop and colleagues,[24] for example, found that of 100 cancer patients surveyed, 33% with metastatic disease believed it was localized, 34% being treated palliatively believed that their treatment would lead to cure, and 10% being treated for cure believed they were being treated palliatively. Yet all of the doctors concerned believed they had given the correct information in the consultation.

Similarly in a study just completed,[48] we found a high level of misunderstanding in 127 cancer patients interviewed prior to their second chemotherapy treatment session. Almost half the patients either did not know or incorrectly identified the extent of their illness. A third of patients did not understand what their treatment was meant to achieve. Fifty-seven percent of patients disagreed substantially with their doctor's estimate of the probability of cure. For example, 6 of 21 patients whose doctor said their chance of cure was zero thought their chance of cure was greater than 50%. There was a clear optimism bias in patients' responses to this question, which raises the issue of the influence of denial on patient "misunderstanding," to be discussed in greater detail below.

Why Communication Fails: Misinformation

One explanation for poor patient understanding is that patients do want to retain information but are thwarted by the fact that doctors present too much, not enough, or poorly organized information. Research in cognitive psychology has established the limitations of human memory. In a famous paper, Miller[49] demonstrated that short-term memory can retain only seven plus or minus two chunks of new material. In a recent study evaluating the use of consultation tapes, our group found that the average amount of information presented routinely by the oncologist in this study was 25 items, with a maximum of 72.[47] Ley and Spelman [50] reported a clear negative relationship between amount presented and percentage recalled.

On the other hand, Simes and coworkers[51] have reported data that suggest that some patients remember more if they receive *additional* information to that presented under standard clinical circumstances. They found that giving patients more information than was standard practice resulted in improved recall of information about randomized controlled trials. Perhaps patients are unable to draw the information they receive together into a coherent, memorable whole because there are holes in their knowledge. Others have demonstrated that various techniques, such as organizing information into explicit categories, summarizing information, and supplementing verbal information with written or taped materials, can result in improved patient recall.[52-54] According to this model, and in line with concerns about informed consent, efforts should be made to improve doctor–patient communication.

Why Communication Fails: Denial and the Assault of Truth

Some authors believe that "patient misunderstanding" is in fact the mechanism of denial operating as a helpful and hope-giving coping strategy.[55,56] According to this view, no matter how well the doctor presented information the patients would screen out those aspects with which they could not cope. Indeed, attempts to improve patient understanding could be described as an "assault of truth" directly working against the patient's preferred coping strategy. Certainly denial is a common response to serious illness. In the study of patient understanding discussed above,[48] we found that 40% of men and 23% of women having chemotherapy scored highly on a scale measuring denial of the impact of illness. Furthermore, the proportion of patients using denial increased linearly with declining probability of cure, whether as judged by the physician or the patient. Similarly, Damian and Tattersall[57] found that patients receiving bad news recalled fewer facts presented by a medical oncologist than those receiving good news. These data suggest that denial is increasingly used as the prognosis grows poorer.

But is denial helpful? Studies in the 1970s demonstrated a positive relationship between denial and survival of patients with serious illness.[58,59] However, some writers have suggested that what is prognostically important in denial may have less to do with the denial itself than with other aspects of the denier's approach to life, such as psychological resilience.[56] Other data have supported the notion that information seeking, rather than information avoidance, may lead to more positive consequences for the patient. Cassileth,[3] for example, found that patients who wanted to be informed and involved in their treatment were significantly more hopeful than others, regardless of medical status. These data suggest that realistic information does not generate depression, but rather assists patients in adjusting to their illness.

Conversely, evasion and secrecy may be associated with uncertainty and unrealistic fears. Patients kept in the dark may well imagine worst-case scenarios and respond with relief when the facts are openly presented. In a study investigating the use of question-prompt sheets before an oncology consultation, we encouraged patients to list and ask questions.[60] The question-prompt sheet had a significant effect in one content area: prognosis. Thirty-five percent of patients who received the question handout asked questions about prognosis, compared to 16% of those who did not. One elderly man with metastatic cancer asked the doctor how he would die. He expressed great relief after the frank discussion that followed. Answers to these questions, often unasked because of social or time pressures, allow patients to marshal together their coping resources on the basis of a realistic and predictable future.

Perhaps a certain amount of anxiety about the diagnosis and treatment of cancer is realistic and appropriate. Our findings support this view. In a heterogeneous sample of 165 cancer patients, use of the word "cancer" in a questionnaire measuring psychological adjustment generated significantly higher anxiety than use of the word "illness" but did not produce any distortion in reported adjustment. The anxiety generated was no greater than that reported by general medical and surgical patients; however, when patients received conflicting messages, such as when reading the word "illness" while sitting in a cancer clinic, they reported increased psychological distress.[61]

Thus, open use of the word "cancer" did produce a moderate increase in short-term anxiety, but it also may have reduced the ambivalence of the patients' situation and enabled them to think more clearly about their illness. Cancer patients may be highly susceptible to any implication that cancer is confusing and frightening to the extent that even doctors or nurses cannot discuss it openly. Conversely, if health professionals are frank and unambiguous in the words they use, the concept of cancer will continue to evoke anxiety in the short term, but patients may feel more capable of coping with it.

Furthermore, while detailed disclosure *has* been shown to increase anxiety in the short term, follow-up reveals that the excess anxiety dissipates within a few weeks,[51] whereas effects on psychological adjustment of limited information may persist.[62,63] Fallowfield,[39] for example, found that anxiety and depression were significantly elevated as long as 12 months after surgery in breast cancer patients treated by surgeons who did not offer a choice between mastectomy and lumpectomy.

Individualized Disclosure

Miller[64] has proposed a model that can explain both the differences observed in information and involvement preferences, and the contradictory results within the denial literature. She suggests that people vary in the behavioral strategy they use to deal with an aversive event, particularly when it is uncontrollable. "Monitors" actively seek information, whereas "blunters" (or in other jargon, "deniers") avoid or distract themselves from the information. Steptoe and coworkers,[65] using this model, found that patients who reported the highest amount of satisfaction with the information they had received were more avoidant in their coping style (i.e., blunters). Monitors had the least satisfaction, but in contrast actually possessed greater factual knowledge. These data suggest that blunters claimed a good understanding of their condition and reported high satisfaction not because they had actually received more information, but because their coping style led them to avoid further information that might highlight their predicament. Thus, forcing information on a blunter may be ineffective and perhaps injurious, and withholding it from a monitor may have equally negative effects.

This underlines the necessity for clinicians to assess individual patients' needs and elicit their information preferences. Good communication skills are essential to ensure that this is done effectively, and that explanations about cancer and its treatment are understood.

The Doctor–Patient Relationship

Perhaps it is not the patient's anxiety blocking full disclosure, but the doctor's. In a recent survey exploring physicians' reasons for not entering eligible patients in a randomized clinical trial, 48 of 66 physicians (73%) mentioned their relationship with the patient.[66] Concern often centered on the issues of discussing medical uncertainty and randomization and the need to obtain fully informed consent. As one respondent in the survey said, "Were I to enter my patients into the trial, I might undermine the patients' trust and faith, which are an important part of the cure itself." Another typical response was "How can I possibly tell the patient that I don't know which operation is better?" Moving away from the traditional advisory role, with the accompanying need to provide fuller and more detailed information, is difficult for clinicians who have developed an often highly skilled consultation style and are anxious about the patient's response if they change it. There is some evidence that changing the traditional style of the medical encounter can stress the doctor–patient relationship. In a study evaluating the effects of encouraging patients to ask more questions, consultations in the experimental group were characterized by more negative affect, anxiety, and anger and by lower patient satisfaction.[67] However, when patients were directly asked about their confidence in their doctor and the quality of their relationshp with their doctor, there were no differences between patients receiving full versus standard disclosure of information during an informed consent interview.[51]

What and How Do Doctors Tell?

While it is established that most doctors in Western countries now tell their patients their cancer diagnosis,[44,68] there have been few studies documenting more subtle aspects of communication. Providing the diagnosis is only part of the story. Whether and how a prognosis is provided, the choice of which facts from the myriad available are disclosed, the language used, and the emotional slant with which the facts are delivered are all aspects that may influence the patient's understanding and well-being.[69] Patient reports indicate that the subsequent discussion about the actions to be taken and what the diagnosis means may be at least as, if not more, important to patients than the circumstances of the disclosure of the diagnosis.[69]

Doctors use a number of strategies to try to soften the blow of a cancer diagnosis. Some avoid using the word "cancer" and instead prefer euphemisms such as "tumor," "growth," or "illness."[69] Others use friendly analogies ("the cancer is out and about"; "that could give you a bit of trouble in the future"; "this is really nasty"[55]) or talk about survival-versus-mortality statistics. Some doctors may talk about patients they have known who have done exceptionally well, or coped well with treatment. Some information, such as side effects and symptoms that are extremely rare, may not be discussed at all, while other information may be given in small packages, with time for digestion between them. These strategies do not usually distort or withhold information and cannot be clearly described as misinformation, and yet they may have a profound influence on the patient.

In an exploration of procedures that influence patients' hopefulness, Sardell and Trierweiler[70] reported that patients have clear ideas about which procedures were most and least hope-giving, and that ratings of hopefulness and favorability were related to overall emotional adjustment to the illness. Patients in this study preferred procedures that did not intentionally disguise a negative prognosis, but that emphasized the positive aspects of that prognosis. Examples of the latter included placing an emphasis on putting up a good fight against the cancer, suggesting to patients that each day they survive allows them to take advantage of new developments in treatment, and focusing on positive aspects of the cancer experience, such as the chance to experience personal growth and family closeness. In some cases, patients asking for more information may in fact be seeking these sorts of positive, hopeful messages, rather than new data.

In a study exploring psychological adjustment following surgery, 100 women newly diagnosed with breast cancer completed, among others, a questionnaire measuring their perceptions of doctor–patient communication during the consultation in which diagnosis and treatment options were discussed.[71] In a multiple regression adjusting for other possible predictors of adjustment (such as level of social support and previous psychiatric status) patient perceptions of physician communication were significantly related to psychological adjustment. A factor analysis of patients' responses indicated that the physician's caring attitude was perceived by the women as the most important dimension. As the previous discussion shows, it may not be what you tell, but how you tell it, that is important.

Conclusion

So what can we conclude from this discussion? The study of doctor–patient communication and patient involvement in decision making is still in its infancy. More research is needed to evaluate the impact of different types of information given under different circumstances on patients with different cancers and from different backgrounds. Despite conflicting evidence, the majority of data support an open, negotiated exchange of information. If doctors can inform patients of the psychological risks associated with full disclosure and involvement in medical decisions, then patients can decide on their preferred role accordingly.

Clearly, patients vary in their preferences and needs for information and involvement, and it is not always easy to determine these in the clinical setting. Because of these difficulties, it has been suggested that doctors should measure patients' information and involvement preferences more objectively, and a variety of questionnaires have been developed for this purpose.[3,45] However, not much is known about the reliability and validity of such measures, and whether information preferences remain stable over time and circumstance. Is an information preference a fixed personality characteristic or behavioral strategy? Should such preferences be measured once, or before every consultation? These issues remain to be resolved.

The evidence suggests that communication skills that allow the doctor to determine how much patients want to know, to deliver the information in a positive, supportive way, and to confirm that patients have understood the information they sought may in the end be more critical than objective counts of the amount of information presented. Back in 1961, in a fascinating study of doctor attitudes and behavior, Oken reported that the most powerful predictor of whether a doctor gave or withheld a diagnosis of cancer was his or her first experience of breaking bad news.[72] If the patient was upset, then a policy of nondisclosure was established; if the patient coped well, then the doctor told all. Oken concluded that what doctors choose to tell patients about their cancer is not usually based on logic or observation, but "on opinion, belief and conviction, heavily weighted by emotional justification."

Properly conducted randomized trials of communication strategies and interventions are urgently required to provide evidence-based guidelines for communication. These would provide the basis for communication training, both for students and senior staff. In the absence of clear guidelines and effective courses in communication, most doctors still base their practice on intuition and personal prejudice.[69,73] In the course of a professional career, an oncologist is likely to conduct between 150,000 and 200,000 interviews with patients and their relatives, but relatively few receive formal training during their student years, let alone as part of a continuing professional development program.[74] Even when communication is included in medical education, it is often undermined by a widespread perception on the students' part, not infrequently reinforced by their seniors, that this is a minor and insignificant aspect of the curriculum. Fallowfield[75] has suggested that training senior physicians and surgeons in communication skills can make them more effective models. Some journals have gone so far as to suggest that physicians should be taught acting as one way of improving communication. Clearly this is an area that deserves both ongoing research and educational commitment.

References

1. Lantos J. Informed consent: the whole truth for patients? *Cancer Supplement* 1993; 72; 9:2811–2815.
2. Goldberg RJ. Disclosure of information to adult cancer patients: issues and update. *J Clin Oncol* 1984; 2:948–954.
3. Cassileth BR, Zupkis RV, Sutton-Smith K, March V. Information and participation preferences among cancer patients. *Ann Intern Med* 1980; 92:832–836.
4. Sutherland HJ, Llewellyn-Thomas AJ, Lockwood GA, Tritchler DL, Till JE. Cancer patients: their desire for information and participation in treatment decisions. *J R Soc Med* 1989; 82:260–263.
5. Giesen D. Legal accountability for the provision of medical care: a comparative view. *J R Soc Med* 1993; 86:648–652.
6. Shelp EE, Perl M. Denial in clinical medicine: a re-examination of the concept and its significance. *Arch Intern Med* 1985; 145:697–699.
7. US Gov't F.D.A. Code of Federal Regulations Ch. 1:50.20–25:191–193. Revised April 1, 1982.
8. Tobias JS, Souhami RL. Fully informed consent can be needlessly cruel. *Br Med J* 1993; 307:1199–1201.
9. Editorial. Your baby is in a trial. *Lancet* 1995; 345:805–806.
10. Segelov E, Tattersall MHN, Coates AS. Redressing the balance; the ethics of not entering eligible patients on a randomised clinical trial. Point of view. *Ann Oncol* 1992; 3:103–105.
11. Smith A. Should a doctor tell the truth when a patient has cancer? *The New York Times*, May 1976.
12. Cancer Research Campaign Working Party in Breast Conservation. Informed consent: ethical, legal and medical implications for doctors and patients who participate in randomised clinical trials. *Br Med J* 1983; 286:1117–1121.
13. Emberton M, Wood C, Meredith P. Informed consent in clinical trials. *Br Med J* 1993; 307:1494.
14. Wong JG. Informed consent in clinical trials: open discussion promotes trust. *Br Med J* 1993; 307:1495.
15. Ingelfinger FJ. Arrogance. *N Engl J Med* 1980; 301:1507–1511.
16. Haynes RB, Taylor DW, Sackett DL, eds. *Compliance in Health Care*. Baltimore: Johns Hopkins University Press; 1979.
17. Kasteler J, Kane R, Olsen DM, Thetford R. Issues underlying prevalence of "Doctor-shopping" behaviour. *J Health Soc Behav* 1976; 17:328–339.
18. Pruyn JFA, Rijckman RM, van Brunschot CJ, van den Borne HW. Cancer patients' personality characteristics, physician–patient communication and adoption of the Moerman diet. *Soc Sci Med* 1985; 20:831–847.
19. Molleman E, Krabbendam PJ, Annyas AA, Koops HS, Sleijfer DT, Vermey A. The significance of the doctor–patient relationship in coping with cancer. *Soc Sci Med* 1984; 18:475–480.

20. Cohen F, Lazarus RS. Coping with the stresses of illness. In: Stone GC, Cohen F, Adler NE, eds, *Health Psychology*. San Francisco: Jossey-Bass; 1979:217–254.
21. Simes RJ. Ethical issues in clinical trials: a review. Unpublished Ph.D. dissertation.
22. Blanchard CG, Labreque MS, Ruckdeschel JC, Blanchard EB. Information and decision-making preferences of hospitalised cancer patients. *Soc Sci Med* 1988; 27:1139–1145.
23. Wiggers J, O'Donovan K, Redman S, Sanson-Fisher R. Cancer patient satisfaction with care. *Cancer* 1990; 66:610–616.
24. Mackillop WJ, Stewart WE, Ginsberg AD, Stewart SS. Cancer patients' perceptions of their disease and its treatment. *Br J Cancer* 1988; 58:355–358.
25. Cassell E, cited in Pollard BJ. Autonomy and paternalism in medicine. *Med J Aust* 1993; 159; 6:797–802.
26. Williamson C. Whose standards? Consumer and professional standards in health care. Buckingham: Open University Press; 1992.
27. Degner LF, Sloan JA. Decision making during serious illness: what role do patients really want to play? *J Clin Epidemiol* 1992; 45:941–950.
28. Gillon R. Beneficence: doing good for others. *Br Med J* 1985; 291:44–45.
29. Connoly TJ. Willing participant or exploited patient? *Med J Aust* 1981; 1:172–174.
30. Gerlis L. Informed consent in clinical trials . . . it's the law. *Br Med J* 1993; 307: 1494.
31. National Health and Medical Research Council of Australia. Guidelines for the provision of information to patients by medical practitioners. 1993.
32. Richards T. Chasms in communication. *Br Med J* 1990; 301:1407–1408.
33. Cassileth ER, Zupkis RV, Sultan-Smith K, March V. Informed consent—why are its goals imperfectly realised. *N Engl J Med* 1980:302:896–900.
34. Simes RJ, Tattersal MHN. Informed consent. *Br Med J* 1983; 286:1972–1973.
35. Kirby M. Reform the law: essays on the renewal of the Australian legal system. Melbourne: Oxford University Press; 1983:75.
36. Oberst MT. Patients' perceptions of care: measurement of quality and satisfaction. *Cancer* 1984; 53:2366–2373.
37. Ley P. Communicating with patients. London: Croom Helm; 1988.
38. Audit Commission. What seems to be the matter: communication between hospitals and patients. NHS Report, 12, HMSO: London; 1993.
39. Fallowfield LJ, Hall A, Maguire GP, Baum M. Psychological outcomes of different treatment policies in women with early breast cancer outside a clinical trial. *Br Med J* 1990; 301:575–580.
40. Butow PN, Maclean M, Tattersall MHN, Dunn SM. Information preferences: how and why they change. Unpublished manuscript.
41. Watson M, Greer S, Pruyn J, van den Borne B. The cancer locus of control scale. *Psychol Rep* 1990; 66:39–48.
42. Gordon D. Embodying illness, embodying cancer. *Cult Med Psychiatry* 1990; 14:275–297.
43. Ali NS, Khalil HZ, Yousef W. A comparison of American and Egyptian cancer patients' attitudes and unmet needs. *Cancer Nurs* 1993; 16:193–203.
44. Charlton RC. Breaking bad news. *Med J Aust* 1992; 157:615–621.
45. Hack TF, Degner LF, Dyck DG. Relationship between preferences for decisional control and illness information among women with breast cancer: a quantitative and qualitative analysis. *Soc Sci Med* 1994; 39:279–289.

46. Fraser AG. Do patients want to be informed? A study of consent for cardiac catheterisation. *Br Heart J* 1984; 52:468–470.
47. Dunn SM, Butow PN, Tattersall MHN, Jones QJ, Sheldon J, Taylor J, Sumich MD. General information tapes inhibit recall of the cancer consultation. *J Clin Oncol* 1993; 11(11):2279–2285.
48. Butow PN, Dunn SM, Tattersall MHN. Communication with cancer patients: does it matter. *J Palliat Care* 1995; 11(4):34–38: in Press.
49. Miller GA. The magical number seven plus or minus two: some limits on our capacity for processing information. *Psychol Rev* 1956; 63:81–97.
50. Ley P, Spelman MS. *Communicating with the Patient.* London: Staples Press; 1967.
51. Simes RJ, Tattersall MHN, Coates AS, et al. Randomised comparison of procedures for obtaining informed consent in clinical trials of treatment for cancer. *Br Med J* 1986; 293:1065–1068.
52. Ley P, Bradshaw PW, Kincey J, Atherton ST. A method for increasing patients' recall of information presented to them. *Psychol Med* 1973; 3:217–220.
53. McHugh P, Lewis S, Ford S, et al. The efficacy of audiotapes in promoting psychological well-being in cancer patients: a randomised controlled trial. *Br J Cancer* 1995; 71:388–392.
54. Hogbin B, Jenkins VA, Parkin AJ. Remembering "bad news" consultations: an evaluation of tape-recorded consultations. *Psycho-Oncology* 1992; 1:147–154.
55. McIntosh J. Patients' awareness and desire for information about diagnosed but undisclosed malignant disease. *Lancet* 1976; 2 (August 7):300–303.
56. Druss RG, Douglas CJ. Adaptive responses to illness and disability: healthy denial. *Gen Hosp Psychiatry* 1988; 10:163–168.
57. Damian D, Tattersall MHN. Letters to patients: improving communication in cancer care. *Lancet* 1991; 338:923–925.
58. Greer S, Moris T, Pettingale KW. Psychological response to breast cancer: effect on outcome. *Lancet* 1979; 2:785–787.
59. Hackett TP, Cassem NH. Psychological reaction to life-threatening stress: a study of acute myocardial infarction. In HS Abram, ed. *Psychological Aspects of Stress.* Springfield, Ill: Charles C Thomas; 1970.
60. Butow PN, Dunn SM, Tattersall MHN, Jones Q. Patient participation in the cancer consultation: evaluation of a question prompt sheet. *Ann Oncol* 1994; 5:199–204.
61. Dunn SM, Patterson PU, Butow PN, Smartt HH, McCarthy WH, Tattersall MHN. Cancer by another name: a randomised trial of the effects of euphemism and uncertainty in communicating with cancer patients. *J Clin Oncol* 1993; 11(5):989–996.
62. Fallowfield LJ, Baum M, Maguire GP. Addressing the psychological needs of the conservatively treated breast cancer patient: discussion paper. *J R Soc Med* 1987; 80:696–700.
63. Devlen J, Maguire P, Phillips P, Crowther D. Psychological problems associated with diagnosis and treatment of lymphomas. II. Prospective study. *Br Med J* 1987; 295:955–997.
64. Miller SM. Monitoring and blunting: validation of a questionnaire to assess styles of information seeking under threat. *J Pers Soc Psychol* 1987; 52 (2):345–353.
65. Steptoe A, Sutcliffe I, Allen B, Coombes C. Satisfaction with communication,

medical knowledge, and coping style in patients with metastatic cancer. *Soc Sci Med* 1991; 32(6):627–632.

66. Taylor KM, Margolese RG, Soskolne CL. Physicians' reasons for not entering eligible patients in a randomised clinical trial of surgery for breast cancer. *N Engl J Med* 1984; 310:1363–1367.

67. Roter DL. Patient participation in the patient–provider interaction:the effects of patient question asking on the quality of interaction, satisfaction and compliance. *Health Educ Monographs* 1977; 5:281–303.

68. Thomsen OO, Wulff HR, Martin A, et al. What do gastro-enterologists in Europe tell their cancer patients? *Lancet* 1993; 341:473–476.

69. Lind SE, Good DM, Seidel S, et al. Telling the diagnosis of cancer. *J Clin Oncol* 1989; 17:583–589.

70. Sardell AN, Trierweiler SJ. Disclosing the cancer diagnosis: procedures that influence patient hopefulness. *Cancer* 1993; 72:3355–3365.

71. Roberts CS, Cox CE, Reintgen DS, Baile WF, Gibertini M. Influence of physician communication on newly diagnosed breast patients' psychologic adjustment and decision-making. *Cancer* 1994; 74:336–341.

72. Oken D. What to tell cancer patients: a study of medical attitudes. *JAMA* 1961; 175:1120–1128.

73. Holland JC. Now we tell—but how well? *J Clin Oncol* 1989; 7:557–559.

74. Fallowfield L. Can we improve the professional and personal fulfilment of doctors in cancer medicine? *Br J Cancer* 1995; 71:1132–1133.

75. Fallowfield L. Giving sad and bad news. *Lancet* 1993; 341:476–478.

14

Clinical Response to Spiritual Issues

MICHAEL J. McCABE

The biomedical model has served medicine well in the diagnosis, treatment, and curing of disease. However, the fact that health care is as effective as it is can obscure the deeper reality of the effects of illness on the personhood of the patient. In overlooking or giving minimal importance to the spiritual dimension of the patient, medicine limits its ability to be an even more effective agent of healing and health.

The purpose of this chapter is to explore the impact of spiritual concerns on the experience of symptoms and adaptation of patients with progressive medical illness. An appreciation of this "lens" of meaning is a fundamental prerequisite and invaluable source of insight for the health care professional. Specifically, these issues will be addressed: spiritual concerns in the context of progressive medical illness; the overlap between suffering and major depression; "pathological" spiritual concerns; assessment by clinicians of spiritual concerns in the context of other potential medical and psychiatric pathologies; and some possible interventions available to clinicians who elicit such spiritual concerns.

Spiritual Concerns in the Context of Progressive Medical Illness

Although there is a common scientific language for the pathophysiology of bodily disease and common psychological phenomena, such as anxiety, depression, and transference, a broad and inclusive definition of the spiritual dimension of the person is elusive. Indeed, the very suggestion of a spiritual dimension inevitably stumbles on obstacles erected by cultural background, religious traditions, and political correctness. For the purposes of this discussion, *spirit* is defined as "the animating or vital principle" of an individual[1] and *spirituality* is defined as the "life principle that pervades a person's entire being and that integrates and transcends one's biologic and psychosocial nature."[2] Every person has a spiritual dimension that influences his or her physical and psychosocial well-being. This quality is innate and distinct from other cognitive and physical abilities. While spirituality differs from religion, a set of beliefs and rituals tied to a specific faith tradition, it may find expression through religious practice.

Kearney considers spiritual experience to be part of a continuum that "results from the particular relationship dynamic between the individual's ego (or personality) and their soul (deepest self)."[3] Spirituality provides an integrative function for the personal narrative and enables an individual to make sense out of life's successes and losses, shadows and achievements. It is this integrative function that gives the health care professional insight into addressing the spiritual dimension of illness.

Kearney's model highlights the fact that *spiritual concerns for the progressively ill center on the question of meaning.* In describing spiritual experience, he locates experiences of "connection, alignment, harmony and meaningfulness" at one end of a continuum, while placing "experiences of disconnection, disharmony, non-alignment and disintegration" at the other. The latter experiences constitute, and contribute to, *"spiritual pain,"*[3] a major source of suffering for the patient with progressive disease.

Because personhood is the result of a complex, and essentially holistic, interplay between body, mind, and spirit, the impact of the experience of illness will necessarily be multidimensional, mysterious, and complex. It takes great skill to assess and distinguish the physical from the psychological and spiritual dimensions. All are causes of suffering for the patient.

To gain further insight and precision in discussing spiritual concerns, it is helpful to consider suffering and its implications for progressive illness. In his germinal work *The Nature of Suffering and the Goals of Medicine,* Cassell defines suffering as "the state of severe distress associated with events that threaten the intactness of persons."[4] Similarly, Callahan describes suffering as ordinarily referring "to a person's psychological or spiritual state"—a state "characteristically marked by a sense of anguish, dread, foreboding, futility, meaninglessness, or a range of other emotions associated with a loss of meaning or control or both." He notes that although suffering may or may not include physical pain, not all pain leads to suffering. For example, the long-distance runner does not suffer from pain but accepts it as part of the pleasure of running in a marathon. Neither does suffering require the presence of pain, as in the case of knowing one has Alzheimer's disease.[5] Hauerwas says that suffering always occurs in an "interpretive context" and has "as its root sense the idea of being forced to submit to and endure some particular set of circumstances."[6]

A key element in all these definitions is that suffering is fundamentally and profoundly personal. It is experienced by persons and can occur in relation to any of the multifaceted aspects of the person. There is no direct correlation between a patient's physical, spiritual, or psychological condition, and the meaning that the patient ascribes to it, as is illustrated by the fact that two patients can present with identical symptoms and respond completely differently to their illness. It is precisely because the patient's meaning system intervenes that spiritual concerns are so difficult to evaluate and assess.

Cassell provides a valuable "topology" of the person to enhance understanding of how the patient's meaning system impacts on the meaning given to suffering. These dimensions of the person have important implications for the role of medicine in relieving suffering. Indeed, Cassell argues that although a person cannot be reduced to any one of his or her dimensions, ignorance of these elements actively contributes to suffering. The salient dimensions are as follows (Table 14.1):

> *Personality and character:* Some individuals have a low pain and suffering threshold, whereas others are able to tolerate a greater level of stress resulting from illness.
>
> *A past:* An individual's past has enormous power to influence the present and the personal meaning given to a particular illness. Memories can "stimulate fear or confidence, bodily symptoms, and even anguish."[4]
>
> *Family:* An individual's experience of family, positive or negative, acts as a filter to the meaning of suffering.
>
> *Culture:* Closely allied to family is the impact of culture. Every person has a cultural background whose values help to shape and reshape personal values and beliefs and, therefore, individual responses to illness.

Table 14.1. Topology of the person: "lenses" of meaning: locus of spiritual concerns[4]

Personality and character
A past
Family
Cultural background
Roles
The ability to relate
The ability to act or create
Political dimension
Regular behaviors
A body
A secret life
A perceived future
A transcendent dimension

Roles: People have multiple roles in life, for example, teacher, nurse, doctor, sister. Progressive illness can lead to the virtual destruction of a person and make the performance of his or her roles impossible.

Ability to act or create: Often the *only* way a person knows himself or herself is through creative acts. A person's concept of self is formed in and through relationships with the self and with others, "even if only in memory or reverie. . . ."

Political being: Illness can interfere with an individual's ability to relate equally to others and enjoy social rights and obligations. This can leave the sufferer feeling marginalized and politically disempowered.

Regular behaviors: Daily habits are taken for granted when health is present and cause suffering when the customary pattern is broken through sickness.

A body: The relationship of a person to his or her body may include identification, admiration, constant loathing, or fear. Illness affects this relationship.

A secret life: Similarly, the response to illness and suffering will be influenced by the fact that everyone has a secret life that includes one's fears and fantasies, past experiences, and current ways of solving problems and arriving at meaning, and so forth. As Cassell wisely notes, "Disease may not only destroy the public person but the secret person as well."[4]

A perceived future: The loss of a future may cause intense suffering because it is within this dimension of personhood that the individual is reminded of his or her transcendent dimension.

Transcendent dimension: The life of the spirit will be expressed and known in a myriad religious and secular ways, but its inherent quality is to locate the individual as part of a much larger landscape. In the presence of progressive illness, the patient perceives that this landscape is reduced or under threat—a profound cause of suffering.

In describing the complexity of personhood, Cassell provides insight into the potential for injury and suffering that exists within the human person. Likewise, he helps to locate the focus and origin of spiritual concerns. However, patients cannot be simplistically reduced to any one of their parts, as all aspects of personhood are susceptible to damage and loss.[4]

Suffering and Major Depression

The multifaceted dimensions of personhood provide a lens through which suffering is interpreted and gives insight into the impact of illness for the progressively ill. However, the pain and other symptoms of disease, and the psychological well-being of the patient, take initial priority in assessment, not least because of their ability to mask the spiritual. Just as ethical issues in medicine are embedded within the particular clinical case,[7] so are spiritual issues. These spiritual issues are delicately intertwined with physical and psychological symptoms, particularly in the most obvious focal points of pain control and depression.

The relationship between tissue damage and pain is complex, and is clarified by further distinction from psychological issues and suffering. The fundamental goal of cancer pain assessment is "to characterize the nociception that is presumed to exist, and simultaneously identify other, non-nociceptive contributions to the pain."[8] Clinical experience consistently highlights the fact that treatment of pain alone is insufficient because of the interrelationship between pain and emotional distress. Nevertheless, the control of the patient's pain is a fundamental starting point in the care of the whole person because psychiatric symptoms may be entirely or partially driven by uncontrolled pain. After the patient's pain has been addressed, his or her mental state can be reassessed to determine the presence of a psychiatric disorder.[9]

The interrelationship of the physical, psychological, and spiritual symptoms is further illustrated through the skills of psychiatric assessment. Unaddressed psychological factors intensify the experience of pain and affect the patient's quality of life. Like existential suffering or spiritual distress, the level of psychological distress will vary according to personality, coping ability, social support, and medical factors.[10] Cancer patients exhibit a pronounced vulnerability. Prior to their illness, most cancer patients are "psychologically healthy." With the onset of illness and aggressive treatment, these patients present with appropriate psychiatric disorders, 90% of which are either reactions to, or manifestations of, the disease or treatment.[10]

A major cause of suffering for the progressively ill is depression. The prevalence of depression in cancer patients is 20% to 25%; this prevalence increases with higher levels of disability, pain, and progression of illness.[11] *Major depression* is defined as a "mental disorder characterized by the occurrence of one or more major depressive episodes and the absence of any manic or hypomanic episodes."[12] The *symptoms of depression* include depressed mood, hopelessness or the sense that everything is getting worse and nothing will get better, preexisting guilt, and decreased energy and concentration.[9,10,13]

The presence of a progressive medical disorder complicates the diagnosis of major depression. Consequently, the diagnosis is based more on the range of the cognitive symptoms of depression: sad mood, feelings of worthlessness and hopelessness, excessive guilt, and suicidal ideation, rather than the somatic symptoms of anorexia, insomnia, fatigue, and weight loss.[9,10,13]

Because it is the key variable in the suicide of cancer patients and those who are not medically ill, and is also a significantly better predictor of completed suicide than depression alone, the sense of hopelessness requires specific attention by the clinician.[10] A pervasive sense of hopelessness, accompanied by a sense of despair and despondency, and exacerbated by isolation, can indicate the presence of a depressive disorder or the presence of profound spiritual pain. Through extensive exploration of these feelings with the patient,[9] the skilled clinician uses the given cues to sift through a complex range of physical and psychiatric symptoms. In gaining insight into the genesis of these symptoms and, therefore, the personal implications of the progressive illness and its attendant goals of care,[14] the clinician is also opening up the possibility for the integration of spiritual concerns by the patient and family.

Before focusing further on the assessment of spiritual concerns it is relevant to address briefly the possible link between the psychological and a "pathological" spiritual concern.

"Pathological" Spiritual Concerns

As are all cognitive and physical abilities, spirituality is capable of growth or distortion and can, therefore, be mature or unhealthy. When spirituality is immature, it may be expressed in excessive dependence or unrealistic expectations on the part of the patient. To the extent that it interferes with the patient's care, or contributes to emotional disorder, anxiety, or the distortion of reality, it can be labeled "pathological." The existence of such pathological spiritual concerns can be a factor in the patient's disease that requires psychiatric treatment, or possibly originate in distorted religious beliefs that may simply require the mediation of a sensitive chaplain or clinician. There is a danger of labeling a spiritual concern "pathological" simply because we do not understand it or it is not part of our worldview. Many rituals or beliefs of religious traditions easily fit into this category. However, as Fins notes, while the sacred and profane may appear to be distinct categories, they are "inhabited by individuals who draw upon both sources" in giving meaning and hope to their lives.[15] An appreciation of these deeper cultural and spiritual realities, as expressed through religious traditions, can assist the clinician in assessing spiritual concerns and distinguishing them from the physical and psychological symptom.[16]

Assessment of Spiritual Concerns in the Medical Context

Assessment of spiritual concerns is a skilled process that begins with a thorough medical and psychiatric evaluation. In addressing the psychological variables that contribute to pain and suffering, such as the perception of control, meaning of pain, fear of death, depressed mood, hopelessness, the clinician is treating the deeper spiritual concern of the patient. Just as relief of pain can result in the disappearance of apparent psychiatric disorders,[10] so it can give greater freedom to address existential and spiritual issues. Pain and unrelieved symptoms of psychological distress have a preoccupying effect for the patient and his or her family. With adequate relief both are freed to address the transcendent dimension.

Careful and adequate spiritual assessment begins by attention to the *context* in which the spiritual concerns are being raised. The context will, in turn, determine the response of the clinician. Although there is a need for specific training in spiritual care, and specialists in this area can be a valuable resource for the clinician constrained by time and caseload, spiritual care is not the exclusive domain of the chaplain. Each discipline brings its own spiritual insight to patient care. Thus, to enhance assessment of spiritual concerns, and to avoid inhibiting the context in which they are being raised, spiritual care should be interdisciplinary and transcend personalities and professional turf.[17]

As Cassell's model provides a paradigm for understanding the context of spiritual concerns, the "7 by 7 model for spiritual assessment" of Fitchett and colleagues can help to organize an approach to specific spiritual concerns. This model addresses the diverse ways in which spirituality is experienced and expressed, and incorporates insights from medicine and the behavioral sciences[18] (Table 14.2).

To recognize the presence of spiritual pain, Kearney suggests that it is often accompanied by a "why" question or expressed as a feeling. The models of both Cassell and Fitchett and colleagues enhance a holistic approach to patient care, specifically by identifying for the clinician how and where spiritual pain might arise. The following case vignette illustrates how spiritual pain is embedded in the physical and psychological condition and how such pain centers around the question of meaning.

A Case History

A 35-year-old man was diagnosed with a primary gastric tumor with widespread metastatic disease to bone and liver. The patient was married and had two daughters aged 2 and 3. Prior to diagnosis he was very physically fit and enjoyed an active social life. As his disease progressed his pain and anxiety

Table 14.2. The "7 by 7" model for spiritual assessment[18]

Holistic assessment	Spiritual assessment
Medical dimension	Belief and meaning
Psychological dimension	Vocation and obligations
Family systems dimension	Experience and emotions
Psychosocial dimension	Courage and growth
Ethnic, racial, cultural dimension	Ritual and practice
Societal dimension	Community
Spiritual dimension	Authority and guidance

increased but were reasonably well controlled with opioid drugs. In a visit to the patient, the psychiatric nurse clinician felt that, although the patient was relatively calm and pain free, he "clearly wanted to talk even though he tired easily." She recorded the subsequent conversation in the patient's notes:

> P [patient]: "I'm very frightened . . ."
>
> N-C [Nurse-clinician]: "What are you frightened of?"
>
> P: "That I'm getting sicker . . . see these pictures . . . (he points to pictures of his two daughters) . . . I'm frightened of leaving them. I don't want to leave them. . . ."
>
> N-C: "What are you frightened of?"
>
> P: "Of dying."
>
> N-C: "You think you're dying?"
>
> P: "Yes."
>
> N-C: He then spoke of having his children remember him as fit, successful, athletic . . . he wanted to "give my children good memories to remember me by . . ."

This case typifies the presence of raw spiritual pain in a 35-year-old man who had everything to live for. While the management of gastric tumors is difficult, and there is little oncological optimism for such advanced disease, the patient's real pain concerned his profound sense of impending loss and departure from his wife and young daughters. The nurse-clinician, through sensitive questioning, allowed him to express his feelings. She did not remove his pain but provided an opportunity for discussion about the "good memories" he wanted to leave to his daughters. To judge his pain as the sole result of an underlying physical or psychological pathology would have meant overlooking this filter of meaning and its profound causal effect on his symptom threshold.

Assessment of spiritual concerns is further aided by a *focus on loss and change*, because progressive illness brings loss and change on a variety of levels, including the financial, social, career, and so forth. Equally important, progressive illness becomes the focal point of all the losses in a patient's narrative and in the narrative of the family. For the family, feelings of loss will be expressed in fatigue and anticipatory grief. Fatigue stems from the exhaustion of physical, emotional, spiritual, and financial resources;[10] anticipatory grief reflects the impact of the "roller-coaster" experience of walking with a loved one through illness. Both feelings are heightened when the dying process occurs over some time. This may lead to a desire on the part of family members to withdraw in order to "protect" themselves from further grief and distress.

Illness also becomes a focal point of loss for the clinician. In response to progressive disease some begin to reduce their visits to the patient. Although the medical role is not identical with the personal, the clinician's response should never include abandonment. A patient's disease may not be curable, but it is still possible for him or her to die "healed" of spiritual distress, as Cicely Saunders observes:

> We aim at maximizing the potential that still remains for each patient and the family in the place of their own choice. . . . We aim to control symptoms in order to give a person freedom to move toward his own aims. Often this will be the resolution of family problems. People move fast in a crisis, and many can resolve longstanding problems within a relatively short time given the right assistance. . . . We cannot ignore the fact that there is a spiritual dimension to this work. The longing for significance and meaning goes beyond our own capacity to fulfil but we can try to create an atmosphere in which others find a freedom to make their own uniquely personal journey.[19]

Possible Interventions

The key to bringing healing to the patient and family is for the health care team to persevere with practical and achievable goals of care. The following list of interventions is not exhaustive, but is provided as a practical aid for clinicians who elicit spiritual concerns in caring for patients with progressive illness.

Know the history: The history is not necessarily limited to medical or psychological symptoms. Given the multiple medical teams, the possibility of fragmented patient care, and the constraints on the time of the clinician, the full history can be difficult to acquire. Fragmented care often means that no one has all the relevant "pieces" of the patient's history, and equally, the nuances of the pieces that are known are misunderstood or overlooked. The asking of open-ended questions can amplify the clinician's knowledge of a patient's history.

Learn the patient's meaning system: Suffering and spiritual distress are highly subjective and distinct from their cause. It is necessary to learn and engage in the patient's meaning system. The medieval maxim "everything which is received is received according to the mind of the receiver" finds in the experience of a suffering patient a unique configuration.[20]

Empathic listening: Careful listening encourages patients to share their narratives, which is central to assessing how the spiritual is impacting on the experienced illness. The telling of the narrative enables patients to articulate answers, responses, and "re-minds" them of previous strategies for coping and transcending experiences of illness and loss.[21]

Articulate spiritual concerns: Spiritual concerns require careful and specific articulation for each patient. This process is inhibited by an exclusive focus on the pathophysiology of disease. Often, the asking of a

patient's religion on admission to a health care facility is equated with
knowledge of his or her spiritual belief system. Obvious cues at the
patient's bedside to assist the clinician in assessing the spiritual, such as
a pair of rosary beads, or a yarmulke, are frequently ignored.

Involve the chaplains: Chaplains are trained interpreters of the spiritual
and are able to help with religious pain. Chaplains are consistently
underutilized members in health care and are often viewed as carriers
of the "last rites" when the scientific has failed and there is nothing
more that can be done for the patient. At the same time, the challenge
for the chaplain is to be so familiar with the medical world and its staff
that they will readily involve him or her in health care.

Offer spiritual care: Advocacy for the patient as a person is not limited to
chaplains. There are times when others from the health care team are
more appropriate givers of spiritual care. An interdisciplinary focus
facilitates appropriate shifts in the discussion and implementation of
the goals of care. The timing and tone of these shifts come with experience, but are essentially simple. For example, "Your medical needs are
very important to us, but we are also concerned about your emotional
and spiritual well-being. Can we talk about this?"[17]

Give information and improve communication: At a practical level, the
giving of information and the improvement of the level of communication can change the degree of meaning for the sufferer. Information is
the "initiation rite" into meaning, but only to the extent that illness or
the causes of suffering are defined in terms familiar to the patient. To
paraphrase the writer Broyard, the articulateness of inadequacy helps
to restore a sense of adequacy to the sufferer.[22]

Spiritual assessment is not problem solving: The patient is not looking for
answers, but rather for a physician who possesses the ability to listen
and serve as a compassionate guide.

Develop a spiritual and affective side: In developing his or her own spirituality and affective side, the clinician is able to view the spirituality of
the patient not only as a "lens" through which to frame the goals of
patient care, but also as a source of inner strength for himself or herself.
The current emphasis on narrative ethics and the humanities is primarily aimed at giving clinicians a variety of perspectives through
which to view their craft and improve coping with the myriad demands
on their professional and personal lives. Just as clinicians develop their
scientific understanding of progressive disease over a lifetime, so the
development of their affective side brings further skill to their profession and enhances their ability to recognize the deeper dimensions
present within the human story.

Understand the dynamics of loss and grief: An understanding of the dynamics of loss and the grief process and the development of skills in

crisis intervention can enhance the clinician's skills in assessing spiritual concerns.[23]

Conclusion

The spiritual dimension plays a central role in a patient's experience of progressive illness. An exclusive focus on investigating, diagnosing, and curing disease overlooks this dimension. When spiritual pain is not recognized, or given appropriate attention, patient care is inhibited. Unless addressed, the impact of spiritual concerns on the pain and symptom threshold can frustrate the clinician's efforts to control the effects of progressive disease. Just as palliative care is not a sudden "soft option" when cure has failed, but is part of a continuum of good medical care, so the spiritual must not be relegated to the boundaries of clinical medicine to be visited only when "nothing more can be done."

References

1. Saunders C. Spiritual pain. *Hospital Chaplain*. March 1988:1. [Reprint]
2. Taylor EJ, Ersek M. Ethical and spiritual dimensions of cancer pain management. In: McGuire DB, Yarbro CH, Ferrell BR, eds. *Cancer Pain Management*. 2nd ed. Boston: Jones and Bartlett; 1995:41-60. [For similar definitions see, for example, International Work Group for Death and Dying. Assumptions and principles of spiritual care. *Death Studies* 1990; 14:75–81; Tournier P. *The Meaning of Persons*, New York: Harper and Row, 1957; Holland EJ. The art of hospice spiritual care. In: Gardener K, ed. *Quality of Care for the Terminally Ill: An Examination of the Issues*. Chicago: Joint Commission on Accreditation of Hospitals, 1985:136–140.]
3. Kearney M. Spiritual pain. *The Way*. January 1990; 30:47–54.
4. Cassell E. *The Nature of Suffering and the Goals of Medicine*. New York: Oxford University Press; 1991. [See also, *N Engl J Med* 1982; 306:639–645.]
5. Callahan D. *The Troubled Dream of Life: Living with Mortality*. New York: Simon and Schuster; 1993.
6. Hauerwas S. *Naming the Silences. God, Medicine, and the Problem of Suffering*. Grand Rapids, Michigan: Eerdmans Publishing Company; 1990.
7. See, for example: Johnsen AR, Siegler M, Winslade WJ. *Clinical Ethics*. New York: McGraw-Hill; 1992.
8. Portenoy R. Pain assessment in adults and children. In: *Why Do We Care?* New York: Memorial Sloan-Kettering Cancer Center; 1992:3–10.
9. Breitbart W, Passik SD. Psychiatric aspects of palliative care. In: Doyle D, Hanks GW, MacDonald N, eds. *Oxford Textbook of Palliative Care Medicine*. Oxford: Oxford University Press; 1993:609–626.

10. Breitbart W. Assessment and treatment of psychiatric syndromes in cancer pain patients. In: *Why Do We Care?* New York: Memorial Sloan-Kettering Cancer Center; 1992:213–228.

11. Massie MJ, Holland JC. Depression and the cancer patient. *J Clin Psychiatry* 1990; 51:12–17.

12. *Dorland's Pocket Medical Dictionary.* Philadelphia: WB Saunders & Co.; 1989.

13. Lederberg MS, Massie MJ. Psychosocial and ethical issues in the care of cancer patients. In: De Vita VT, Hellman S, Rosenberg SA, eds. *Cancer: Principles and Practice of Oncology.* 4th ed. Philadelphia: JB Lippincott: 1993:2448–2513.

14. Lane NJ. A spirituality of being: women with disabilities. *Stauros Notebook* Summer 1993; 12.

15. Fins JJ. Across the divide: religious objections to brain death. *Journal Religion Health* Spring 1995; 34:33–39.

16. Andrews MM, Hanson PA. Religious beliefs: implications for nursing practice. In: Boyle JS, Andrews MM, eds. *Transcultural Concepts in Nursing Care.* Glenview, Ill.: Scott, Foresman/Little Brown College Division; 1989:357–418.

17. Holland EJ. The art of hospice spiritual care. In: Gardener K, ed. *Quality of Care for the Terminally Ill: An Examination of the Issues.* Chicago: Joint Commission on Accreditation of Hospitals; 1985:136–140.

18. Fitchett G. Linda Krauss and the lap of God: a spiritual assessment case study. *Second Opinion* 1995; 20:41–49.

19. Saunders C. The evolution of the hospices. *Free Inquiry* Winter 1991/92:19–23.

20. Breton S. Human suffering and transcendence. In: Dougherty F, ed. *The Meaning of Human Suffering.* New York: Human Sciences Press; 1982:55–94.

21. Bowers CC. Spiritual dimensions of the rehabilitation journey. *Rehabilitation Nursing* 1987; 12:90–91.

22. Broyard A. *Intoxicated by My Illness: and Other Writings on Life and Death.* New York: Clarkson N. Potter, Inc.; 1992.

23. Eaton S. Spiritual care: the software of life. *J Palliat Care* 1988; 4:91–93.

Index